Electronic Data Processing in the Cerebral Cortex

By Eugene Olney (1925 - 1981)

Published By

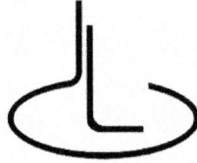

Olney Labs, LLC

Sammamish, Washington

ISBN: 978-0-9903478-1-1

$25.95
ISBN 978-0-9903478-1-1
52595>

9 780990 347811

...so little time

Electronic Data Processing in the Cerebral Cortex

CONTENTS

Electronic Data Processing in the Cerebral Cortex

PROLOGUE

We read science fiction about computers that think and tend to
dismiss the idea that a machine could perform as a human brain.
After all, we are conscious and we are taught from day one that we
exist, we are real. So it must be true; we are really in here.
Machines can't believe like that. They can't be as different as
each of us are and yet maintain collective beliefs about the world
we live in. Machines can't relate today's events to last week's.
They cannot reach conclusions formed from all such events. They
cannot use such conclusions to shape their environment; better,
safer, more colorful. Surely a thinking machine would be able to
talks to us about those things; if it were possible. What happens
in our heads that is so unimaginable, so complex, so mystical that
a machine can't be made to do it? What does the human brain
actually do?

Brain science is but slightly further along than it was when this
book was originally written in the 70's by my late father, Eugene
Olney. He used research results available at the time and his
incredible intellect to piece together how the brain must work. It
must do and does everything it seems to. His postulated unique
data processing architecture aligns with the physiology and
psychology that we see. He sorts out past experimental evidence as
clincher arguments for his model and his case becomes compelling.
He writes for everyone; defining and explaining uncommon terms and
prior conditions. The illustrations are his. Later, I developed a
mathematical model for a machine that thinks better than a human

that is based on some of his ideas. That model is described in my
book, Indeterminate Cognitive Automata.

INSPECTING THE PROBLEM

"Cortex" means "rind" or "bark". The gray and outermost layer of the cerebral brain system is the cerebral cortex. For thirty years or more, it has been a matter of settled argument among brain experts that the cortex is an electronic data processor. Whether it takes guts, art or innocence, there has never been as explanation of the way it works. In so far as I know, this is the first attempt to set out the overall circuitry and schema of the cortex. We have here an early overview, a first trial approximation of the way this marvelous computer (probably) goes about its exacting computation.

This book is speculative writing, it has to be. It is speculative because the cortex is not a convenient network to study and because I am an electronics technician and only modestly qualified to do all of this. Ideally it should be done by someone better qualified than myself, since no one better qualified has so far stepped forward, I am undertaking the project myself.

Starting as a hobby, I have been working on this study or playing with it, as the case may be-- for about 25 years. I am satisfied; and inspection alone should have told us, years ago, the cortex is not, cannot be, the complex and baffling mechanism it has been said to be. The cortical nerve cell, roughly comparable to the diodes and transistors in factory made computers, is the active element in the cortical system. I do not doubt nor minimize the physiological sophistication of the cell. The cell, in its role as the active element in the cortical computer is a different story; here, it is only capable of computing operations of limited sophistication.

The 16 billion cells in the cortex are spread so thin and the
capabilities of the cell are so constrained that the cortex is
flatly incapable of performing every fancy computing operation
temptation would want to include in the system. The circuit
philosophy of the cortex can be worked out and, in working it out,
the very real limitations of the cortical cell are not to be
scorned.

Though speculative, this study is based on the outcome{s) of
hundreds of experiments on nerve cells and a few on the cortex.
Our treatment of the cortex intimately depends on our respectful
regard for these experiments and, more-so, upon the inferences that
have a way of becoming attached to experimental findings. This
circuit for the cortex is my own idea and not (especially)
confirmed experimentally. I show as much experimental support as I
am able and to the extent the available information is applicable.
Happily, for electronic purposes, there is no need to discuss
experimenters reports in depth.

Experts, usually the cytologist (studies cells) and the
neurologist, are not sure they understand all of the signal
conducting parameters of the nerve cell and experimentation leaves
a lot to be desired.

While it is not my intention aforethought, I am reasonably
confident I have found a few experimenters mistakes and some
experimental inference that could stand to be reworked. My field
is electronics and I am more or less an outsider in some of these
areas and not the one to give them the house cleaning they deserve;
the study of membrane parameters is one of those. A few bum

experiments and a few shortcomings on our understanding of the
nerve cell are not insurmountable, even with inexact knowledge of
the cell, we still have a pretty good idea of the way the cell
behaves as the active electronic element. I do the best I can with
the nerve cell. One of the problems goes like this; the nerve cell
conveys a <u>D.C. analogue signal</u> from one of its ends to the other
and, in myelinated nerves, the D.C. analogue is converted to a
<u>pulse rate</u> coded signal. This conversion is fairly simple and is
explained later. This strange conversion has been poorly
understood and has brought all sorts of confusion to the study of
the nervous system. According to me, the analogue signal is
translated to a pulsed code solely as a noise immunity measure.
This being the case, the pulse rate code is an ancillary matter, a
technique of last resort, entirely devoted to overcoming noise.
Save for the noise problem, it could be dispensed with altogether.

(Here we can explain a couple of terms. "Noise" in not to be
construed as an irritating sound. Throughout the book, "noise" is
to be understood as an unwanted pulse, or a stray signal, with a
bad habit of ingratiating itself in places it is not wanted and
ending up superimposed on the desired signal being carried by the
nerve cell. The D.C. analogue is explained in the text.
"Analogue" simply means "analogous to". The deflection of the
indicator on a bathroom scale is an "analogue" of the weight of the
person standing on the scale. Factory made computers are "digital"
and the active element is an all-or-nothing device that flip-flops

from one state to another. The smoothly graded response of the
analogue device contrasts with the patterned "flip-flop" of the
digital.)

(The animal of nature is under the supervision of a D.C. analogue
computer from the foremost drip of its runny proboscis to the
southernmost whisker on its ever-loving tokus: trust me. If there
are those who are persuaded the cortical system is a digital
system, I wish them well, may they find whatever it is they are
looking for and may they enjoy it in health.)

   If the nerve cell was a factory made device, it would be enclosed
in a braided copper shield to protect the signal from noises in its
surroundings and the confusing pulse rate code (a variation of the
FM radio signal) would not be needed. The nerve cell,
conspicuously, is not shielded. In the text, I pass along my own
theories with regard to the radical measures that are needed to
shelter the unshielded nerve from stray voltages, stray currents
and crosstalk (all noise). I take possession of the <u>Node of
Ranvier</u> and another device: the <u>electrotonic junction</u>, as key
elements in a wondrous, system-wide, noise immunity scheme. The
need for these extensive and drastic noise immunity measures will
be clearer in the item: "The nerve cell as the active element".

   The problem of maintaining rigor in laying out the cortical
circuit is, at least, manageable. For my own satisfaction, I am
following what is called a "critical path". I do not want a
missing or doubtful experiment, or an avoidable assumption, to
become a key vulnerability; that is, I do not want them to fall on
the, must-be-right, critical path.

4

Inspecting the Problem

Assumptions are to be as few as possible and defendable on grounds of concrete necessity and the realities of the system. I make only one critical path assumption. With sound justification, and plenty of it, I point to where the cortical memory device has to be physically sited and explain its general characteristics. The proposed memory unit is a molecular device and I assume, or hope, the electro-chemistry of the memory device does not outrageously contradict the known laws of chemistry. Otherwise, I am able to show a fairly non-critical critical path. This book is speculative writing; nevertheless, I try to bring into it as much rigor as conditions will permit. I doubt if I have made and, frankly, I doubt if it is possible to make, a mistake so serious it wholly disqualify the entire circuit philosophy. The problem of rigor will fall into place after we delve into the nuts and bolts of the mechanism.

The cerebral cortex is a special and very ingenious D.C. analogue data processor. It is utterly unlike present factory made analogue machines. For one thing, factories do not have a comparable analogue memory device. The cortical memory device is of molecular dimensions and it has enormous storage capacity: it is fast and it is precise. The cortex is also an extraordinarily efficient computer and it processes the cortical throughput statement with millions of individual elements (symbols) in the statement with an incredible economy of apparatus. The living cortex has the consistency of raw egg. After it has been preserved and prepared for anatomical study, it is somewhat firmer, about the same as hardboiled egg. In gross anatomy, the 16 billion or so cortical cells (gray) are confined to a thin layer (about 1/8 inch) which constitutes the outer "bark" of the hemisphere. The remainder of the hemisphere, most of it, is made up of the white "fan-in" fibers that carry information to and from the cortex and arcuate fibers running between lobes.

The white "fan-in" fiber attaches to a cortical module. (Only recently has the histologist been able to delineate the cells as a module.) There is one module for each fan-in fiber. In so far as I know, the number of fan-in fibers has never been counted. As a guess, there may be about 1500 gray cells for each radial white fiber. There are two halves to the module, so there will be about 800 or so gray cells per half. The apparent abundance of gray cells is so easily used up if they are fairly allocated to the modules that there are not enough active elements (gray cells) to permit a large number of complex computing operations in the cortex. "Estimating Memory Capacity" explains why the apparent abundance of cells has to be spread so thin. Additionally, the cortical system is known to be intrinsically free of a type of vulnerability where a dysfunction in a few key cells would put it out of business. The gray cells route the cortical statement through recursive channels as it moves through the cortex and, if the cells are in redundant usage, they are not functioning in a format that would make them available for more sophisticated computing operations. Cortical computation must be simple and straight forward: "bare bones", so to speak.

Inspecting the Problem

There is even a relationship between the formative processes that assemble the cortex and the level of sophistication we can expect to find in the system. Early formation of the cortex is a drawn out process with most of it completed by the second year postpartum. The remnants of this process, which began with the embryo, are not completed until the tenth year or later. These formative processes are interesting and more speculative than the circuitry. It is not possible to code enough hereditary information in the genetic code (information coded in the cell's nuclear DNA) to write instructions for the formation of the individual cortical cells, much less the thousands of connections between the cell and its neighbors. The disparity between the information the hereditary code is able to carry and the information required to dictate the assembly of the cortex on a cell-by-cell basis is far too great. Since highly critical, site-specific formative codes are out of the question, the hereditary code must dictate a gross formative subroutine for forming the cortical module. The module is universal: any module fits anywhere. Formative factors argue against sophisticated operations in the cortex because the operations, would require complex inter-cellular connections and, hence, highly site-specific hereditary codes.

The nerve cell, with its limitations, can only be used in five electronic applications. The applications are: repeater, summator, transducer, inverter and comparator. (I try to keep jargon at a

minimum. This list is virtually all of the jargon we can expect in
the text and it goes easily once we start to work with it.) The
nerve cell has two kinds of terminals: inputs and outputs, the cell
body is the input terminal and hundreds of connections from
neighboring cells are attached to it. The cell axon (the
elongation of the cell body) carries the signal to hundreds of
output branchings at its distal end. The co-axial cell ("co-
axial", an inner signal conductor surrounded by an outer "ground")
will only permit the limited computing operations on our short
list. The co-axial nerve cell itself restrains our expectations of
complex computing operations with the nerve cell for the computing
element.

The essence of the cortex is finesse: to do a moderately complex
computing job with a minimum of apparatus, operations and
vulnerabilities. (If I had to choose one adjective to describe the
cortical finesse, it would be the word "slick".)

Experiments and tissue studies are the main sources of
understanding of the cortex we have realized to the present. The
cortex itself is sparely amenable to experiment and tissue studies,
to the extent they expose cortical circuits, have temporarily
reached a point of diminishing returns. Cortical studies are
almost sure to be a sort of log-rolling movement where a small
advancement is made at the theoretical end, followed by another
step based on experiment. Tissue studies have reached something of
an impasse and the later text points to a need to work out the
electronic circuit in order to figure out the cellular organization

of the cortex. For the moment the only open and attractive avenue
to a better knowledge of the cortex is not being used.

A reliable circuit theory is central to better knowledge of the
cortex. The circuit theory has not been forthcoming because there
too few electronics specialists working on the study. The worst
mistakes that can be made with circuit theory is trying to write a
theory without actually studying the tissue of the cortex first.
Up to now, too much of cortical electronics has been in the hands
of dabblers who are eager with opinions that are not based on a
personal study of the cortex, and, up to now, the dabblers have
left us with the usual pedantic over conceptualizations, ad hoc
"model building" and a scattering of high sounding but otherwise
nincompoop ideas believed only by the parties who proposed them.

There is a conventional wisdom of sorts, perhaps a "pop" wisdom,
with regard to the cortex and we will try not to collide with the
conventional wisdom any more often that we have to. I see
avoidable contention as a profitless encumbrance. The most
engaging conflicts follow immediately.

The cerebral cortex does not have access to the subject matter of
the information it is processing. The conventional view would
probably insist the cortex must deal with the subject matter, as
subject matter, in order to function. Traditional opinion non-
withstanding, there is no operational need for the cortex to
concern itself with the subject matter on its throughput (This is
true of any computer); it serves no useful purpose as far as the

9

computer is concerned and there is a far better technical procedure.

Throughout, the text uses the visual system as a typical system. The input to the system, in this case: the retina, writes a coded statement derived from the phenomenology of the visual image, rather than the subject matter, and uses this for the cortical statement instead if the incredibly complicated, if feasible, procedure that would be required to extricate the subject matter of the image. The text explains how the input statement is written. Be it an input or an output, or both, a coded statement is the throughput statement for the lobe. In all cortical lobes, a coded electrical replica of the phenomena the lobe is assigned to, rather than subject matter, is the throughput statement.

Coding the phenomenology of the throughput and by-passing the incredibly complicated rigamaroles of sorting out subject matter is a far better technical process and it is fast, precise and uses a minimum of apparatus. The input statement is initially written in the phenomenal format anyway and is already available to the cortex so it is only reasonable for the cortex to process it in this form. The phenomenal statement is exquisitely compatible with internal cortical procedures, nothing is sacrificed, and, due to the elemental precision of the phenomenal statement, there is a gain with respect to the psychological "grasp" of the behavior of the world outside of the cortex.

The phenomenology of the visual image refers to the detailed, element by element, variations in the intensity of light falling on the microscopic receptors in the retina. The retinal coder generates an electrical replica, a million element "analogue", of these light events in the visual image and presents it, simultaneously and entirely, to the visual cortex for its input statement. This contrasts with the suggestion the visual cortex interprets the image by classifying it as edges, slanting lines, rounded forms and processes of that general nature. This sort of interpretation is not to be found anywhere in the cortex for reasons explained in the text. Why do all of this. All we need is a retrieval instruction and an instruction in phenomenal language is just as useable as one that sets out the subject matter. The retrieval instruction allows present experience to interrogate memory or enables one lobe to command another. An instruction in the language indigenous to the lobe, its phenomenal language, is an unestimatable simplification of the retrieval procedure. The lines, edges and forms suggestion throws away image detail that would be preserved in the element-by-element phenomenal statement. The phenomenal statement, is the cheap way, the only way to write the cortical statement, and we have the fastest and most precise way of retrieving information as a bonus. As far as I am concerned, it is technically impossible to isolate and classify the subject matter of the cortical statement or to write the retrieval instruction in any other way if we confine ourselves to a practical system and a reasonable amount of apparatus.

In claiming the cortex does not have access to the subject matter of its throughput, I had better be able to back up my point of view. I am. I back up this view if I accomplish nothing else.

Throughout the text I have a running series of strategically placed

arguments: arguments I call "clincher" arguments, supported by less

rigorous arguments I call "bonus" arguments, all arguments that

(should) conclusively demonstrate the cortex does not have access

to the subject matter of the information it is processing. (The

summit "clincher" argument is the retinal coder. The retinal coder

"homogenizes" the subject matter in a way that forbids sorting it

out and recognizing it as subject matter later on in the cortical

process.) The brain-body mechanism can be thought of as a behaving

mechanism in closed loop of behaving mechanisms. The brain/body

mechanism is one segment of the loop. The behavior of the

environment that surrounds the corticated organism is the other,

the complementary segment of the loop. Information (coded

behavior) moves from "sources" of information to "sinks" for

information as it circulates within the loop. The cortex keeps

track of behavior: the cortical input, and delivers behavior as an

output. Perception is the "source" and articulation of the body is

the "sink" for behavior in the brain/body segment of the loop. The

body moves around, does things, transacts with its environment and

the environment reflects this articulation as perceived behavior.

The environment again becomes the source and the body the sink for

the circulating information and the loop is closed back to the

input cortex. Somewhat simplified: the cortex makes positive

contributions to the behavior circulating in the loop by accepting

inputs, delivering outputs, forming trial associations within the

input, within the output or between input and output in any
combination, present or remembered.

The subject matter of this circulating behavior is only
meaningful, valid, operative (whatever) within the environment.
The environment is where we observe it, enjoy it, classify it with
our fine sounding categories and descriptions. Merely that the
cortex is dictating the body's behavior, forming these
relationships between inputs and outputs, without access to the
subject matter is not a big deal: as long as it gets the job done,
it makes no real difference how the process is managed within the
cortex. Writing instructions in the cortex is an uninterrupted
process. As long as the retrieval instruction is unique one and
only one instruction will elicit the same response, both the
recipient lobe and memory will have all of the information it needs
to respond forthwith. Given an instruction that uniquely
replicates an input or an output, the system can relate inputs to
outputs quite handily without a highly fretted treatment of the
subject matter of either.

We now move on to another small conflict with traditional ideas.
The fashionable idiom of contention and convenience implies an
ideational system. The language itself presupposes certain basic
identifications about ourselves, the world around us and the way we
behave in that world. The fashionable typology regarding the human
personality implies a perspective--entire philosophies for that

matter--and we can hope these ideas are not such a monopoly they preclude a reasonably factual description of ourselves.

Unfortunately, a lot of what is said about the human mental personality boils down to linguistic inventions--to "animisms" of language. A special agent, a special operator or operation, an animated something-or-other, is either overtly invoked or wrestled into existence by means of a metaphorical use of language. These fictionalized, these animized, views of the human and his world become so commonplace we accept them uncritically, hardly paying attention, and after a while the archetypes become so familiar we are not likely to question them.

These fictions of language, these "animisms", are easier to see when they refer to the mechanisms in our surroundings. "Water seeks its lowest level", metaphorically "animises" water. Here, a fiction of language gives water human qualities: the ability to seek, to make and carry out decisions, to anticipate and prosecute its deliberate actions. Factually stated, the water will be propelled to its destination by the usual forces whether the water intended that destination or not.

The posited operator is often less conspicuous when it is a frank linguistic construction, a named idea, a traditionally accepted label. Almost any psychological factor could be used as an example. "Motivation", if it is said to be a mental operation, is an example. We watch someone else behave. Confessedly he is a creature of habit. As we watch him, we tell ourselves we are seeing patterns, extra exertions, in some of his habits and we classify this selectively observed behavior as "motivated". This is a conventional idea and innocent enough as long as we do not mislead ourselves into assuming there must be a special process somewhere in the brain dedicated to bringing about what we call motivation. A habit is a habit. There are no special operations in the brain, over and above, the normal processes responsible for all habitual behavior. There is no mechanism that would select some habits as "motivated" habits, as such. There are operations in the cortex that might suggest the appearances of motivated behavior. While it is true there are emotionally reinforced habits, it is also true there is no mechanism responsible for motivation, as such. "Motivation", per se, is a fiction of labeling and not a cortical operation as such.

This imagery is endless and touches everything. It enhances an observation here, distorts an important appreciation somewhere else. The idea of an "abstract" mental process, which is said to be different than "concrete" thinking, is another fine example of this sort of imagery. (I have noticed one thing about abstract thinking: in its most reaching transports, in its most awesome subject matter, somehow it is always accompanied by a very concrete physical statement: a spoken word, a graven image and so on. I venture to say, without the visible image and the spoken word, there would be no abstraction.) Separate and distinct processes are posited. Peeling a banana is a concrete activity and involves "concrete" thought: designing a suspension bridge is an abstract process and requires a different, an "abstract", thought. Peeling

a banana, the cues are present and only hand eye tasks are needed.
Designing the bridge, the cues are recalled from memory and the
process is spread out over time and distance and takes in a lot
factors not immediately visible to the observer. As far as the
cortex is concerned, it is the same computer that figures out how
to both peel the banana and design the bridge. The computer
doesn't know which it is doing and couldn't care less; the
technical operations within the cortex are exactly the same.
Designing the bridge is a grand enterprise, a greater diversity of
relatable tasks are involved, the scale is bigger, with more of it
accomplished by thinking and less by visible body movements; there
are, however, no special cortical operations employed in the
"abstract" task that are not equally used for "concrete" thinking.
This is a complex and specialized area and merits more than the
mention in passing I am able to manage here.

The worst pitfalls in defining the human personality derive from
the use of the metaphor, from posited but otherwise nonexistent
processes, and from out-and-out fictionalizing the definition of
the human. These inventions have a useful suggestive value and
probably enrich our lives with imagery where a more factual
description of ourselves and our behavior might be less
interesting, less graphic and probably somewhat more monotonous.
Imagery loses its innocence when it obscures fact. Most of it is
trivial and can be safely disregarded. On the other hand, if we
say there must be a cortical operation for every assumed
psychological factor, for every alleged component of behavior, for
every fashionable opinion that comes along, we will never close the

already abysmal disparity between what the cortex is said to be doing and what it is actually does.

The cortex deals with the minutia of behavior: its underlying phenomenal substrate made up of the thousands of finely detailed physical events so minuscule and commonplace are un-noticed. An input to, an output from, the cortex must be stipulated as a detailed physical statement. The minutia of this statement is the only "handle", the only "purchase" the cortex has on the world outside. The business of reducing behavior to the minutia of the physical input and output statements, as perceived, as articulated, by the cortex, is a problem for the psychology people. It is not an easy job to begin with which probably accounts for the traditional dependency on so many posited operators assumed to reside in the brain somewhere.

Sooner or later, cortical theory, psychology and, I suppose, the study of language, will converge and explain the human capacity to verbalize. As a matter of fact, explaining the verbal process has been emerging as something of a new and oncoming art in recent years.

We humans, with our more elaborate vocal mechanism, and more sophisticated use of the temporal cortex (where vocal motor instructions originate). Have a much needed edge over our animal friends who are not able to verbalize at all.

The speech lobe is set off to the side of the mainstream of data flow in the cortex. Here it is able to function in its own regimen and, not needed to maintain the posture of the body, it freely devotes itself to remembered information regardless of immediate cues and present tasks. Set off to the side, it is able to function as an independent cortical system, more or less.

We verbalize as we experience, unvocalized, it is an inner and continuous, running commentary concerning the things we perceive and the actions we will take. The temporal cortex associates this inner, running commentary with worldly experience. A combination involving the freedom of the temporal lobe and its verbal annotation of experience, the physics of the speech system (with its capacity for silent vocalization), along with persistent environmental encouragement and elaboration of the speech process, allows the human to commemorate his experience with a verbal mnemonic "flag" which surely consolidates and expedites the thinking process.

This remarkable scheme renders it possible to appreciate, to manage, to "exercise" experience on a surrogate basis. Past and anticipated experience become a relevant part of immediate experience. The surrogate "flag" allows trial relationships between experiences where the relationship can be formed and silently "exercised" without the effort and delay of moving the body.

The problem is not so much how we think abstractly but, simply, how we think. For the most part, we think verbally. Just what it is we do when we think verbally has been studied by experts over the years and questions such as this are usually answered in small bits and pieces over a span of time and by contributions from a large number of specialists. Drawing a diagram of the cortical computer will not have a direct bearing on these problems, problems that had best be left to the experts.

Some of the things the expert must take into consideration as he studies vocal skills and their verbal outcomes are mentioned in the item: "Habits and Strategies that Augment the Raw Machine Intelligence". Our concern is the computing module. A better understanding of the module should make it easier for the people who work in these fields to assess the cortical contribution to the thinking process. Some of the following suggestions may be helpful;

1. The verbal throughput is processed in the form of a vocal motor skill. The way it is silenced is explained in the text. The temporal cortex, like all other lobes in the system, processes its throughput statement without access to the subject matter of the throughput.

2. No special cortical procedures or formats are to be found in the temporal cortex for verbal computation that are not standard in the rest of the cortical system. As we become more familiar with cortical tissue, it becomes unignorably evident there is only one type of module and one processing format for all cortical lobes. As I see it, an alternate mechanism is neither possible nor necessary.

3. The problem for the speech expert is stipulating the minutia of the vocal task, and there are a lot of subtleties and unknowns

involved. Once the specifics of the vocal task are worked out, I am confident the computing module we have, with its speed and flexibility, will be entirely adequate to provide the computing substrate underlying the vocal skill. Again, a more complex or more specialized module is neither possible nor necessary. We now move on to another major point of contention with the conventional wisdom as it accounts for the human personality. The traditional wisdom, already sprinkled with more posited operators that it really needs, culminates in a grand and total fictionalization of the human. This time, he in infested with a posited non-physical agent, an animism (again), an incubus (the little green spook that lives in the head and evidently spends its time trying to get its lantern lit). All of this is fine conjury and topical too; it does, however, draw attention away from the scarce possibility the brain might have something to do with the things that go on in the head.

The spook gets the axe--better still: Occam's razor--on grounds there is no evidence there is such a thing and no common sense reason to suppose one either. It is not one spook but a genre of spooks and assorted non-physical agents, all disguised by a number of colorful names and all abroad in our midst. They originate in the tribal incubania and are variously named: the "psyche" (as it is called), the "mind" (as it is called), and the "ego" (in the sense of it being a personal, or "subjective", non-physical agent).

If this book is to be a serious treatment of the cortex, it had better anchor down the phenomena it purports to be dealing with "up front". Having made these first and basic identifications, we had better remain consistent throughout. If we neglect to do this, we will have nothing but mud.

A decision has to be made: either the spook or the computer runs the show; it can't be both. There is no need to belabor the spook; the incompatibility between cortical procedure and the spook is pretty much self-evident in the text.

Such cavalier dismissal of ideas as cherished as these ought to be accompanied by a few words of explanation. Most dictionaries list the word "mind" as an all-purpose, all inclusive, word for just about anything having to do with mental activity. It does not seem to be anchored to a specific phenomenon and the breadth of its definitions include mental activity that should be more precisely named by a more appropriate and already extant term. "Mind" (as it is called), in so many of its definitions, denotes a mental "mechanism" or its equivalent. (The mechanical appreciation of "mind" is in fashion with fiction writers. They speak of: warped minds, twisted minds, broken minds, mind bending, and so on.)

The active mechanism in the cortex is the memory mechanism and the mistake is made when "mind" (as it is called) is given credit for performing mental operations that are, in fact, carried out by the memory mechanism. The memory mechanism is the cortical mechanism that thinks, combines, builds up habits, accepts inputs and dictates action. This is done by the cortex and the cortex alone.

(If I am reading a book which frequently refers to the "mind", I have found I can upgrade the good sense of the discussion immeasurably and make it infinitely more careful of fact if I take a felt tip pen and draw a line through the word "mind" whenever I see it and substitute "memory mechanism" or "memory". Try it.)

The first paragraph of a dictionary definition of "mind" usually suggests the "mind" is an operator or a mechanism of some sort in the head. The second paragraph of a dictionary account of "mind" is often not in keeping with its first. The idea of an internal operator is abandoned and the "mind" is defined a second time. This time it is: learning or training, habits or habituation, activities or components of behavior that can only be acquired from the environment. The sense of the definition drifts from internal matters and the situs of the "mind" moves out to the world....out there.

Semantic problems become more intractable than they, at first, appear. It is not easy to argue the meaning of a word that is not clearly attached to a "thing" or a "process" on the one hand, and is so commonly used in such general and diffuse usage, on the other, that it could include any convenient invention as long as it speciously referred to the human personality. "Mind" in its pure and original understanding, intends a genuine, card carrying, non-physical incubus. It is a fiction of language. It is a figment of the tribal incubania.

We are born to a province somewhere in the world and we inherit the pre-existing language, ideation and philosophies indigenous to the province and the era. This is not necessarily a fair and sensible arrangement; the question of fairness arises because we inheritors have little choice but to accept the ideas of the distant past, such as they are, with no consultation regarding their relevance or validity. Acceptance of these ideas, dubious ideas that were slung together--ad hoc, by ancestors far less knowledgeable, perhaps less contentious that ourselves, is the price we have to pay for the privilege of harvesting the accumulated tribal wisdom without which human existence would be pretty grim indeed.

The tribal incubania is a part of that heritage. A frank incubus, such as the idea of a "mind", is fairly easy to expose and kindly protest. Seen personally, there is no great personal investment in the outcome of a dispute over the existence of this particular spook.

The personal "subjective" (the posited "subject" in the "subject/object" relationship), the "ego" (as it is called), the "me" notion and a few related ideas are also figments of the tribal conjury and cold exposure may require slightly more detachment and objectivity that we normally expect of ourselves. The egocentric conjury has been handed down from antiquity, an enduring monument to an almost atavistic bad logic. The logical predicament is given a name: the "egocentric predicament".

The language is overwhelmed with egocentric ideas; perfuse with egocentric assumptions and apologetics. The language suggests and enforces its suggestion. On the other hand, the language: the most intense ideational monopoly of all, does not suggest, may even be incapable of expressing, its antithetical corollaries. It certainly does not suggest, nor contra-argue , alternatives to egocentric ideas with the same monopoly and resounding effectiveness. The user of the language tends to be "linguistically blind", hence, philosophically blind, to a less egocentric view of himself or able to appreciate his surroundings unless his surroundings are accounted for within a framework of egocentric assumption. This is the egocentric predicament.

The language, biased with egocentric assumption, strong in sparing embarrassment to the "ego" it invents and defends, is not the best tool to use in demonstrating the fictitious nature of the notions of a personal "subjective", or a personal "spook", or whatever it may be called. This is difficult enough to manage as a philosophical issue and the philosophical issue is the smallest part of the problem.

We verbalize as we experience: the silent running commentary noted earlier. This is an inner verbalization and, as we do this, we habitually fictionalize a transaction wherein we mentally comment on something we recognize in the world "out there" followed by mentally artificing a relationship between it and a habitual "me" notion....here, inside. Logically we recognize the mechanism of the body and the mechanisms of the physical world are involved in the transaction and then, illogically, we habitually fictionalize a third participant to the transaction: a personal non-physical agent, the "me" as we are wont to think of it. We are indoctrinated with this ritual (it does not come naturally, it is a cultural matter) at a very early age in life, long before our critical faculties have been sharpened to the extent it would take to question the validity of the ritual or inquire about the possibility the whole shebang might be falsified to begin with.

Counter arguments to the egocentric rigmarole, surely personal counter arguments, however diligently and carefully reasoned, are almost totally ineffective in opposition to the powerful and ceaseless habituation of the "me" notion. (Egocentric doctrine is not especially amenable to prima fascia argument. To deal with the problem at all, on a personal basis or otherwise, it is almost necessary to be a "buff" who studies the egocentric predicament or one or more of its ramifications: psychological, philosophical or linguistic.)

Let's face it, the "me" notion is the most deeply set habit we have and there is a lot more to it than a simple habit. It is an extensive repertory of habits, an enduring personal legend of interdependent and intervalidating habits. The "me" habit is so repetitively suggested, so emotionally nurtured and so inflexibly (personally) defended that, as the years go by, the habit becomes so deeply set, it is taken for granted the habit cannot be interrupted. We make a mistake when we take it for granted the "me" habit is so necessary, so immutable, that it is beyond interruption.

We should allow there may be spontaneous pauses in the "me" habit. Maybe these pauses are so common we fail to give them

special notice or fail to verbalize an acknowledgment of the pause
while it is in progress. The free processes of the cortex can and
do suspend habits from time to time, however deeply set they may
be. The belief there is an object--out there, and a "me"--in here,
is a habitual notion that can also be voluntarily suspended, but it
takes training and practice to do it.

With training and practice we can train ourselves to deliberately
bring about a suspension of the "me" habit. Zen buffs will
recognize this as the central preoccupation of Zen. Zen is a
rather distilled form of Buddhism indigenous to Japan. There is no
straightforward and predictable gambit that will assure the
suspension of a habit. It is more a matter of arranging for, and
encouraging, a memory accident to take place. The accident we are
arranging for is a 10 to 20 second suspension of the silent and
habitual "me" verbalization, or personal variations of the same
thing.

If we go to the trouble of training ourselves to do this, we also
want to be alerted and prepared to grasp whatever psychological and
philosophical implications that may turn up if and when a brief
period of dehabituation should occur. I say this because so much
is written about this experience by writers under the influence of
dope. They unerringly spell out the psychological aspects and
seem utterly unable to attach any philosophical significance to the
experience. I never use booze or dope and see it as a hindrance in
trying to bring about this odd experience.

The recommended technique, per Zen, is to relax and meditate.
Here, meditation is understood to be unrestrained free recall, to

be unpreoccupied thinking: free of distraction, free of a focused thread of thought. The meditating novitiate, caught with his guard down, caught less alert and facile at defending his idea of his personal "subjective", is surprised by the abbot with a sort of practical joke called a Koan.

The novitiate asks: "How long will it be before I attain enlightenment?". The master answers the question with a question. "Who is making the inquiry? " The student, a little defocused and caught off guard by the unexpected question, is now hard pressed to account for and defend the "I" or "me" he just referred to. If things go on schedule, he will discover, in an unexpected lunge of spontaneous understanding, the idea he perpetually persists in contriving--his "me" notion-- is a falsification to begin with.

Meditation has brought him to a freer, less egocentrically biased mood, the unexpected insight was on accident. Practice makes him less up-tight about relinquishing his cherished beliefs about himself including his unshakeable belief he is a special phenomenon in all of its prickly uniqueness. He is now free to discover, or is jogged into discovering the fictitious nature of his personal version of his "me" notion. (Depending on how uptight he is, he may resort to a panicked defense of his cherished beliefs and the opportunity for "enlightenment", as they say, slips past him one more time.)

The whimsy and spontaneity of the Koan have caught on easily in the western world and the whimsy sets the fashionable impression of

Zen. The practice and noodle work required to become adept at
suspending the "me" habit are less appealing, so it often passes
un-noticed. Acquiring this skill is the central purpose of Zen.
To learn more about this technique, I recommend The Way of Zen by
the late Alan Watts. Even with Watts, it is necessary to read the
pertinent paragraphs in The Way of Zen a couple of times in order
to discover becoming adept at dehabituation, not the Koan, is the
purposeful objective of Zen.

If a master is able to accumulate, say, seven minutes of
dehabituation, in 10 to 20 second fragments over a lifetime of
practice, it is said to be all that can be achieved. I have
trained myself to do this and probably have about as much luck as
anyone. I do this without meditating and, as I see it, technique
is unimportant as long as the objective is achieved. I have a
feeling the seven minute goal can be greatly exceeded, though, I
cannot say how it should be done. I am not able to dehabituate
predictably and, after playing at trying for a while, it loses its
edge and I forget to practice. About 95% of becoming adept is
merely being alerted to the fact the "me" habit will suspend itself
from time to time. To a first timer, the abrupt suspension of this
long standing and faithful habit can be thoroughly irksome. So,
enjoy the irksomeness.

Acquiring this skill is not thought to be gainful. It does not
make anyone happier or wealthier nor does it make anyone's sky a
little bluer. It does wise one up a bit and that is all it does.
No philosophies or perspectives are directly derived by cultivating
this skill. Those of philosophical bent should see it as a takeoff

point, a thought and experience to be investigated, before writing philosophies that pertain to the egocentric predicament.

The "spook" in the head allegation has had credibility problems throughout its long history. The burden of demonstrating there is such a thing (after explaining what it is supposed to be) and dealing with the credibility problems is up to the proponent of the idea.

I think this short dialogue on Zen has been worthwhile because Zen demonstrates the foolishness of the spook business with an authority and finality seldom equaled in settling arguments. The trouble with Zen is that it only interests the Zen buff, even so, the Zen buff needs a certain amount of luck. The egocentric wisdom and the spook in the head are side issues, as far as I am concerned. I can only point to the existence of the issues and move on to the electronics of the computer,

We have one small, final difference of opinion between the folk wisdom and the practical cortex. As the folk wisdom comments on the brain, it fails to notice two computing mechanisms are needed to produce the personality and intelligence we have come to know and love.

One mechanism has to be an "iterative" mechanism and the other an "associative" mechanism. Now then, there is a wondrous cortical finesse which permits one physical apparatus to be operated in two modes thereby enabling one cortical computing mechanism to do both jobs.

An iterative mechanism repeats ("iterate", to do again). It learns and makes use of what it learns in a "parrot-like" fashion, nothing more. It is not an intelligent mechanism as such. In addition to doing its own work, this parrot-like cortical mechanism provides the guidelines essential to the intelligent mechanism and without which it could not function at all.

Oddly enough, it is the parrot-like iterative mechanism which does most of the brain work that gets done in day to day living, If we are fortunate enough to live in an informative environment, we learn from our environment and the iterative mechanism is all that is needed for this parrot-like learning. We can learn and use what we need to learn by rote and get along without critical or urgent need for intelligence. Each day is a lot the same as the last and the things we will be doing shortly are predicated on the things we have been doing recently. If the environment will indicate the guidelines, the iterative mechanism will accumulate them, convert them to habits, and intelligence will only be needed in small contributions.

(The iterative mechanism never ceases to function, even in the damaged brain, and, while the loss of intelligence is sorely missed, it is the still functioning iterative mechanism that makes it possible for the mentally impaired to get on in life.)

A throughput is a series of input or output statements, usually both. The iterative (only) mechanism enters or delivers throughputs or builds them up in memory: "as acquired": it does nothing toward modifying the throughput. The throughput recalled from memory is the same one that went in.

Inspecting the Problem

Merely that a mechanism can be trained to do something, merely that it is "conditionable" or "habituatable" does not make it a "smart" mechanism. In other words: "conditionable" and "intelligent" are not the same thing. We have to define a mechanism that (only) iterates as a "dumb" mechanism in order to avoid contradiction in a spectrum of interdependent definitions and understandings in this area--already a trifle blurred the way it is.

Cortical intelligence manifests itself as an intelligent contribution added to a guideline provided by the iterative system. The iterative process always provides the guideline by dictating the core of the throughput statement.

Cortical intelligence is a computing service; it does not function independently and self-sufficiently. Intelligent procedure differs from iterative procedure because it _modifies_ the throughput where iterative procedure does not. There is a further stipulation; intelligent contribution must modify the throughput on a _free_ basis. Since it is a free basis, intelligent procedure can only be a trial and error business and, this being the case, the outcome of an intelligent process is not predictable.

Suppose we have a system and, as a test, we ask it a question. If the system has the answer in its memory inventory, it simply looks it up and uses it. Nothing needs to be "figured out". Here, an iterative capability is entirely adequate. Even if the system is "figuring out" a targeted answer, that is, an answer confirmable within the system (or an equivalent procedure), it is still a "dumb" system though it may have used intelligent procedure to "figure out" the targeted answer. Iteration and intelligent procedure complement each other. The outcome of iteration is always predictable, intelligent contribution is not. Iterative systems will function self-sufficiently. Intelligence must always be accompanied by an iterated dictation from some other source.

(The later text takes a look at intelligence in its original function and suggests the cortex initially evolved as a computing service added on to the then extant reflex and instinctive systems. The cortex was, and still is for most animals, an accessory computing service which overlays and supplements a primordial "core" system of reflex and instinctive capabilities. Without the evolution of the cortex, evolution of animal life would have arrested with fairly simple creatures, perhaps insect like, with stiff mechanical movements and with its livelihood always in doubt due to the inflexibility pre-programmed in its behavior, its life style and even the conformation of its body. The evolution of the cortex brought forward a greater diversion of animal species, allowance for variations in the somnatype within the species, plasticity in the animals life style and an assortment of related factors. Cortical intelligence does not originate throughputs: it can only manifest itself as an add-on contribution to a throughput that originates in some other source. In its original function, cortical intelligence is a strategy for rapidly manipulating and modifying old and rigid throughputs to fit new situations.)

Inspecting the Problem

A short preview of intelligent procedure might be helpful.
Either real experience or memory can be the source of a "core", or
"backbone" throughput which is used for a retrieval instruction.
The present retrieval may not be, probably is not, in exact
agreement with one that has been used before. Intelligent
procedure is a technical procedure, rapidly repeated if necessary,
to adapt, to modify, an extant memory response so it is "tailored"
to the requirements of the present retrieval instruction in the
time permitted. It becomes a true "procedure" when the instruction
is repeated for the special purpose of computing the intelligent
"add-on". It is this incessant technical embellishment, this add-
on, made more elaborate by human formalization, that ultimately
underpins intelligence as it is observed in the human personality.

We must also allow: starting with a core throughput as a
guideline and with repeated trial efforts, the cortex modifies the
core throughput to such an extent we can fairly say it has emerged
with an original and genuinely synthetic throughput. At this point
intelligent procedure is concluded: it has contributed all that is
technically feasible for it to contribute and its participation in
the game is over

The cortical contribution is entirely a trial and error matter,
therefore, the outcome of the trial synthesis must be confirmed as
useful, or appropriate, or whatever test is needed, by sources of
information other than, and outside of the cortex itself. Of
inescapable necessity, it is the milieu of worldly experience, the

surrounding sensorium, that must ultimately confirm or repudiate the outcome of cortical synthesis. Since the worldly environment does not methodically and immediately indicate the validity of everything we do, a certain amount of good fortune probably helps.

Our gung ho logical positivism is almost an atavistic affliction; unfortunately its enthusiasm for the potential of human intelligence puts more emphasis on the positive that it does on the logical. We are mistaken if we believe a system with intelligent capability should be able to examine a problem it has never seen before, expressed in terms and language not in repertory, and to positively and predictably deliver the correct solution, on sight, on the first try.

Here are a few practical and limiting truisms with regard to intelligence

1. Intelligence cannot make use of information never presented to the system or information that does not exist. Intelligence does not pick information out of the air. The imaginings of cortical intelligence all begin with "real" information derived from encounters in the past. Intelligence is riveted to the beginning state of the information it has to work with: it can neither escape nor transcend this informational substrate.

(While we may think it is one of our wildest flights of unconstrained imagining, on closer look it turns out to be, not the way-out synthesis we thought it was, but a new arrangement of old experiences and perceptions. However original we may think our imaginings to be, they never escape the familiar world. This fact even penetrated the density of the mediaeval inquisition. The inquisitors, after hearing thousands of confessions, some volunteered, some forced, began to notice the confessions never seemed to report experience beyond the bounds of the victim's day to day knowledge ability. Expecting tales of incredible midnight sport in the unimaginable worlds of the devil, the confession always turned out to be an eclectic fabrication of ideas and experiences easily within the demonology of the province and the world close to the confessee.)

2. The presence or absence of the substrate information is the first concern. The second concern it the quality of that information. If "soft" information is presented to the system, it will not become "hard" information merely for having passed through an intelligent mechanism. The "garbage in/garbage out" rule for all computers also applies to the cortex.

Intelligence cannot answer questions that do not have answers nor questions that are paradoxical. Intelligence does not resolve irresolvables or clarify ambiguities if they are presented to the system as irresolvables and ambiguities. If there are problems in our surroundings to be solved, it will be helpful if our surroundings will clearly state the terms of the problem free of credibility difficulties or contradictions and, better yet, tell us how to solve them. These are environmental matters and constitute a never ending limitation of the potential for intelligence.

3. Communication and information processing schemes are intrinsically unable to traffic novel throughputs. The throughput

must be stated in a language, a format, and a continuum indigenous to the system. This restraint is absolute and unconditional to the same degree the novelty of the traffic is absolute and unconditional. This blindness to novel throughputs is a reality of system logic and restrains not only systems but problem solving philosophies as well.

When the cortex generates its own synthesis, the synthesis amounts to a novel throughput by reason of its trial nature. It is generated in the dark and passed on to the next step in the process. The trial needs to be confirmed. Since the trial has heretofore not been in inventory, a prior way to confirm it will not be in inventory either, therefore the cortex must ultimately depend on its environment to confirm the validity of its trial outputs. If it could confirm its own trials internally it would be an iterative rather than an intelligent procedure and there would be no synthesis, nothing new and original.

(The cortex is a practical mechanism. The inability to predict the outcome of its trial throughputs logically follows its blindness to novel throughputs. This is another way of saying the cortex is denied both the gift of prophecy and the gift of omniscience. Intelligence is a strategy for dealing with problems that can not otherwise be dealt with. It is simply a strategy that works. It gets a job done, it does not work miraculously.)

4. We have two mechanisms at work; the intelligent mechanism and the iterative mechanism, both are needed in the cortex. If neither seems to be working in quite the way we expected it to, it is because, up to now, we have been looking at the mechanisms as they

would function in isolation from each other. In isolation, an intelligent (only) brain would be all trial and so much error its output would be unusable. With the iterative (only) brain, working in isolation, intelligence is not a part of the system and, if we are relying on the iterative procedure to answer a question for us, we must remember the iterative mechanism is "stuck" when there is no prior answer in inventory.

The two systems must work together. The underlying cortex is confronted with roughly the same decision making impasse we face in the behavioral sense. When we make a decision, we gather the terms and values that will influence the decision and we weigh them. If there is an imbalance in the weighing, a direction for our future actions is indicated. In keeping with the guideline, we interrogate memory and come forth with a disposition for this decision based on experience we have had with this problem at some time in the past. Whether it is the underlying computed substrate or gross behavior, this is a matter that can be iterated and intelligence is not required.

If we recognize nothing in the outcome of the weighing that would tell us how to decide, we have no basis for making a decision. Nothing is accomplished by paralyzing the decision making machinery with endless attempts at making a decision that cannot be made. We can only toss a coin (the cortex resorts to an equivalent strategy) and the outcome just of necessity be a trial, uncertain and unpredictable. In this case, we have an impasse. Whether it is efficacious or not, the only recourse for intelligent procedure is to keep plugging away with repeated trial solutions since it has no real basis for making a decision.

(Making a big decision by dividing it into smaller decisions, deciding not to decide and this sort of strategy changes nothing fundamental about making decisions. Smaller decisions, subroutines and sub-decisions, are still 'small' scale versions of the same decision making predicament.)

Allowing the character of decision making changes with the presence or absence of a guideline, given the decision making milieu and the complementary nature of the iterative and intelligent procedure, there is only one way to employ these two processes. A parlay must be worked out with lubricous switching, rapidly and ad hoc, from one procedure to the other in keeping with the indicators of the moment. The cortical "smart" engine is a single physical mechanism. It is capable of functioning in either its iterative mode or its intelligent mode (called the "associative" mode in the text) and it is continuously and rapidly switched, ad hoc, perhaps several times a second, as the instant and task require. (The format for judging when to switch and when not to switch is a cortical finesse and discussed in the item on the "Finesse of the Exalted Data Stage".)

5. An inventory of throughputs builds up in cortical memory over the years. These are "core" throughputs which are modified by add-on contributions from intelligence. The outcome is both a new entry in memory and a corollary of one of the "core" throughputs. This parlay combined an old, tried and true, throughput with a

smaller "trial" component, forming a "near" corollary of a throughput already in inventory. Intelligence works its way from one throughput to the next by generating "near" corollaries of the throughputs involved. This is not a bad arrangement. By using inventory as a backbone and guideline, by allowing intelligence to make its contribution as an "add-on" so intelligence can hedge its bet, intelligence is never in a predicament where it must "jump off the deep end", so to speak. With this parlay, there is always a rational core for each trial throughput.

Drawing the relationships between observed behavior and the underlying cortical computation is a study in itself. There are at least two obstacles to the bridging the gap between behavior and the underlying cortical computation. One is the scale of observation problem with its need for constant reminding the behaving event is dictated by the computer as a detailed instruction to the muscles of the body. The second obstacle is the tendency to believe there is a special and unique computation for each category of behavior.

The underlying cortical computation is entirely a technical matter based on the blind manipulation of the minutia of this or that throughput statement. The cortical output is "blind" because the cortex does not have access to the subject matter of the throughput as the text so conclusively points out. The subject matter of end behavior is entirely an environmental matter. End behavior is contrived in the environment, acquired from the environment, enforced by the environment and whatever is said about it, it is only meaningful in the environment.

THE "SMART" ENGINE AND THE MEMORY THROUGHPUT LEDGER

The mechanism I am showing for the cortical intelligent mechanism bears a distant family resemblance to another intelligent mechanism which was proposed by British mathematician: Alan Turing (Alan Turing, code expert, mathematician and logician, did pioneer work on artificial intelligence in England. He was killed in an automobile accident in 1954 at age 42.) This is not a Turing machine. There are significant differences between the two mechanisms. I will explain these differences in the summary of this item.

The neurologists and researchers studying the cortex have an almost standing objection to the intelligent machines that have been proposed up to now. The logician contrives a fine model of cortical computer, one he has a fondness for, and proposes it as the only and true cortical mechanism. He then leaves all questions about the way it fits into the histology of the nervous system for someone else to answer.

I approached this problem from the opposite direction. A study of the nerve cell will give us a pretty good idea of what the nerve cell is, and is not, capable of doing as the active element in the computer. Some of the topology of the cortex can be worked out with general principles and common sense. I did this about 20 years ago and concluded the smart engine has to be the mechanism we will be analyzing presently.

In the intervening years I have been unable to either evolve or discover still another mechanism that held any promise of working at all. In so far as I am concerned, this is the only device compatible with the nerve cell and capable of both iteration and intelligence in the same unit. I point this out because is so easy to invite the stigma of trying to promote a "pet" model for the cortical smart mechanism. When we discuss the nerve cell, we see it is clearly not a matter of promoting a pet and special mechanism but a genuine scarcity of alternatives.

It takes a sympathetic looking and some imagining to visualize the way the machine functions in the cortex. One does not embrace this mechanism on sight: it has to "grow on you", so to speak.

The mechanism is not understood on sight either, so it will be necessary to devolve the explanation of the beast somewhat. We will start with the common tape recorder as a mechanical analogue of the cortical memory mechanism and work our way into the only slightly more sophisticated engine in the cortex. A tape recorder, hybridized as a memory device in the visual cortex would look like Fig. 1. Both the sensor and the coder are in the retina of the eye. (The sensor is the sensitive element in the special senses: sight, sound, touch, taste and smell. The individual sensor is found in an array of sensors: the retina is such an array. The sensor is

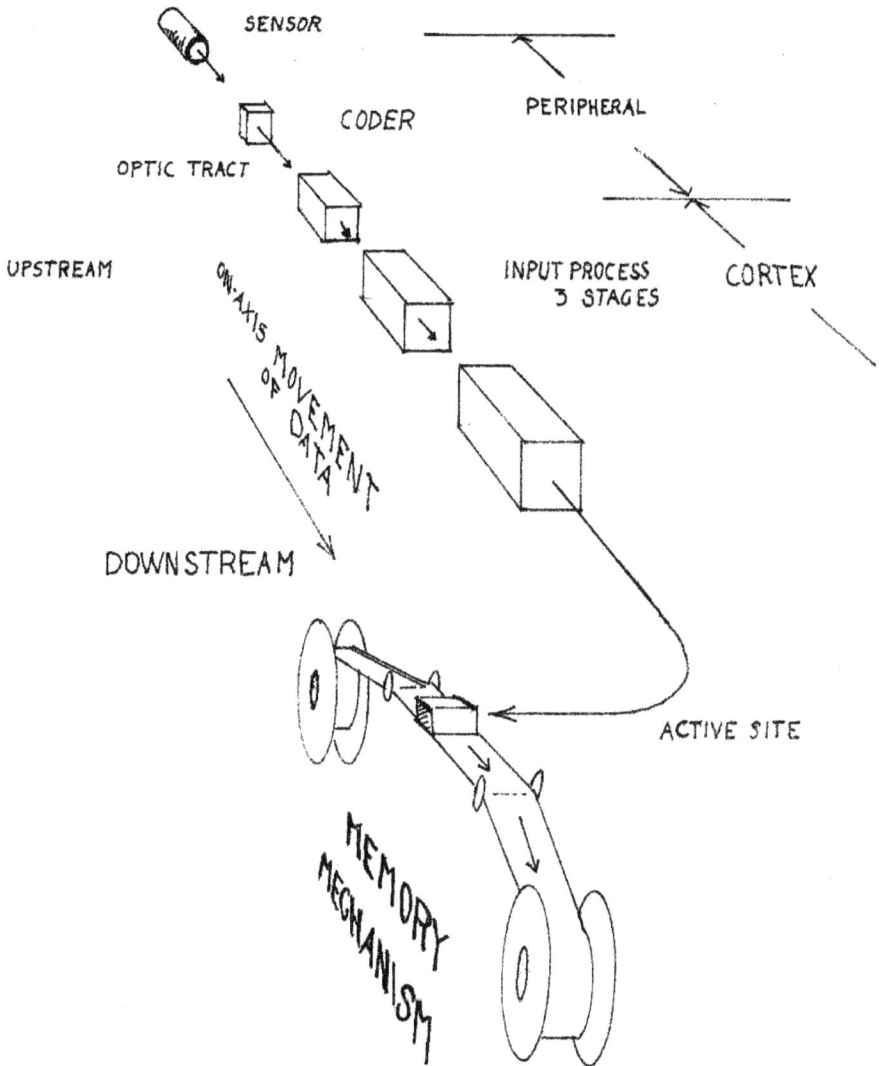

Figure 1

usually described with its generic name; photoreceptor in the

retina, hair cell in the organ of Corti in the hearing array and so on. The sensor transduces (or translates) the physical stimulus

which falls on it to an electrical equivalent: a voltage or

current. The voltage is a direct function of, or proportional to

the intensity of the stimulus. (The voltage is an electrical

"analogue" of the physical stimulus.)

   The combined action of the more than 100 million photoreceptors

in the retina, along with the processes of the coder, has

translated the entire light image to an electrical replica of the

light image and put it on board the optic nerve.

   The optic nerve (or optic tract) is the link which carries the

signal from the retina to the cortex. There is another system, a

reflex system, which picks off visual information in the middle of

the optic tract that is used to aim and focus the eye. This system

has been omitted.

   After the electrical replica of the visual image has been erected

at the retina; it moves down the optic tract toward the cortex and

ends up in memory. This is the "on-axis" movement of data in the

network. Fig. 1 is a single "on-axis data bus". A "data bus"

picks up information somewhere and delivers it to its destination.

There are a million data buses carrying visual data to one lobe of

the visual cortex. Two million data buses for the two hemispheres.

   Fig. 1 shows the data bus straight through and has the data bus

in isolation, this arrangement is not used in the cortex. There

are also "lateral-to-the-axis" processes, omitted here for clarity.

   The combined output of the million data buses in the visual

system is a statement, written in visual system language, where an

electrical event has been substituted for a light event that took place at a particular photoreceptor. (Since there are more photoreceptors than there are optic nerves, each data bus reports to memory with a composited signal which was originally impressed on about 125 photoreceptors.) This is an analytical statement, an alalysand, which replicates the perceived image in all of its detail; the visual system is typical of the several perceptual systems.

A similar electrical statement is written in the motor cortex. The motor statement originates in motor memory and flows out of the cortex as a motor instruction to the muscles of the body. Each lobe of the cortex writes one of these statements which is entered in memory at the site where it is written. Taken together they constitute an overall cortical statement which is continuously delivered to all active sites from memory. Each statement is a memory throughput and each throughput is entered in the memory throughput ledger.

When memory scan takes place, the active site will select a particular throughput as a cortical statement. Mindful of keeping jargon at a minimum, I will call these active sites the "exalted data stage". When the active site selects a throughput for the cortical statement, the throughput is "exalted".

There are millions of elements in the throughput statement. An element is an instantaneous sampling of the stimulus on the sensor. The elements are entered on the tape one at a time. Entry takes place while the stimulus is still present which is a leisurely rate compared to memory delivery. The entry site is also the "read" site. On memory delivery, memory "dumps" the tape and data elements pour through the site on the order of millions per second. The exalter process will select the element passing through the active site at any instant determined by the exalter finesse. The data element selected is raised in rank from one merely in memory to one that is in active use. (A factory made system would probably call it a "gated" stage. There are enough differences to merit a new term.)

When the eye looked at a visual image, one throughput was entered in memory. Upon entry, we say the throughput has received one reinforcement. When recalling from memory, the system will deliver a throughput and upon delivery, it will make an additional copy of the throughput which is re-entered in memory. The throughput receives one reinforcement each time it is used. This is self-reinforcement.

This business of enter, deliver, copy, enter again, is the "iterative" process of the mechanism. Throughputs are built up in memory as a result of two processes; one it the iterative process, the other, the associative process which we investigate later on. Fig. 2 is a closer look at the tape and illustrates the technical need for a means to separate
the entries on the tape.

Fig. 3 follows the progress of one of the million-data events that constitute the statement, this is the contribution made by one data bus.

THE "SMART" ENGINE AND THE MEMORY THROUGHPUT LEDGER

In Fig. 4, at an instant of inspection, there are coherent data entries (capital letter "A") and noise events (symbol, *). The coherent date event is coherent because it is a part of a total statement which is, in itself, coherent.

(There is always a certain amount of noise in the system in spite of vigorous noise suppression measures. The noise can be seen with this simple experiment. With the eyes closed, recall a letter of the alphabet. The solid, most stable and best defined part of the image will be in the center of the recalled visual field. Around the periphery of the central image, there will be a black and white scintillation resembling "snow" on a weak TV channel. The snow can be so dense it looks like blotches or fingerprints on a photograph. This is the "on-axis" noise, or simply "noise", in the visual system. With practice, this experiment can be used for insight into other aspects of the visual process.)

METAL FOIL ——————————

MAGNETIZED PARTICLES ——————

SUPERVISORY EVENT

DATA EVENT

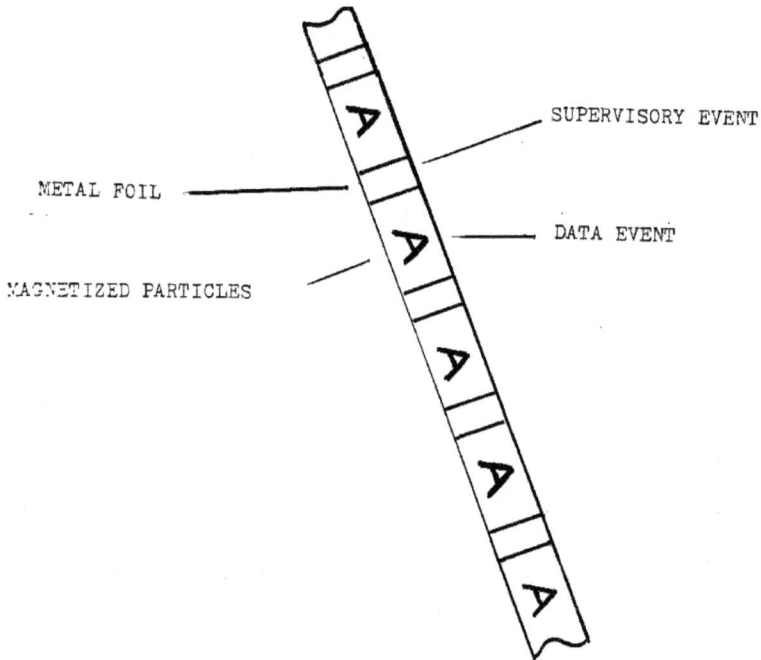

Taking a closer look at the tape, a means must be provided to separate the entries and, with this way of doing things, to insure the tape control system will not scan back and land in the middle of an entry. If we actually used magnetic tape in this apparatus, we could glue a piece of metal foil between the entries to meet these requirements. The foil becomes the "supervisory event" and the magnetization of the particles on the tape becomes the "data event". The two events are needed to make a single entry.

Separation of data events on the cortical memory device is brought about by a variation of this arrangement. We can disregard the supervisory event for the time being. (See summary of this item)

Figure 2

A signal originates in the
environment and, disregarding its
specific nature (light, sound, etc),
we will "flag" it with the letter
"A" in order to follow it in
memory.

A

ENVIRONMENT

· ·

DELIVERING

Unlike the tape recorder,
the cortical memory mechanism
makes a copy of everything it
delivers. The copy is then
re-entered in memory. The repetitive enter, deliver, copy,
sequence is called "iteration"
(iterate, to repeat).

SENSOR

CORTEX

Odd as it may
seem, on recall,
the recalled data
physically termin-
ates in the enter/
read site.

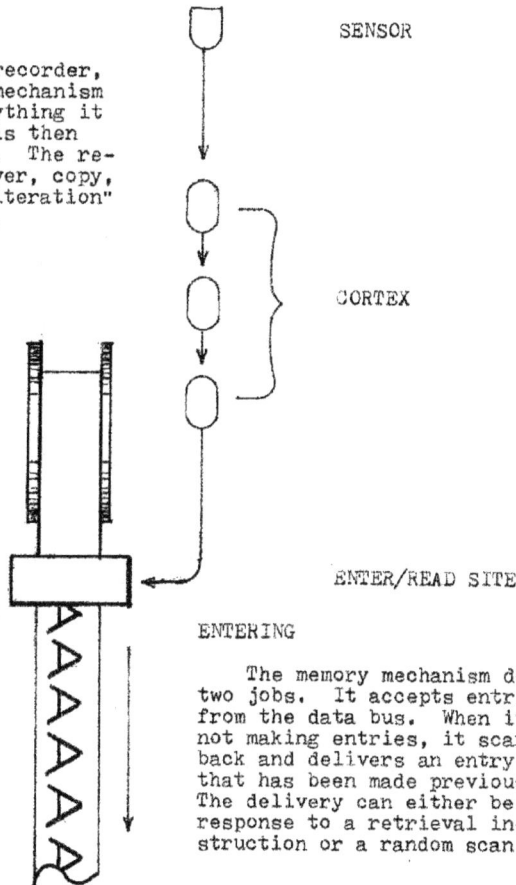

ENTER/READ SITE

ENTERING

The memory mechanism does
two jobs. It accepts entries
from the data bus. When it is
not making entries, it scans
back and delivers an entry
that has been made previously.
The delivery can either be a
response to a retrieval instruction or a random scan.

With a tape recorder, the tape must be moved back and
forth to place the recorded data under the record/playback
site, a process much too slow for the cortical memory mechanism. In the cortical memory, the "tape" is physically advanced one position for each entry. Delivering, the tape is
held stationary and the data event is moved back up the tape
by electronic means--a much faster process.

Figure 3

COHERENT DATA

MIXED ENTRIES OF
COHERENT DATA AND
NOISE (This is
the probable ar-
rangement.)

NOISE EVENTS

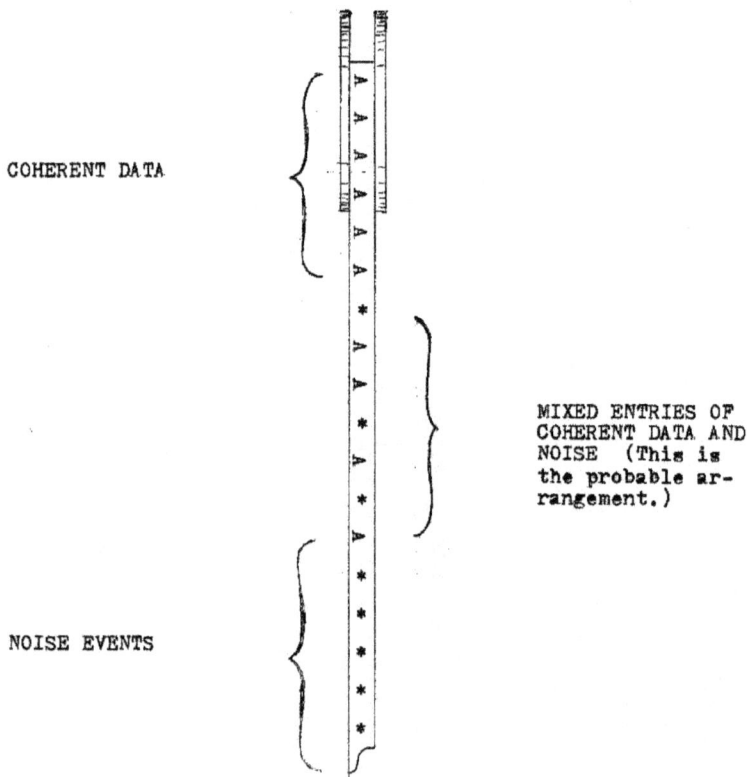

As used here, the word "noise"
means "electrical noise" and refers
to a stray voltage, not an irritating sound.

Figure 4

"Referencing" is the name of the game in the cortex. A coherent

data event is coherent because it can be referenced to the cortical

statement. A data event which is not a part of a coherent cortical

statement is a noise event. Physically and electrically, the event

is the same for noise and coherent data. In other words, a

technical analysis of the event would not tell us whether a

particular event was coherent or noise. This can only be

determined by the way the event fits in with the rest of the cortical statement.

Intelligent procedure fills in its contribution to the cortical statement with random events so the procedure needs a generator of random events and noise provides just such a generator. A noise event is characterized by its random frequency and random amplitude. During the recall cycle, memory is responding to a retrieval instruction. With its random component, it is not possible to write a retrieval instruction for noise and noise can not be recalled by deliberate means. Since noise will not respond to a retrieval instruction, noise cannot be self-reinforced. The cortical memory device incorporates a "fade" provision where the distal end of the tape is dissolved and seldom used throughputs and noise are removed from memory. The memory mechanism, by itself, contributes to noise suppression within the system by letting it fade from memory.

Noise also helps with necessary housekeeping. When memory scans back looking for a throughput, there is an enriched probability it will stop on a throughput that has received a great deal of reinforcement and a diminished probability it will stop on a lesser used throughput. Since a new copy of a throughput is entered each time it is used, the process, if allowed to run unchecked, would result in hyper-reinforcement. As we see later, hyper-reinforcement is done at the expense of intelligence. Noise counterweighs the tendency to hyper-reinforce and contributes to preserving intelligence. Noise does not disappear from memory altogether. While old noise is fading from the tape, new noise is being entered continuously along with the coherent data. Noise assumes a permanent residual value in the throughput ledger.

Fig. 5 is the memory ledger for the data bus in Fig. 4. The vertical line is proportional to the number of copies of the data event stored in memory. The letter "A" is merely a flag for the data event. Each time a visual image carrying this event appeared in front of the retina, another copy of the event was added to the ledger. Each time the visual image containing this event is recalled, the event is also recalled, and new copy of the image and, perforce, the event is made and re-entered in memory. This is the iterative process where throughputs, or more accurately: the data events that constitute a throughput, are built up in memory either by new "real" entries or self-reinforcement when a new copy is made with each recall. Entries attributable to both of these sources are added together and constitute the total reinforcement the data event has received. Iterative reinforcement expands the throughput ledger in the vertical direction.

SPECIFIC DATA

REINFORCEMENT
(Attributable to
entries only.)

MEMORY SURVIVAL
THRESHOLD

A

COHERENT
DATA

*

NOISE

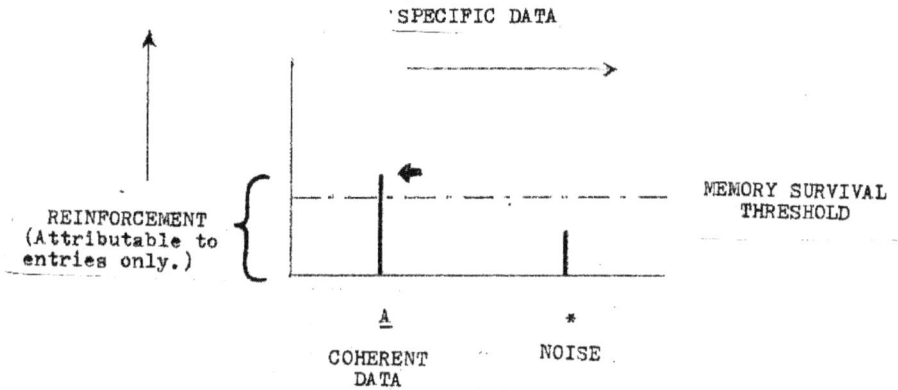

(Height of line is proportional to the number of copies
of a specific data event that have been entered in memory)

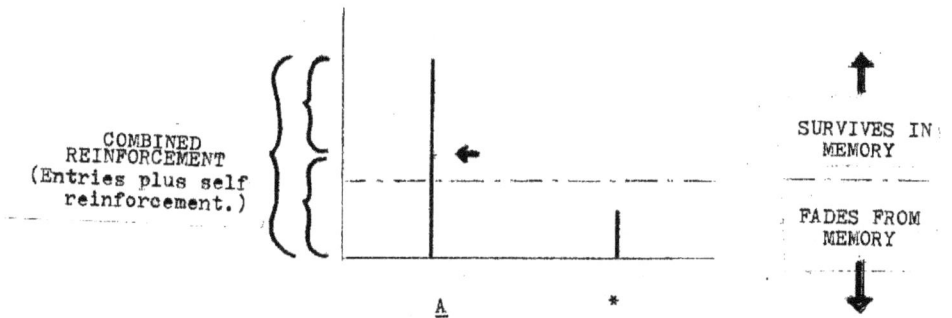

COMBINED
REINFORCEMENT
(Entries plus self
reinforcement.)

SURVIVES IN
MEMORY

FADES FROM
MEMORY

A

*

Coherent data gains reinforcement in memory
by the self reinforcement process of the cortex.
Noise can not be self reinforced. It does not
entirely fade from memory either. Some noise is
being entered continously so it assumes a permanent residual value.

Figure 5

MEMORY THROUGHPUT LEDGER FOR THE DATA BUS IN Fig.

There is a fade provision built into the tape. The recent entry is

entered at the front end of the tape. As the tape lengthens, the entry moves toward the distal end of the tape. The distal end of the tape is destroyed, destroying the distal data in the process. The data event must be recalled and re-entered frequently enough at the front end of the tape to compensate for the losses at the distal end. With enough reinforcement to maintain a build-up above this line, the event will be conserved in memory. Below this line, the event will be forgotten.

Second by second, or spread over decades, an endless process is at work: enter, reinforce, and, in the absence of reinforcement, fade. Then a throughput is entered, or when it is recalled and re-entered, we may say the throughput has been "exercised". Then we could say there is a rule: "Exercise or perish". Exercise on a current basis or be forgotten. Obsolete and seldom used throughputs, if they can be exercised on a current basis, are brought forward and re-entered in memory and the re-entry assures they will not be dropped from the memory ledger. Otherwise they fade.

When memory is responding to an instruction it responds in kind if it has the throughput in inventory. In addition to a direct response to a retrieval instruction, the cortex also scans at random. There is an enriched probability scanning will bring forward frequently used, frequently reinforced, throughputs at the neglect of lesser used throughputs. This is the "habituation" of memory. (It is also the "Markov" build-up discussed in the summary of this item.) Frequently used throughputs tend to be frequently used because they are enriched by habituation.

THE "SMART" ENGINE AND THE MEMORY THROUGHPUT LEDGER

By itself, reinforcement alone (or habituation) would follow a straight-line, frequency-of-use parameter. The reinforcement process (operationally, the _iterative_ process) de-randomized memory inventory. The other activity of the cortex, the _associative_ process, _re-randomizes_ inventory and, in doing so, defeats the straight-line, frequency-of-use parameter. We deal with the associative process next.

The associative process is the intelligent process of the cortex. Serving several functions in addition to making intelligent contributions to the throughput, it protects the habituation of memory and prevents it becoming monolithic. The self-reinforcement process cannot be allowed to operate on a run-away basis. If it did, a very limited range of throughputs would shortly be selected and hyper-reinforced to a point where they would monopolize memory.

Unused, seldom used throughputs fade because they are infrequently exercised. Fading throughputs can be rescued before fading if they can be exercised in association with another throughput that is being exercised on a contemporary basis. Parts of an old throughput are combined with parts of a recent throughput and the combined fractions entered in memory in the associated form. When the cortex is scanning, fading throughputs are recalled, combined in newly formed associations and newly entered in memory by the associative process. This work goes on both awake and asleep. Retaining fading throughputs also defeats hyper-reinforcement.

The two processes, the iterative process and the associative process, cooperate with each other in building up and sustaining the memory ledger. The iterative process builds up the ledger in the vertical direction and the associative process builds out the ledger in the horizontal direction.

In Fig. 6 we have the same mechanism we have been discussing; nothing different, we have simply added more data buses. Each memory tape is carrying its own data event. A supervisory system assures the data events move down the data buses in a precise and synchronized movement. This synchronization is preserved while the memory tapes are scanning and delivering. Flagged here with an unlikely letter of the alphabet to aid diagramming, the data events correspond to visual events in the visual image.

The data events in Fig. 6 are presented to the active site at the same instant and should be collectively thought of as a fraction of a visual image. The fraction of an image appears as a data line in the drawing. Starting with Fig. 6 and mentally adding more layers to the data line, it takes but little imagining to visualize the data events fitting together in a data plane. The cortical network is a three

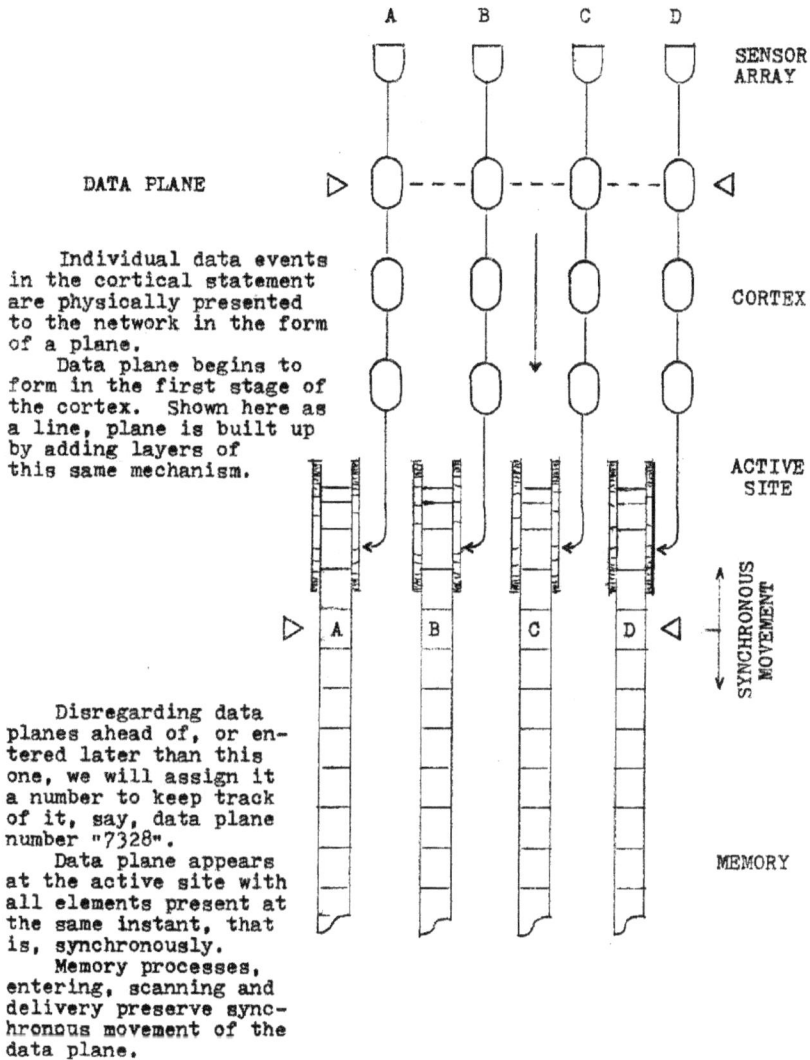

DATA PLANE

A   B   C   D

SENSOR ARRAY

CORTEX

Individual data events in the cortical statement are physically presented to the network in the form of a plane.

Data plane begins to form in the first stage of the cortex. Shown here as a line, plane is built up by adding layers of this same mechanism.

ACTIVE SITE

A   B   C   D

SYNCHRONOUS MOVEMENT

Disregarding data planes ahead of, or entered later than this one, we will assign it a number to keep track of it, say, data plane number "7328".

Data plane appears at the active site with all elements present at the same instant, that is, synchronously.

Memory processes, entering, scanning and delivery preserve synchronous movement of the data plane.

MEMORY

Figure 6

dimensional lattice (sketched in a later discussion) and the cortical statement moves through the network in the form of a plane.

(The visual system "takes a picture" of the visual image. It is essential that the physically scattered and separate pieces of the image be processed by the network simultaneously. Suppose, with an ordinary photograph in one

hand and a paper punch in the other, I punch out a small piece of the picture. I lay tiny round piece on the tip of my finger and then throw the rest of the picture away. My take is to make use of the information contained in the small piece that is left. I am not able to do this without the remainder of the picture to refer to. This fragment of the image is data in isolation, unreferenced data, and unreferenced data is not usable for anything. The need to process the entire visual image all at the same instant for referencing purposes is often overlooked in visual theories. This is a key point with regard to the timing and geometry of the network.)

There are barely enough gray cells in the visual lobe to process the million element visual statement in a physical plane. Understandably, a neat, right angled geometry is not seen in the anatomy of the cortex. The geometry is there, it has been folded in the middle to make its input and output terminals accessible. The convoluted topology of the cortex is mostly to satisfy the physiological rather than the operational needs of the system.

Ignoring the data lines (or data planes) that preceded or followed the one we have here, we will give this data plane a number so we can keep track of it. This is data plane #7328 in Fig. 6 and 7.

Now, instead of entering single data events in the throughput ledger, we will still use the same throughput ledger and change our scale of observation this time an entry is a complete data plane. Data plane #7328 has been entered in the ledger in Fig. 7 and given one reinforcement upon entry (dot raised above baseline in Fig. 7). This data plane is a replica of a visual image. If this image should again appear in front of the eyes, or it is recalled, it has a chance to build up in memory via the iterative process.

Now we have the cortical statement presented to the active site in the form of a data plane and established the need for a synchronizing mechanism to prevent the individual data elements from drifting out of plane. Before we go on to the associative process, a couple of small digressions are needed because this alphabetic model of the cortex is becoming a problem.

As set out here, we have a straight through data bus (or buses) and we have the data bus in isolation. If this model, with the data buses in isolation was actually used in the cortex, the data buses would leave a permanent artifact in the memory throughput ledger, this is explained in Fig. 8.

Figure 7   61

SPECIFIC DATA ———————————>

REINFORCEMENT   SURVIVAL
                                                 THRESHOLD
(Attributable
to one entry)

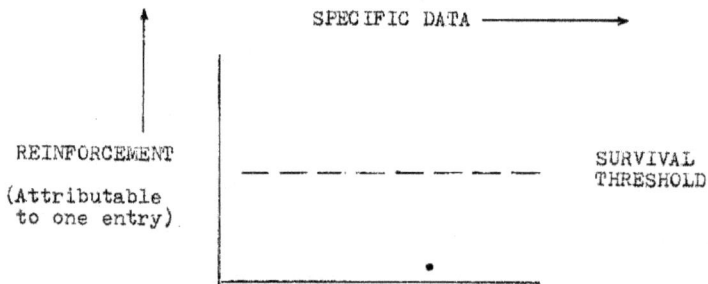

DATA PLANE #7328

Data plane #7328 is given one reinforcement
upon entry. (Dot above baseline)

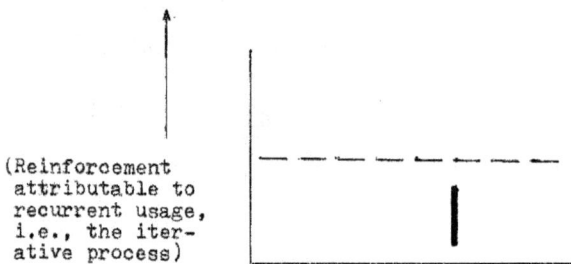

(Reinforcement
attributable to
recurrent usage,
i.e., the iter-
ative process)

DATA PLANE #7328

        The data events in this data plane constitute a replica of a
particular visual image. If this image should appear in front
of the retina at a later time, additional entries will be made.
If the image is recalled and re-entered (exercised) it may
also gain reinforcement by the iterative process. If it is
If it is reinforced above the survival threshold, it will become a permanent entry in the throughput ledger.

MEMORY THROUGHPUT LEDGER FOR FIG. 6

        Figure 7
The   ier to see in Fig. 8, also applies to the cortical

ledger.   In the cortex the data buses are re-

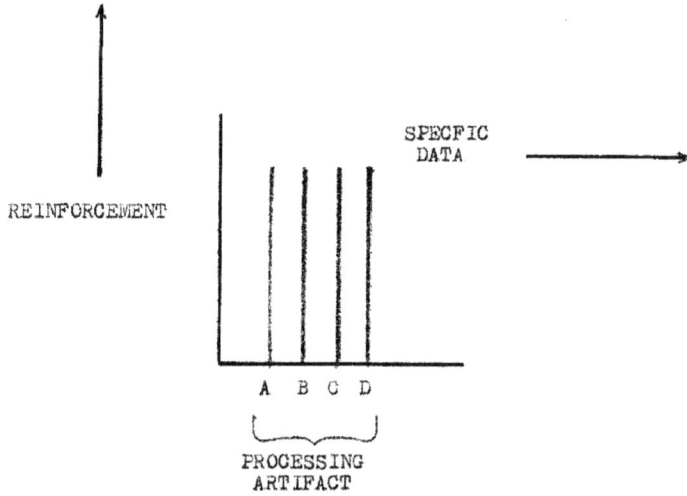

REINFORCEMENT

SPECFIC DATA

A B C D

PROCESSING
ARTIFACT

(1) A problem comes up when we use the alphabetic model.
The alphabetic letter carries no information; its specific value
is invariant regardless of the stimulus on the retina. Since
the data bus reports continuously, the alphatebetic data events,
logically, would reinforce to the same height in the memory ledger without entering useful information. In the real cortex,
the data event in in an analogue format and each data event has
a specific signal value, a value that is a function of a specific intensity of stimulus that fell on a particular sensor in
the retina. It is this analogue "font" that carries the specific visual information.

(2) We still have the data plane being carried down the
network on discrete and independently functioning data buses.
With this termination, the physical structure of the network
will leave a processing artifact in the memory ledger per this
sketch. This artifact is eliminated by a number of techniques;
particularily the lateral reorganization of the network. All
data buses are terminated at several sites and the analogue
data events are arithmetically added together in such a way
that the artifact is "added out".

Figure 8

organized laterally, that is, cross connected lateral to the axis

of data flow. This terminates the data buses in a way

that eliminates the artifact. (It takes millions of gray cells to move the cortical statement on-axis. The remaining billions are allocated to the lateral re-organization of the network and the elimination of artifacts. See, "Lateral-to-the-axis Re-organization of the Network".)

Our model has been writing its statement in the alphabetic font, making it easier to follow the data flow through the network. The real cortex writes its statement in an electronic font instead of the alphabetic font we have here. Without simplifying with the alphabetic model, it would be impossible to demonstrate on paper just where a particular data event is positioned at a given inspection because the data event is "buried" in several sites in the lateral re-organization of the network. We also would not be able to show how associations are formed between events and groups of events. The cortical statement is, by its nature, in an electronic (analogue) font in the cortex. In electronic font, data events are added together arithmetically and artifacts are "added out".

Any mechanism of nature is an analogue mechanism. The length of a shadow is an analogue of the height of the sun, the impact of a raindrop is an analogue of the height of its fall (minus aerodynamic losses). With man, making analogue machinery, though not necessarily analogue computers, is an ancient and venerated art dating back to antiquity. (A sort of classic man made analogue mechanism that comes to mind is the gas gauge in the automobile where the deflection of the indicator pointer is an analogue of the fluid level in the tank.)

THE "SMART" ENGINE AND THE MEMORY THROUGHPUT LEDGER

With the interest in digital computers being what it is there is a tendency to pass over analogue computers as quaint relics of interest only to the specialists who work with them.

Analogue processors usually express the analogue as a D.C. current or D.C. voltage. D.C. refers to "direct current", The amplitude of the D.C. signal can, and does, vary; but the sense of the signal excursion is always unidirectional. This contrasts with A.C. (alternating current) where the current in the circuit reverses direction periodically. The nervous system, including the cerebral cortex, is a D.C. analogue system throughout.

Our model, with its alphabetic font, has served well in demonstrating where the data event originates, where it is positioned and how it moves through the network. The letter of the alphabet carries no specific information about the visual image; its value is invariant regardless of the stimulus that falls on the photoreceptor. We have reached the point where we must abandon the alphabetic font in favor of the analogue font. The circuit in Fig. 9 may look a bit farfetched to be an equivalent of a retinal photo sensor. This is a "legal" equivalent circuit.

The light stimulus falling of the retinal photoreceptor is translated to a D.C. voltage. The D.C. voltage is an "analogue" of the light stimulus on the receptor. Since the optical image is the source of the stimulus, the D.C. voltage is a function of a bit of information contained in the visual image.

Fig. 9 and Fig. 10, show step by step, how the data event is derived, The voltages in the drawing are for illustration only and suggest relative voltages during the signal excursion. They are not representative of the voltages inside of the cell membrane. The voltages on the inside of the cell membrane can be almost diabolically confusing, Zero is at minus 70mv and maximum signal excursion is at minus 20mv. We can get around this problem by expressing the signal as so many units of amplitude, without specifying the units.

In making the change from the alphabetic font to the analogue font, nothing whatever is changed in our view of the "smart" engine. The only difference is a type of change in the type of event we are using.

The memory can only accept entries that come in discrete pieces. The input lobe of the cortex is a "chopper" and "chopper" is the correct word for this function. The normally continuous D.C. signal is "chopped" into discrete, instantaneous samplings. This is the "analogue event" or

66

LAMP AND
BRIGHTNESS
CONTROL

PHOTO-
ELECTRIC
CELL

DC
VOLTMETER

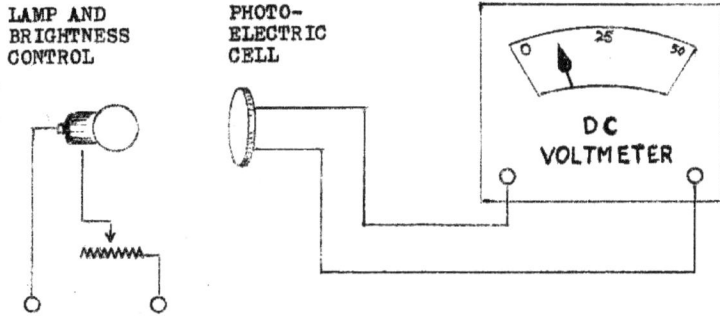

Simple analogue apparatus. Lamp illuminates photo-
cell and photo-cell generates a voltage proportional to
lamp brightness. Voltmeter indication follows the brightness of the lamp and the voltage is an "analogue" of
brightness. Voltages within the nerve cell are measured
in millivolts (1/1000 volt). The useable signal excursion
is 50mv and, to simplify things, we will say the signal
excursion is 50 units of signal amplitude.

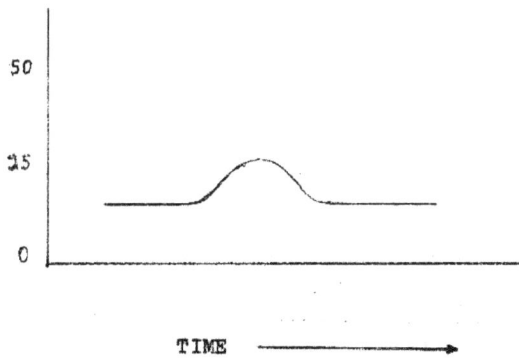

50

25

0

TIME ⟶

Someone has turned the brightness control up, then
down again. Brightness started at less than half value,
increased to about 25 units of brightness, then back to
the starting value. The analogue voltage follows these
changes in brightness.

DC ANALOGUE FORMAT

Figure 9

67

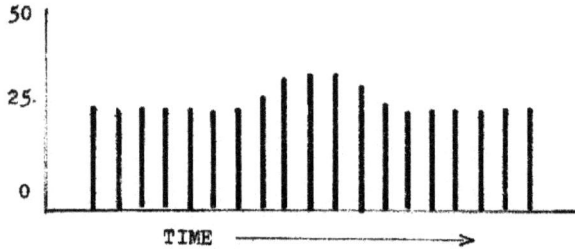

Information from the sensor array is carried to the
cortex as an uninterrupted and straight forward D.C. signal. Within the cortex, a mechanism makes instantaneous
samplings of the D.C. signal. The technical name for this
mechanism is: "chopper".

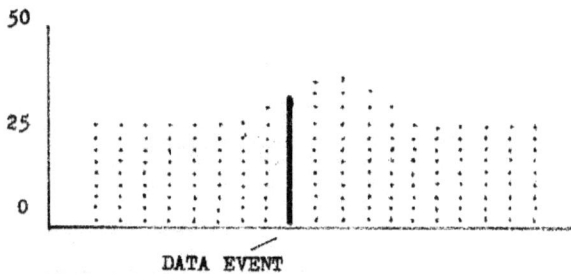

Disregarding instantaneous samplings made before and
after this one, we will set this one out as a typical
"data event". It has a specific amplitude which replicates, electrically, the intensity of light stimulus which
fell on a particular receptor in the retina at the instant this sampling was made. The light stimulus was evidently about 30 units of brightness.

D. C. ANALOGUE "EVENT" FORMAT

Figure 10

"D.C. analogue event" format and the format used in the cortex.

The "event" format is not used anywhere else in the nervous system.

It is confined to the cortex where the enter/deliver cycle of the

memory unit must have the entry chopped into discrete "events".
The real-time lobe of the cortex is the "chopper" and one of its
functions is to record the rate of movement of information in the
visual image.

All data events in the data plane are entered on their respective
memory tapes synchronously and at corresponding positions on the
tape. Fig. 11 is a part of a data plane, as usual, shown as a data
line. Fig. 11 is a repetition of the memory units we had earlier
in Fig. 6. This time the alphabetic letter has been removed and
replaced with the analogue data event. The number indicated the
amplitude of the data event. The units of amplitude are left
unspecified all we need here is to suggest relative amplitudes.

The visual input system has constructed an electrical replica of
a particular visual image; the chopper makes sure it is just one
image. The electrical replica is presented to the network and to
the memory system in the form of a "data plane". The data plane is
made up of D.C. analogue data events (about a million of them in
each lobe of the visual cortex). Neglecting lateral contributions,
the data event is an instantaneous sampling of a D.C. signal
originating at the receptor and the signal at the receptor is a
function of the light intensity stimulating the receptor.

In fig. 11 we have selected a data plane and, by implication: a
visual image. We will give it a number: data plane #7328 or image
#7328. In Fig. 11 and Fig. 12, the

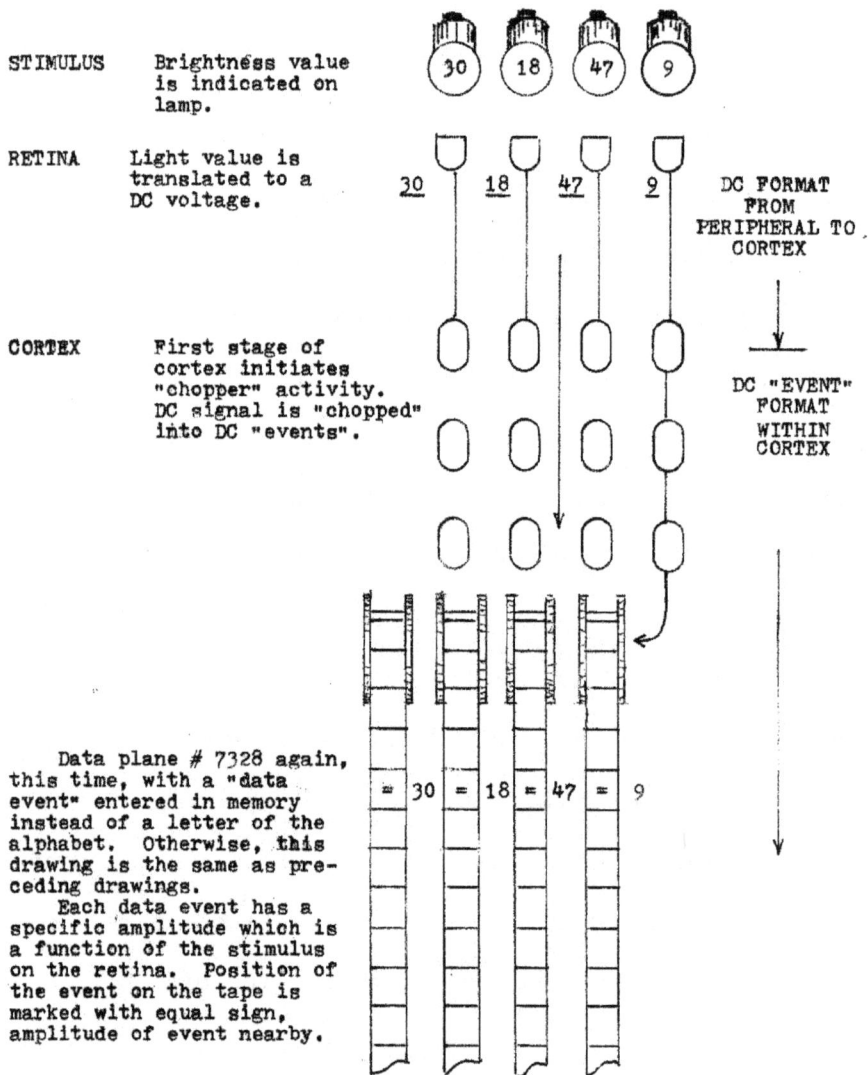

STIMULUS   Brightness value
           is indicated on
           lamp.

           30   18   47   9

RETINA   Light value is
           translated to a   DC FORMAT
           DC voltage.   FROM
                     30   18   47   9   PERIPHERAL TO
                                        CORTEX

CORTEX   First stage of
           cortex initiates
           "chopper" activity.   DC "EVENT"
           DC signal is "chopped"   FORMAT
           into DC "events".   WITHIN
                                         CORTEX

     Data plane # 7328 again,
this time, with a "data
event" entered in memory   = 30 = 18 = 47 = 9
instead of a letter of the
alphabet. Otherwise, this
drawing is the same as preceding drawings.
     Each data event has a
specific amplitude which is
a function of the stimulus
on the retina. Position of
the event on the tape is
marked with equal sign,
amplitude of event nearby.

Figure 11

SPECIFIC
DATA

REINFORCEMENT
(One entry)

SURVIVAL
THRESHOLD

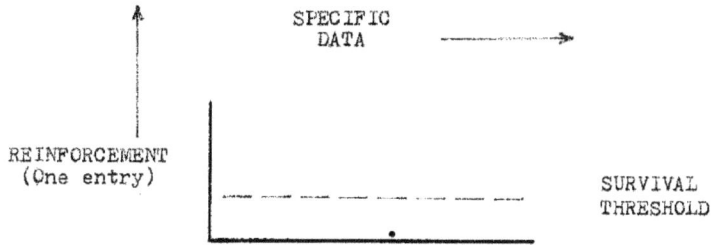

Data plane #7328 is given one reinforcement upon entry. (Dot raised above baseline)

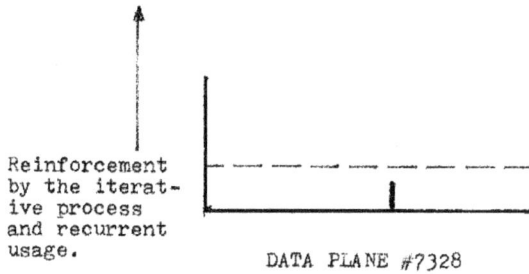

Reinforcement
by the iterat-
ive process
and recurrent
usage.

DATA PLANE #7328

This is the memory ledger for the madules in the last drawing. The change from a letter of the alphabet to the analogue
event format does not require any change in our understanding
of the memory throughput ledger.
     The data events in this data plane constitute a replica of
a particular visual image, say image #7328. If this same image should appear in front of the retina at a later time, additional entries will be made.
     If the image is recalled and re-entered (exercised), it may
also gain reinforcement by the iterative process. If it is reinforced above the survival threshold, it will become a permanent entry in the ledger.

Figure 12

memory throughput ledger is the same as it was for the data plane

in the alphabetic font.

Fig. 13 is the cortical module. Again the lateral processes have been omitted. The upper half of the drawing

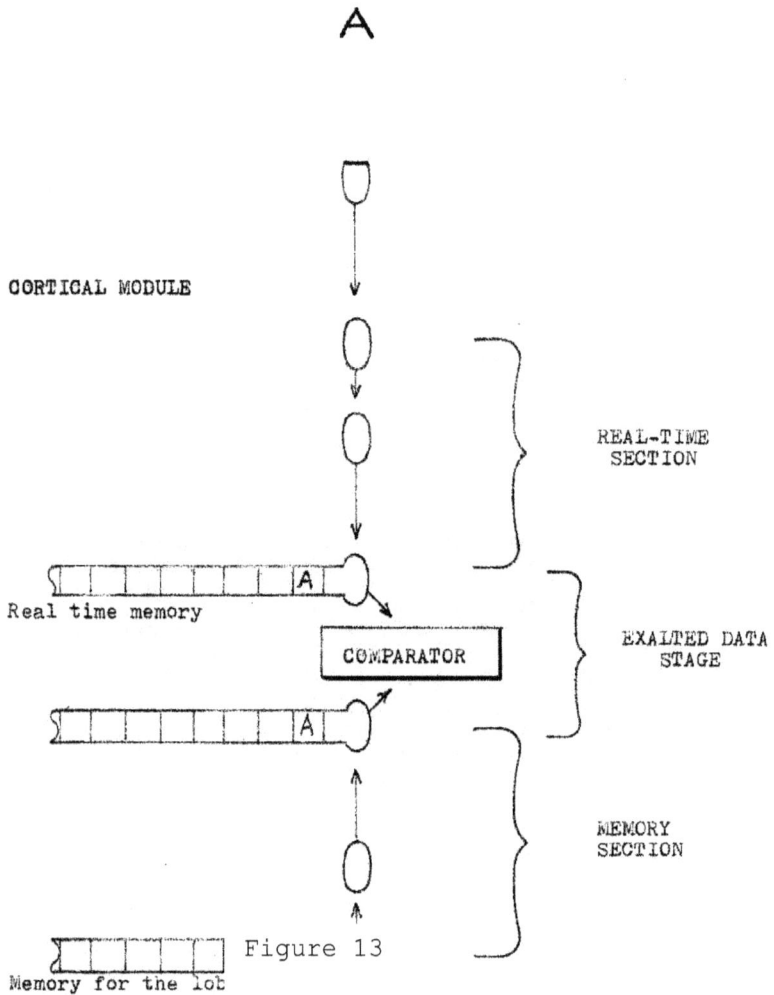

A

CORTICAL MODULE

Real time memory

COMPARATOR

Memory for the lot

REAL-TIME
SECTION

EXALTED DATA
STAGE

MEMORY
SECTION

Figure 13

Fig. 13

is the on-axis data bus we had earlier. This bus (upper half of

the drawing), along with millions just like it, make up the real
time section of the cortical lobe. The real-time section processes
the visual image while it is still on the retina. The memory
section is capable of recalling the visual image it need not be on
the retina. I think the cortical lobe is divided, both
operationally and anatomically, into two lobules: one "real-time",
one "memory". The real-time section of the lobe terminates in the
real-time memory. This is a technical memory only and the circuit
is organized this way for technical reasons. The lower half of the
drawing is the memory for the visual lobe. Here, visual
information originates in memory and flows toward a common
interface between the real-time system and the memory system
(arrows).

The memory for the lobe is able to either "pay attention to" or
ignore the instruction coming from the real-time system. When it
ignores the real-time instruction, it writes its own instruction
and does so by free-scanning. (If we close both eyes, the real-
time instruction is removed from the visual lobe. We then see
visual images recalled from memory on a "free" basis. When memory
free-scans it free associates.)

Considering the uncommon and special nature of the cortical
computer, it is, overall, a fairly straight forward system. The
drawing of the module presents a kind of circuitry that is
complicated enough to merit a little extra noodle work. The "A"
indicate the need for a scheme to match the data event at the real-

71

time memory (upper "A") while, at the same time, entering a
corresponding data event in the memory-for-the-lobe (lower "A's")
against the normal conducting direction of the nerve cell. The
"smart" process does this. This is one of the slickest finesses in
the system and is explained in the item: "Finesse of the Exalted
Data Stage".

(Anticipating a discussion of the exalted data stage later on,
the exalter process is the core active process of the cortex and,
of necessity, the thematic core of the cortical circuit philosophy.
The exalter process is responsible for a surprising number of
overlaying finesses, yet it is a simple operation with a minimum of
apparatus. A look at the intricate structure and physiology of the
nerve cell and we have no doubt about its sophistication; its
versatility as an electronic device leaves a lot to be desired,
however. Since the cell has terminals that are either input
terminals or output terminals and signal flow on one direction,
there is the problem of entering the data event in the permanent
memory via the same terminal it must come out of. One of the
finesses of the exalted data stage gets around this problem. When
a factory builds a computer, it designs its components to fit the
circuit of system; with some truth, it is the other way around in
the cortex.)

The major divisions of the cortex do not function in isolation.
They are referenced with respect to each other. They talk to each
other by matching data events in paralleling memory mechanisms.
The memory mechanisms are opposite each other, one on each side of
a common interface. The comparator, a part of the exalted data

stage, is the common interface. (If the lobes or divisions are physically separated, half of the exalted data stage is in one lobe and half in the other.

An event for event match is attempted and the comparator decides if the match was successful: that in, both memory units are delivering data events with the same amplitude. Since "exalting" a data plane requires matches at a large fraction of the million sites in the lobe, the exalted data plane "attempts" a data plane.

For purposes here, we will say slightly more than 50% of the events in the data plane must be matched before the exalted data stage will "fire". When a major fraction of a data plane (say, 60%) has been matched, the exalted data stage "fires" and, upon firing, the data plane is committed to the cortical statement. During the firing cycle, a new copy of the data plane is made and entered in the memory ledger. (Nerve cells "fire"; this is explained later. In myelinated nerves, the firing is a pulse in a pulse rate code. The cortical cell is a D.C. cell. It is fired as a part of exalter procedure and the firing controls memory entry.)

A test is made with the outcome indicating enough elements in the data plane, say, 60%, have been filled in and matched to constitute a competent cortical statement. It would take more time than can be allowed to fill in and match all of the million participating sites; it might take forever, for that matter, so an adjustment has to be made. An agreement is reached in trading off the time available against the number of sites that must be matched.

Typically, the real-time system is looking at a visual image and the visual memory is attempting to match it. The statement presented by the real-time system is a retrieval instruction originating in the real-time system. Let us say visual memory is not only able to match 50% of the data plane specified in the retrieval instruction, but is also able to supply an additional 15% all in one data plane. This meets the firing requirements and the stage fires. <u>When the exalted data stage fires, all sites in the stage are fired in unison</u>. Upon firing, the data plane is entered in memory, the sequence of events in the exalted data stage has been completed, and the exalter is ready for the next attempt.

Up to now, in these examples, only the iterative process has been considered. There were data events standing in the remaining 35% of the active sites. These were the sites unable to respond to the match of data events requested in the retrieval instruction, but were fired anyway when all of the sites in the exalter stage were forcibly fired in unison.

Recalling our two kinds of data events, there are coherent data events which respond to the retrieval instruction and the noise event with its random amplitude and its cavalier way of always being present in the active site in the absence of coherent data. When the exalter fires, the noise events become a part of the data plane because of the requirement that all sites in the stage must fire in unison.

In our example, we considered 60% to be a major fraction of a data plane. (These percentages can only be guesses.) The stage fired when 65% of the sites were filled in. The remaining 35% of the sites, all carrying noise events, also fired in synchrony with the firing of the stage. Now we have a major fraction of a data plane supplied, in one chunk, by memory in response to a retrieval instruction: and we have a smaller fraction of a data plane, an "add-on" chunk, which was filled in with noise events. This is sketched in Fig. 14.

In Fig. 14, a trial association is formed when a major fraction of a data plane, made up of coherent data elements (equal sign) and a smaller fraction of a data plane, all noise events (asterisks), are presented to the exalted data stage at the same instant. The two fractions are fixed, frozen and entered in memory as one data plane when the stage

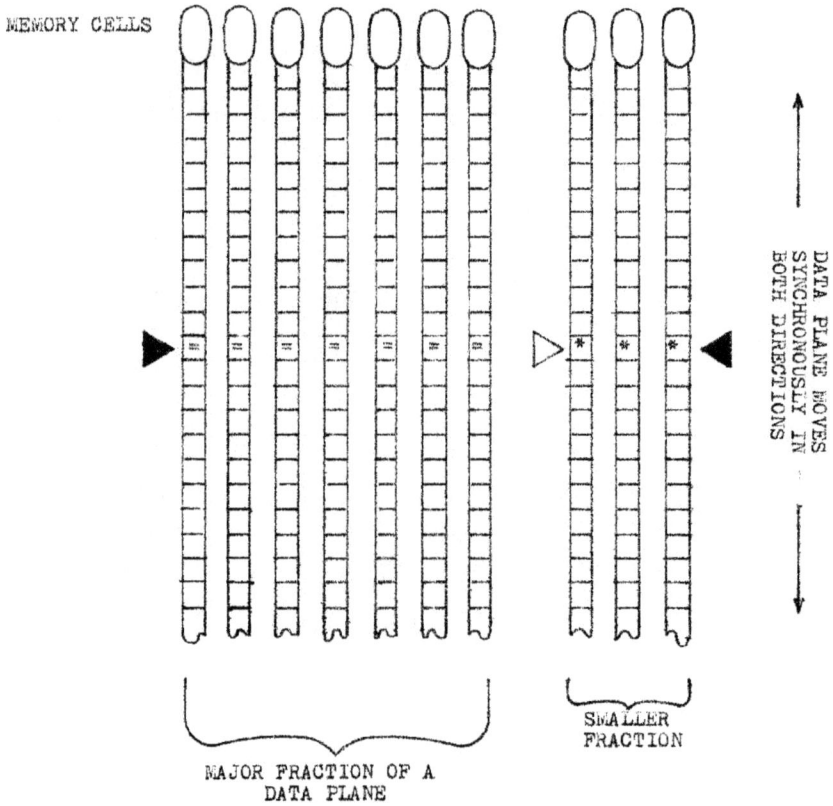

Figure 14

fires. The exalter process commits this new data plane to memory

with the trial components (small fraction) fixed in their newly

associated form (attached to the big fraction). Fractional data planes, between arrows, are collectively entered, moved and delivered synchronously. The equal sign for coherent data indicates all upstream arithmetical summations have been completed prior to reaching this point.

The arrows pointing up and down the tape are to suggest the synchronized movement of the data plane in and out of memory. The ladder like tape is physically manufactured at the active site and, with each entry, it physically moves one position away from the entry position down in Fig. 14. The rate of movement of the memory molecule varies from 10 positions, or entries, per second to 40 or 50 at its most rapid. On memory delivery, only the signal event moves from its distal position on the tape and toward the active site. The delivery rate is on the order of billions per second. Since two distinct physical processes are involved, the inbound and outbound memory rates are different. Synchronization of the scattered memory units is enforced by several means.

Fig. 15 is the throughput ledger for the new data plane formed in Fig. 14. This is a new and original throughput and it contains components that were not in response to a real experience and have never existed elsewhere in the memory ledger. Unlike any other throughput in the ledger, it must be entered as a separate and unique entry. The ledger has gained one new entry by the associative process and it expands horizontally.

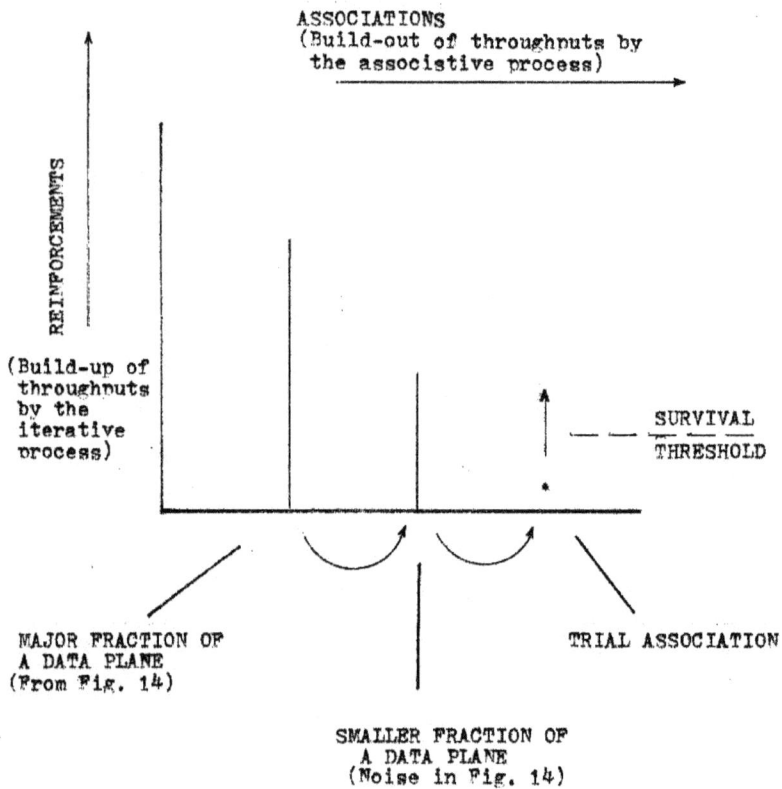

Figure 15

Figure 15

The new throughput is given one reinforcement upon entry (dot above ledger baseline) and the arrow indicates a potential for growth by the iterative process, if ongoing experience exercises the new throughput in the associated form. The potential for growth in the associated form may exceed that of the components from which is was made. Furthermore, parts of this new throughput may be the precursors of further expansion of the ledger by the associative process.

An odd activity has taken place, the ledger has a new entry that was never dictated by the environment or any other rigorous source for that matter. The cortex is now attempting to advance its own synthesis: a throughput that was generated by the cortex itself.

The throughput is novel, alien, heretofore unknown, and, being novel, the cortex has no way to validate the trial throughput using only internal resources. Trial usage, measured against the requirements of experience, will ultimately confirm or discard the throughput. I may figure out a new way to move my hands in a hand/eye task, say. I cannot know if this new way will work without trying it in a real hand/eye trial. If it does work, the trial movement is "validated". The cortex has no internal way to validate its own trial throughputs.

Whatever "validation" may entail, "validation" perfuse right down to the individual data event. When the trial throughput is validated, the noise events that make up the trial fraction are also validated and raised in rank to "coherent" data events

When the body is in motion, or when we are at a real task, cortical memory "locks up" with the real time system. Here, the cortex is running fast (to keep apace of on-going events) and the system is functioning essentially in the iterative mode. While the associative process is not entirely discontinued in high speed running, this is a time for memory to confine itself to tried and tested throughputs and not fool around with a lot of innovation. There is not enough time for elaborate attempts to fill in missing or improvable throughputs and keep up with on-going activity at the same time.

With the body at rest, the real-time task (say, a visual task) can be relinquished and the visual system permitted to free-scan. When the cortex free-scans it, free associates. The visual system alternately "pays attention" to the real image or "pays attention" to memory. Running slower, "time out" can be taken for the specific purpose, or pleasure, of generating trial associations.

(The shift from the iterative mode to the associative mode is made solely by shifting the exalter firing rate. The physiology of the nerve cell forbids "switching" as such, where switching is understood to be the physical opening or physical separation of circuits. The activities of the nerve cell cannot be paused for any length of time because it gets out of calibration. This speed-up/slow-down procedure is a finesse of the exalted data stage for getting around the restriction on switching.)

With no preoccupying task at hand, there is time for reverie: the exalter shifts to slow running, scanning is protracted, and memory begins to free scan. Recent experience tends to prejudice the randomness of the scan and reverie will probably begin with recent visual experience. (While the visual system is our typical system,

it is almost a cinch the other lobes of the cortex do this same
routine.)

During reverie, the large fraction of the data plane is recalled
from memory. The trial fractions are filled in, and the new
throughput is entered in this form. This is a "near" corollary of
whatever had been brought forth in reverie. This "near" corollary,
just entered, is again recalled. On this recall cycle, it may be
competent in 60% of its sites, but not necessarily the same sites
that were competent in the original entry. Using random noise for
data events, another attempt is made to fill in the unmatched sites
and the outcome of this attempt is entered in memory. We now have
a "near" corollary of the preceding "near" corollary. The scan
shifts from one throughput to another by re-stating the recalled
image, generating a corollary, repeating the corollary, generating
a further corollary, and so on. I call this process "intelligent
procedure". The throughput ledger in Fig. 15 sketches the basic
process. The associative process generates these corollaries and
expands the memory ledger on its associative axis (horizontally and
to the right in Fig. 15).

The associative process moves from one throughput to another by
generating a series of corollaries: a "segue", bridging the
differences between the throughputs. (A "segue" is a bridge
between musical selections without a pause.) This is accomplished
by generating corollaries "near" a starting throughput and ending
"near" the final throughput. The throughputs are relatable to each

other because they are relatable to the common fractions they contain. The associative process, working with either whole throughputs or major fractions, forms new combinations of old throughputs by computing a "segue" (pronounced: seg way) between them. The new trial associative, or trial segue, will be retained in memory if it fits in with experience and continues to be exercised on a contemporary basis. There are not one, but two data processing operations in the cortex. They are: the iterative process and the associative process. The two processes overlay and collaborate with each other as they alternately expand the throughput ledger. (If I want to remember something, I have two strategies: I can repeat it over and over, reinforcing it is memory by the iterative process, or I can form a lot of associations with it, enriching the likelihood it will be retained in memory by the associative process.)

Running in high speed, the cortex is in the iterative mode and builds up the ledger by forming (mostly) reinforcements (vertical expansion of the ledger). Running in low speed, it forms associations and "builds-out" the horizontal aspect to the ledger. The associative process is never suspended; there are always a few "very near" associations formed even in high speed running. A few reinforcements must always accompany associations; without reinforcement, the association will be forgotten.

SUMMARY OF THE ITEM ON THE "SMART" ENGINE

1. Throughputs are selected for build-up by reinforcement because they are frequently "exercised" by the environment or because they

can be exercised in association with another throughput that is being exercised. Once selected and exercised, the iterative process will reinforce and self-reinforce the selected throughputs at the expense of lesser used throughputs. The buildup of information in memory will take on a sense and pattern dictated by the environment; this is habituation.

We can say the iterative process <u>de-randomizes</u> the memory inventory. (The associative process re-randomizes it.) In a poker game where the deck is shuffled each time before the cards are dealt, probability alone will set the pattern in cards when they are dealt. In a strange poker game where the deck was never shuffled before dealing, patterns would begin to appear when the cards were dealt and the patterns would "stick" over a great number of games. The patterns are attributable to previous hands where the players retained the combinations they liked and discarded the un-patterned cards. The accumulation of these patterns is not re-randomized by shuffling so the patterns are always present and will have an influence on the way the next game, and future games, will be played. A chance process, where the probability and character of the next event has a dependency on events that have already taken place is a "Markov" process, a Markov "chain" of events. The things we will be doing in the next several minutes start with the present state of affairs as a beginning state. This beginning state is predicated on the things we were doing in the last several minutes. Restrained by the situation at the moment and long

83

standing habits, if I insisted my next act had to be utterly
random, I would be hard pressed to do this.

We are habituated by our environment. The problem is: the
environment is hesitant and wishy-washy about indicating which
experiences are to become habits. To the extent this problem can
be dealt with, Markov accumulation in memory is one of a number of
cortical processes that bring resolution and clarity in the
habituation process

2. Fig. 16 is a sketch of a Turing machine, the original and
classic version as set out by Turing. There are differences
between the Turing and cortical machines. (The chart explains the
differences.) In analyzing data processing schemes, it pays to keep
one eye on what is transpiring as far as "data" is concerned and
another eye watching what is going on as far as "process" is
concerned. The cortical machine forms associations within the
"process". The cortical machine forms associations within the
"data". These are abysmally disparate ways of doing things.

Mathematicians design smart engines to solve problems on a trial
and error basis. When the trial is successful, the machine is
"rewarded"; for wrong answers it is "punished". (More likely,
correct answers are "flagged", incorrect answers dropped from
memory.) The system depends on a cooperative environment to tell
it which answers are correct.

It is a felicitous occasion when the environment tells the cortex
which of its answers are correct without delay. The cortex has an
internal "reward" system and trial "rewards" are attached to the
throughput on a probationary basis. Rather than scan back through

a mass of undifferentiated data, the cortex can expedite things by

scanning to

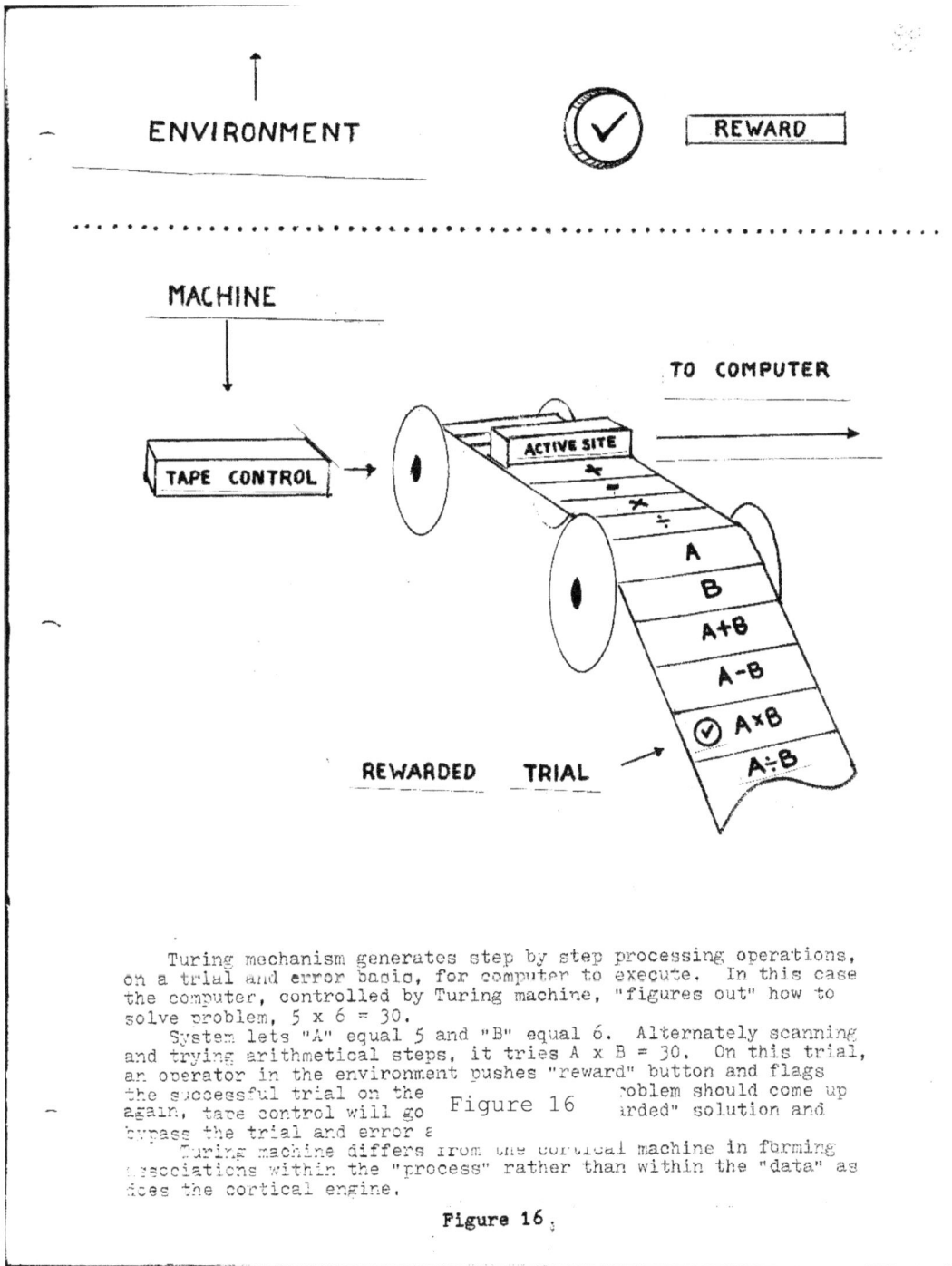

ENVIRONMENT   REWARD

MACHINE

TO COMPUTER

TAPE CONTROL   ACTIVE SITE

A
B
A+B
A-B
A×B
A÷B

REWARDED   TRIAL

Turing mechanism generates step by step processing operations,
on a trial and error basis, for computer to execute. In this case
the computer, controlled by Turing machine, "figures out" how to
solve problem, 5 x 6 = 30.
    System lets "A" equal 5 and "B" equal 6. Alternately scanning
and trying arithmetical steps, it tries A x B = 30. On this trial,
an operator in the environment pushes "reward" button and flags
the successful trial on the   roblem should come up
again, tape control will go   Figure 16   irded" solution and
bypass the trial and error a
    Turing machine differs from the cortical machine in forming
associations within the "process" rather than within the "data" as
does the cortical engine.

Figure 16

"rewarded" information. The reward scheme tends to enforce patterned build-ups in the memory ledger, Fig. 17.

The Turing machine does not incorporate accumulation or Markov build-ups in the smart part of the machine operation.

At a passing inspection, the Turing machine and the cortical mechanism resemble each other. At a closer inspection, the dissimilarities overwiegh the similarities. Here is an outline of the differences between the two systems.

TURING ENGINE	CORTICAL ENGINE
1. Mathematicians make a distinction between "trivial" and "non-trivial" devices. A single element of a Turing machine is a non-trivial device because a single element is all that is needed to form associations.	A single element of a cortical mechanism (the cortical module) would be regarded as a trivial mechanism because it merely iterates a data event. It becomes a non-trivial device when it is used in gangs and with the data association being formed between the outputs of a great number of devices.
2. Trial associations can be formed either within the "data" or within the "process" Turing forms associations within the "process". Furthermore, the Turing scheme forms associations serially and on the axis of data flow in the system.	The cortical system forms associations within the "data" (the major distinction between the two devices). Associations are formed simultaneously rather than serially. They are also formed "lateral-to-the axis" of data flow in the system
3. It is not likely accumulation, per se, would be incorporated in a Turing system. If it was, the machine would scan for an enriched probability of finding a problem solving step rather than a particular, and known to be valid, step it had generated earlier.	For better or worse, the enrichment of selected throughputs by the iterative process is an essential characteristic of the cortical engine. Patterns build up in memory that are added to patterns that were built up in memory at an earlier time.

Figure 17

Figure 17

I suppose Turing could have incorporated Markov build-ups in his mechanism; it would have slowed things down. With the Turing machine, the beginning state begins when the problem is presented to the machine and the outcome has no dependency on what the machine had been doing previously.

3. Fig. 18 is a schematic of our (proposed) cortical memory device. It is a ladder shaped, long chain molecule which is discussed in the next item. The spacer between the rungs serves the same purpose as the metal foil in the tape recorder model. When a new entry is made, a new rung is added to the ladder and the entire memory molecule moves away from the entry position, moving one rung at a time. When the data event is delivered, the signal propagates down the molecule toward the read position. This arrangement is different than our tape which moves back and forth on both entry and delivery. The end performance is still the same, though the mechanics are different. On memory delivery, the molecule is stationary and the signal, with nothing to accelerate and de-accelerate, does all of the moving. There is no way to accurately estimate the delivery rate. It should be able to deliver one data event, if not several per micro-second. A micro-second is one millionth second. This refers to scanning only: it takes longer to erect the data plane because time is required to "fire" the stage. Ultimately <u>noise</u> is the primogenitor of all activity in the

The memory molecule physically moves
one step away from the entry position
after each data event is entered.

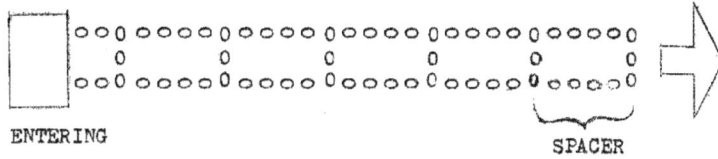

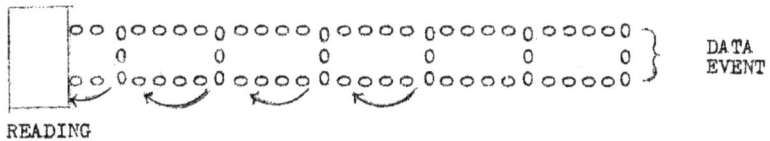

ENTERING   SPACER

READING

On delivery, memory molecuse remains
stationary and the data event propag-
gates down the molecule toward the read
position where the data event is read.

Figure 18

cortex. The data event at the real-time face of the comparator is

a "real" D.C. event. Here, at this stage in the system, is the

last contact with "real" data events. From this stage downstream,
intelligent procedure must "figure out" the amplitude of the data
event by trial and error. Noise provides the physical source for
these data events. Noise events provide the original internal
"currency" of these internal stages.

Sometime in the third trimester of fetal development, at a time
in life when the coherence of data in the throughput is
unimportant, noise gets the cortical memory ledger started
initially. The data planes in inventory are probably mostly noise
at first and are replaced at a later time with coherent
throughputs.

The cortex makes up the outer layer of the telencephalon, the
gross hemispheres of the brain. The rudiments of the telencephalon
have begun to form in an embryo of 10 weeks. At about 30 weeks the
gyri have begun to form and forming carries on to term. The cortex
is not completely formed at birth and fetal brain development
trails off to the second year postpartum. It is not entirely
assembled until about the tenth year.

The brain weighs 300 to 400 grams at birth, more than doubles its
weight in the first year (1000 grams), and reaches its final
weight, about 1500 grams, in late childhood. It would be hard to
set the earliest time when enough of the cortex has been formed and
connected so it is capable of writing competent throughputs in the
first year of life. A large part of the cortex may be functioning
in the first months of life with the balance becoming functional in
the first two years. The cortex of an infant probably writes
throughputs that are technically only marginally competent. In the

hierarchy of reasons for retaining or dropping a throughput from the ledger, technical competence of the throughput will be at the top of this list. The marginal throughputs are dropped from the ledger and replaced by more competent throughputs as soon as cortical development has progressed to the point where this is possible. I think this is the reason we are able to recall so little of these early years of life.

Random noise is the primogenitor of all intelligent activity in the cortex. The smart engine must have a random signal generator built into the system to make original thinking possible. If the noise generator was not built into the active site, it would still be necessary to have one, even if it had to be a separate apparatus and attached externally.

5. The eye aiming system first chases, then fixes the foveal retina on an interesting area of the visual image. The eye is capable of remarkable acceleration, 3600 degrees per second getting started, 500 degrees per second in pursuit. In the few milliseconds preceding fixation of the target, the eyeball is slowing down, and, in the process, the visual system is entering a few, say - 3 or 4, irregular data planes in memory. The relationship between the image and the slowdown rate has to be unique; so unique, we can say the first 3 or 4 data planes are a technical preview of the visual scenario about to follow. The visual "scenario" is the "burst" of data planes required to state the serial changes in a short visual experience. The system is

probably capable of processing two or three, perhaps four, visual scenarios per second. The shortest scenario will probably be about 10 data planes.

We will call these first 3 or 4 irregular data planes the "scenario index". When the index is recalled, the control system will assure the remaining data planes, perhaps - 10 or 15, in the visual scenario, will follow immediately.

Our conceptual juggling of the throughput ledger can be greatly simplified if we arbitrarily let the leading data plane "sign" or "commemorate" the entire sequence of data planes that constitute a throughput. For purposes of showing the throughput ledger, we can discard the follow-on data planes altogether. Our concept of the throughput ledger is not altered if we let the lead data plane be a short abbreviation for the oncoming scenario. The control system itself uses this same strategy when it uses the scenario index as a sort of shorthand "flag" and saves the time it would take to deliver the entire scenario before deciding if it was responsive to the retrieval instruction or not. The follow-on data planes follow-on in due course because they have a fixed relationship to the lead plane and the control system preserves this relationship on delivery.

The retrieval instruction has an index and, it too, is a serial burst of data planes. The retrieval index interrogates memory at the comparator first, immediately followed by the remainder of the data planes in the scenario. Starting with the index, memory is requested to match the retrieval instruction plane for plane. If the attempt is successful, the incomplete and irresponsive fraction of the responding data planes is filled in by the trial process as required. The attempt can result in one of two outcomes. The plane for plane delivery converges on the same data and the delivery continues to the end of the scenario. If there is a divergence, memory failing to match the instruction, the lobe is becoming incompetent and the control system will either scan for a new instruction, or it will re-assign dominance in search of a more competent instruction, a more competent response, or both. The control lobe has its own instruction, also led with a scenario index. The control system tries to preserve harmony within the cortex. The chances are, the control system would try the first few data planes in any response, detect a growing divergence, and, rather than going deeper into the scenario, cancel the attempt and try something else. We will let the first data plane in the scenario be entered in our drawings of the ledger, a marker for the remaining data planes in the scenario. This is not greatly different than the way the control system handles the same problem.

ESTIMATING MEMORY CAPACITY

Estimating memory capacity can only be mostly guesswork because there are so many variables and unknowns involved. Here, I will show some of the factors that have to be considered by anyone aspiring to estimate memory capacity.

The cortical memory makes entries continuously, asleep or awake. What proportion of all entries is made while asleep? How many entries are made in unit time? Are there operational routines which conserve memory space?

While the cortex does not have access to the subject matter of the throughput, it can decide whether it has an incoming throughput in memory or not. If it is not in inventory, the cortex speeds up to make the acquisition. The speed-up can be detected experimentally and experimenters refer to this as the "alert" status of the visual cortex. A similar speed-up in the motor cortex just before sending out a motor instruction to the body is called the "intent" status of the motor cortex. If the memory already has the incoming throughput in inventory, the cortex slows down and withholds reinforcement of the redundant information and, at the same time, conserves memory space. The upper limit of the (motor) speed shift should be about 50 data planes per second. The overall cortical rate may fall to about ten entries per second during sleep.

The average entry rate is not a simple arithmetical average half-way between the fastest and slowest rates. It is also necessary to know the length of time it dwells in high speed running versus the

length of time it dwells at a rate less than the simple average.
Unknowns being what they are, and with habit and experience
influencing the unknowns, for purposes of estimating memory
capacity, we will tentatively set the average rate at 25 data
planes per second. Experimenters should give us a firmer opinion
at a later time, 25 per second should be near the ball park.
Knowing the entry rate is important because the memory device
records one data event each time an entry is made and uses up one
storage position on the memory device for each data event.

Many years ago a few theorists suggested the cortical cell might
be the storage element in the cortex. Consistent with this
proposal, one cell has to be allocated to store each data event.
There was also a variation of this idea where a synaptic junction
would be formed to store data and one junction would be formed for
each data event.

(Synaptogenesis is a growth process. The junctions form far too
slowly to keep up with incoming data. The synapse is the junction
between nerve cells and there have been estimates as high as 30,000
synapses per cortical cell. It takes a number of discrete
junctions to make an operational junction. We will use 100 for an
average discrete junction and 300 operational junctions per cell.)

Here are the requirements that would have to be met, set out in a
way that favors the cellular level of storage proposal. The visual
information from the retina is impressed on the million fibers of
the optic nerve and carried to the cortex via a million data buses.

The information is delivered continuously. Our average entry rate is 25 data planes per second: to use an expression: the visual cortex "takes a picture" of visual experience 25 times per second. 25 entries per second times one million data events in the entry (entered as a data plane, an operational necessity) uses 25 million storage sites per second. One and one half billion sites (cells) are consumed each minute. The 16 billion, or so, cells in the cortex, all assigned to storing the visual image, would last about 10 minutes in memory service. If the synaptic proposal was an admissible proposal the time would be stretched to about 50 hours with an average of 300 junctions per cell. Perhaps the 300 junctions per cell estimate is low. If there were 3000 junctions per cell available for data storage, the time would extend to 500 hours.

It might be argued, to stretch storage capacity, all of this information need not be entered; some of it might fade before permanent entry is made. A 50% fade factor, where memory refuses as much as it retains, would compress 1000 hours of visual experience into the 500 hour memory. Fading, with any reasonable fade factor, will not stretch memory capacity enough to help the cellular theory. Again, it could be argued that it is not necessary to enter all of the visual image in its entirety. To do this, there would have to be a prior way of knowing whether the information at, say, the upper right corner of the image is more important than the information in the lower left corner which, being less important, would presumably be sacrificed. In order to do this, it is necessary to invoke a massive supervisory mechanism to decide which parts of the image are to be retained and which parts to sacrifice. The supervisory mechanism requires a greater number of brain cells than would be needed for straight-forward entry of all of the information on all of the optic nerve fibers. This particular trade-off has already been made at the retina on a fixed basis. There are fewer photoreceptors in the periphery of the visual field than there are in the center, or foveal, area of the retina. Whatever sacrifices of visual information that can be made have already been made before the visual data is put on board the optic nerve.

To further favor the cellular level of storage proposal, visual data might be composited or converged in order to save memory space. Compositing does save memory space; however, the visual data has already been both composited and converged at the retina before delivery to the optic nerve. Further compositing downstream of the retina is out of the question because it requires greater resolution (that is, precision) in the already heavily committed resolving capability of the nerve cell. The compositing format and the resolution problem are discussed in the item on the retinal coder.

Unstinting generosity toward the cellular level of storage proposal will not make it a viable storage system.

<u>We will take it as established: the memory device must be of molecular rather than cellular dimensions.</u>

Almost predictably, our thoughts drift to the nuclear DNA of the nerve cell as a candidate for a molecular storage device. A data memory in the nucleus is out of the question for the following reasons:

1. A voltage is always impressed across two terminals, with D.C. voltages, a positive and negative terminal. The signal voltage appears across the cell membrane with its positive terminal just outside and its negative terminal just within the membrane. The nervous system is a positive ground system. The ground voltage is the invariant voltage of the fluids that surround the cell and the signal voltage, just inside the membrane, varies its amplitude with respect to ground. The nucleolus, containing the DNA and deep within the center of the cell, has access to only one signal terminal, the negative terminal. If the nucleolus is participating in the data storage process, it would have to be in communication with the signal voltage across the membrane, and this would require contact with both the inside and outside of the cell membrane. Intimate contact is mandatory because the active and operational depth of the signal active cellular fluids is confined to a very thin layer (10 angstroms) in the immediate vicinity of the membrane. Fig. 19 is a sketch of this problem.

2. Fig. 20 carries on with the same problem. The cell axon, the long tubular extension of the cell body, carries the signal away from the cell body and delivers it to a downstream cell via the synapse. The output terminal of the cell, the "synapse", is the bulbous, also called "button-like", device in Fig. 20. The signal is expressed as a D.C. analogue voltage in the upper drawing. One

way or another, the signal has to be translated to a chemical
analogue and sent to the next cell downstream via the synapse.
(The output signal from the nerve cell is always expressed as a
precisely modulated flow of chemical neurotransmitters which
control the ion permeability of the downstream membrane.) Merely
that the nucleolus would have communication with the membrane of
the cell that contained it is not enough to make is a viable
element in the memory process. The memory device

106

Precision D.C. analogue
signal voltage is impressed
across membrane and confined
to a very thin layer just inside membrane. The nucleolus
is the organelle within the
cell. It assumes the voltage
of the surrounding cellular
fliuds. (Negative sign)

Data memory can not be
in the nucleolus because it
would require a low resist-
condiction path to the fluid
layers on both the
inside and the
outside of the
cell membrane.

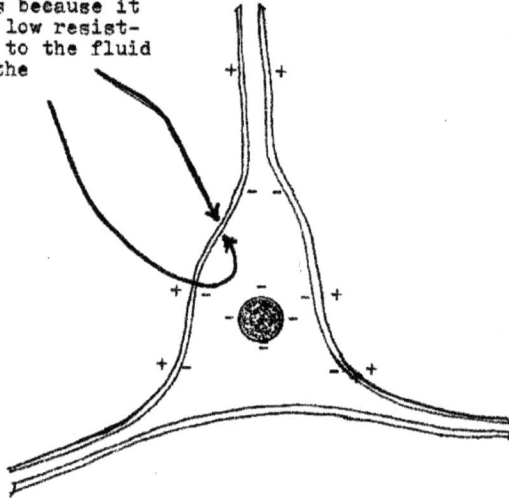

The DNA of the cell is encapsulated
within the membrane of the nucleolus, the
organelle in the center of the cell. It
assumed the voltage of the surrounding cyto-
plasm.

Figure 19

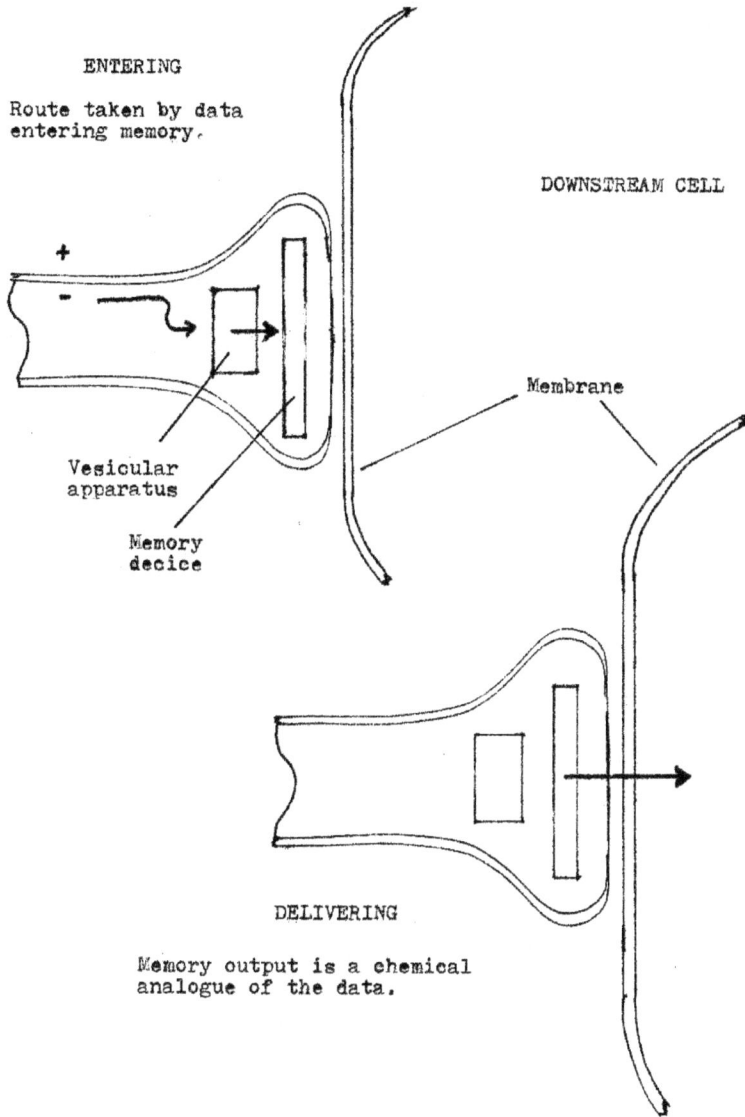

ENTERING

Route taken by data
entering memory.

DOWNSTREAM CELL

+

−

Membrane

Vesicular
apparatus

Memory
decice

DELIVERING

Memory output is a chemical
analogue of the data.

Figure 20

must accept data from one source, the cell membrane, and deliver it

in an entirely different direction to the next cell downstream via the synapse. The synapse itself is the only physical site in the cell where the memory device has access to both routings. (I have a feeling the DNA in the cell nucleus has an unflexing hereditary commitment to the formative, the metabolic and mitotic processes of the cell and for these reasons it cannot be used for data storage.)

We will take it as established fact that the memory device is of molecular dimensions and is physically sited in the synapse of the cell, furthermore the nucleolus is not involved in data memory activity.

Allowing it is my idea, I am convinced this general view of the electronic requirements of the memory device is substantially correct and, furthermore, the device is physically sited in the synapse. I agree to accept the blame if the idea is wrong, I know of no contra-indicators. The apparatus is too small to be resolved with present electron microscopes.

I am not a chemist, about all I can do is pass along a layman's impression of the way the molecular memory system ought to work and I hope there is no need to annul any of the known laws of chemistry.

Nuclear DNA is a source of fixed hereditary information. The DNA scheme is put together with an entirely different plan than that suitable for data memory; however, certain aspects of the DNA molecule can be used for a rough guideline and may help us estimate memory capacity.

(The hereditary master plan of the cell is coded on long-chain deoxyribose nucleic acid molecules. The DNA molecule is a ladder like arrangement where paired DNA molecules, phosphate linked deoxribose groups (ribose is a sugar) form the sides of the ladder and a sequence of four nitrogenous bases, in complementary pairs, form the rungs. The sequence of bases is a code directing the manufacture of protein enzymes which control chemical reactions within the cell. The DNA ladder spirals, 36 degrees for each rung, in a right hand spiral forming a double helix. The helix is coiled in turn, a "coiled coil", so to speak. The exact micro-architecture of the molecule is inferred: it is not visualizable with the electron microscope at its greatest magnification.)

The knowledgeable and dedicated people who devote the best years of their lives studying the cell nucleus periodically revise their estimates of the length of the long chain nuclear molecules. A recent estimate of the length of the nuclear DNA in a single cell is 5 meters, over fifteen feet. I take it, the individual molecules of DNA would have to be added together, end to end, to reach this length. The total length is the important factor.

The cortical memory molecule I am proposing, neatly coiled on a supporting structure, makes more efficient use of the length of the molecule than is made in the nucleolus. Hereditary DNA stores its information in a "codon" which requires three rungs of the ladder to store one coded "word". Our long chain polypeptide "ladder" stores one data event at each rung of the ladder, giving it three times the storage space per unit length.

Fig. 21 is the micro-architecture of the memory device I am proposing. For compelling technical reasons there has to be a large number of memory molecule strands. We will set a figure: say, 5000 to 6000 strands of memory molecule in each memory unit with a strand length of several feet. Each strand of memory molecule originates standing astride one of the openings in the aperture mask (the mask is the middle structure). The memory molecule strands are brought out to the edge of the mask in rope like bundles where they are coiled in a space saving annular ring.

All of this apparatus is in the synapse of the nerve ending. I think it is possible to cram 5000 to 6000 strands of memory molecule, each several feet long, into this small space because, compared to the DNA in the nucleus, the memory apparatus makes more efficient use of the volume available than does the nucleus. The nuclear DNA strands are physically scattered; I suppose to keep them from tangling during the upheaval of cell mitosis. Mitosis is cell division. The DNA strands, forgive the expression, "unzip" and half of the strand goes with each off-spring cell.

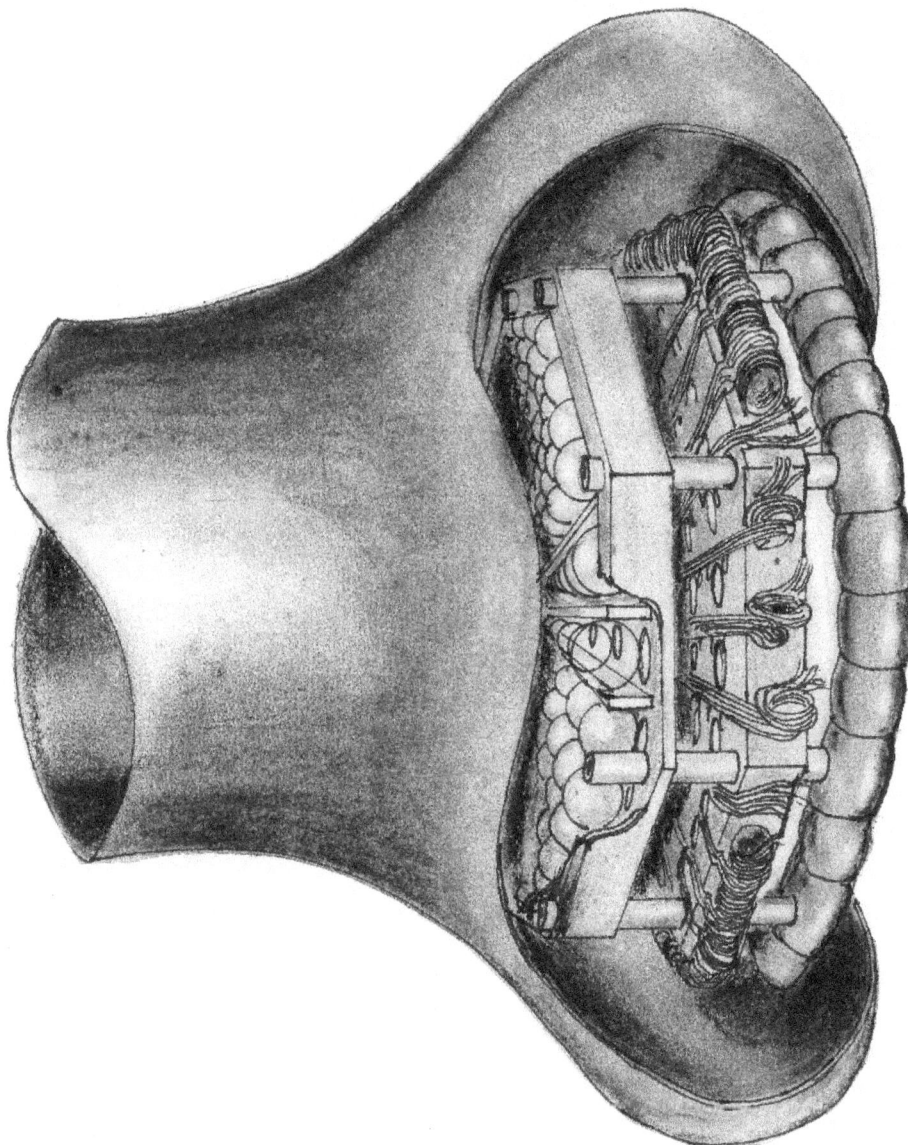

109

Figure 21

There are several thousand strands of memory molecule in each

memory unit. There is an inescapable reason for these multiple memory molecule strands. The signal cannot be expressed as a membrane voltage, then applied to the memory molecule. If the membrane voltage (70 millivolts) was applied to the molecule or a device of molecular dimensions, it would not withstand this comparatively enormous voltage. The signal must be translated from a signal expressed as a voltage to one that is expressed as a current. The current can be divided into small pieces. There is one strand of memory molecule for each of these small currents. The signal is divided into 5000 to 6000 much smaller electrical events which are entered in memory or delivered from memory simultaneously. The assembly, with its thousands of memory molecule strands, functions as a single unit. The multiplicity of strands is a technical necessity because of the voltage to current translation. (There is also an electrical to chemical translation of the signal at this point. The "current" here is a chemical current. Incidentally, the precision of the signal is a function of the number of holes, hence the number of strands, in the aperture mask. There are tens of millions of memory units in the cortex and thousands of memory molecule strands in each unit. The important factor in estimating memory capacity is not the number of memory units or the number of strands. Storage capacity is set by the length of a single strand of memory molecule.) There is a rule that governs the uniformity of nerve cell synapses; the synapses must be all of one kind. If one synapse has a memory unit, then all synapses in the cell must have memory units.

Fig. 22 is a single strand of the thousands of strands that make up the memory unit. The molecule is at the center and resembles a

ladder. The outer covering is the vault. Perhaps the vault is
built of fibrillar proteins (possibly the inner and outer surfaces
are waxy). It should be a mechanically rigid and chemically stable
structure to prevent the memory molecule being dissolved by the
intracellular enzymes and to generally protect it for the 70 or 80
years of life. Understandably, the memory molecule may be coiled
inside the vault and the vault coiled in the annular ring around
the mask. I am showing the memory molecule casketed with a lipidic
(fatty) membrane to suggest the molecule must freely slide into the
vault. Perhaps the electric field around the molecule rather than
the jacket would be adequate to assure its free movement. To
estimate memory capacity, we only consider one memory unit. The
rest of the memory units are entering their respective data events
at the respective sites they occupy, and --again--it is the length
of one strand, not the number of strands that sets storage
capacity. The spacing between the rungs of the DNA molecule is
three nanometers. A nanometer is one/billionth of a meter. If we
take the DNA rung spacing as typical, there will be 1/3 billion
storage positions on a meter of molecule. There are

112

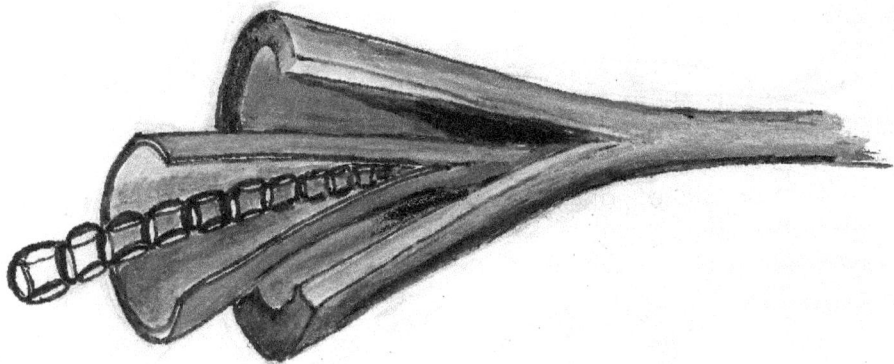

Figure 22

5/3 or 1 2/3 billion positions in the five meters of DNA molecule

in the cell nucleus. Starting with this --the maximum conceivable

storage capacity: a five meter strand-- we will work our way down

to a more realistic estimate of capacity.

ESTIMATING MEMORY CAPACITY

At the 25 entry per second data rate, we are using 1500 storage positions per minute, 90,000 per hour, about 3/4 billion per year. The 1 2/3 billion positions will be filled in 2 1/4 years.

We now have the hours of running time for the memory tape; 2 1/4 years = 19,000 hours maximum. If we "dumped" the tape as a test, and, if dumping the tape required erection of the data event: that is, the exalted data stage must fire as each event is delivered, it would take slightly over two years, dumping day and night at the 25 per second rate, to dump the tape.

When scanning (only), the data event only passes through the active site; it is not "exalted" and there is no delay while the cell completes its firing. Two technical problems become important here.

The first problem is scanning two billion data events in a time short enough to memory can respond to the retrieval instruction and still not have the data rate so high it exceeds the high frequency roll-off of the synapse; just the synapse, the cell membrane is not a factor on memory delivery.

Computers are miniaturized to reduce capacity effects. A capacitor is two conducting surfaces with opposing voltages on them and an insulator between. The memory tape has to be scanned in a reasonable length of time and the device we have here is scanning on the order of billions of events per second. There could be occasions where the signal voltage would have to rise or fall in a billionth of a second. Capacity effects, which limit the high frequency response of the system, tend to resist these fast signal excursions. To avoid this trouble, the extreme miniaturization of the active element is helpful; it is about 1/10,000 the size of active element in a factory computer. To further get around capacity effects, the memory devices face each other with only a comparator cell between, so the distance the very fast, very precise and easily degraded memory signal is kept microscopically short. This face to face delivery of the signal is one of the neater finesses of the exalted data stage. The memory device can probably manage tens of millions of data events per second, but can it deliver billions per second?

There is another technical problem with the billion event storage probe. The cortex must pause firings while scanning. If the cortex fires for any reason, the scan is reset to the "recent" end of the tape and scanning of the distal end is interrupted. The longest allowable pause sets the longest scanning time. I doubt if it can be paused much longer than two seconds, if that much. These two technical problems: the signal voltage rise rate and the length of time the cortex must hold off firing, vigorously argue for a much shorter memory tape, one with a capacity on the order of tens of millions, rather than billions of data events. Memory space is recycled periodically so the absolute length of the tape is less a factor than scanning problems in setting total memory capacity.

Looking at our memory estimate from the "hours" point of view, we said we could store a maximum of 19,000 hours of entries. The actual capacity is probably a lot less than that.

ESTIMATING MEMORY CAPACITY

The visual system takes "pictures" of visual experience. We have to allow ten to fifteen "pictures" may be needed to record one visual experience. Looked at from the "pictures" point of view, the 1 2/3 billion storage positions, our maximum estimate, will give us about 160 million "pictures" for a lifetime storage visual information. One would think this ought to be more than than enough storage space; it will surely be more than enough when recycling memory storage capacity is allowed for.

Another problem comes up now. This abundance of storage capacity can be a liability. The reasoning goes like this: once the memory molecule has reached a certain length, further lengthening it tends to become contra-productive and an encumbrance. The scanning process may have to scan the entire length of the memory molecule for a particular retrieval. If the incremental length of the memory tape--that is, a length beyond a minimum, a practical and necessary length--contains information that is redundant, obsolete or not being recalled at all, then the superfluous entries are slowing down and encumbering the recall process without contributing anything of positive value. For this reason, and to use efficiently whatever storage capacity there is, the memory molecule is recycled. We have the following agreeable outcomes;

1. Information does fade from memory and it fades permanently; it is necessary to account for this curious trait of memory.

2. Storage positions are being recycled and recycling brings an enormous expansion of storage capacity with a given length of memory molecule.

3. Obsolete and fading throughputs are permanently removed from memory and no longer encumber the retrieval process.

Fig. 23 explains the mechanics of recycling the memory molecule.

Fig. 24 is the enter/read terminal of the memory molecule. The rungs of the memory molecule are the molecules shaped like bow ties, the black dots are the molecules. The middle rung is spanning the opening in the aperture mask and monitoring the flow of neurotransmitter chemical flowing

Memory molecule is formed
and inserted at input end of
of the vault.

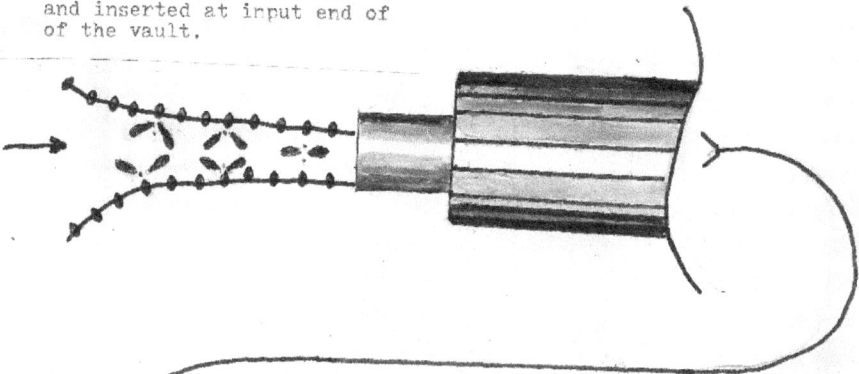

Memory molecule is extruded
and dissolved by intracellular
enzymes at the distal end of
the vault.

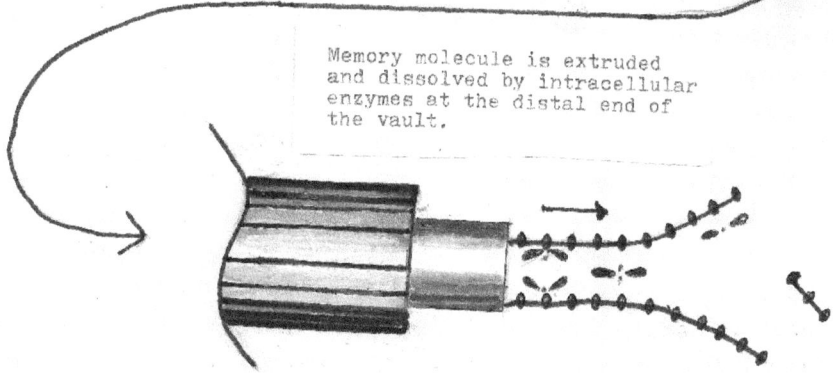

Figure 23

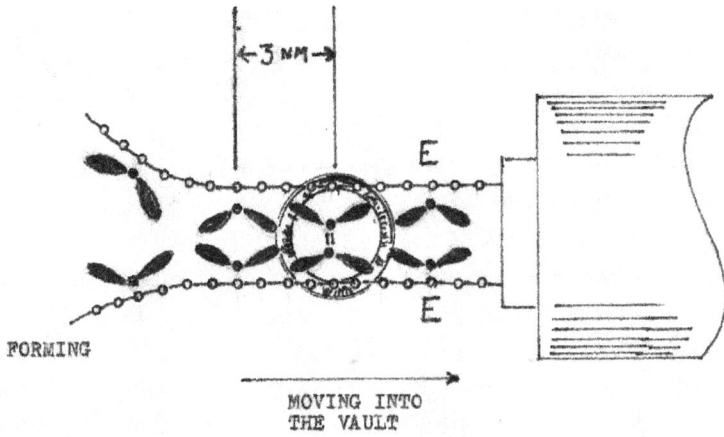

Figure 24

through the opening (into the page). The quantity of

neurotransmitter in the chemical flux modifies the ground state energy of the rung molecule. Possibly special chemical bonds are formed to commemorate the energy change accompanying the data event or perhaps a subunit is flipped from one configuration (cis) to a mirror image configuration (trans). It is also possible the data entry is stored as an internal magnetic realignment of the atoms in the molecule. This will need better opinion than mine.

Whatever the underlying chemistry is, it appeals to me to think the signal event leaves a peizo-electric stress in the memory molecule which is a function of the data event at that rung. Piezo-electric substances have the property of generating a voltage when placed under mechanical stress.

The piezo-electric idea is attractive to me because it may be possible for the stress to propagate, rung by rung, accompanied by the piezo-electric voltage in a high velocity backward movement of the data event when memory is commanded to deliver. The piezo electric effect may make possible a reciprocity where chemical current flow controls a voltage on the memory molecule during the entry part of the cycle and the memory molecule voltage controls chemical current flow on delivery. The stored signal voltage appears between E and E in the drawing and this is the voltage that will move backward down the memory molecule on memory delivery. When the backward moving signal voltage arrives at the opening in the mask it will be in a position to control current flow through the opening. If only the electric field of the piezo-electric voltage is used to control the current, the system may not need an additional energy supply for the delivery part of the cycle.

Memories fade and fade absolutely, a process not utterly devoid of redeeming value. (I spent two high school years studying Ivanhoe. Try as I will, I am unable to remember-anything about the book other than it was written by Sir Walter Scott.) It is only reasonable that provision should be made for removing certain throughputs from memory inventory altogether. For an example, the motor memory, back at age two or three, carried an inventory of motor instructions for a smaller body with clearly different skeletal dynamics that the present body. If these obsolete motor instructions linger in memory beyond their time, they become a hazard. There is a possibility, through cortical inadvertence, for one of these incompatible motor instructions to find its way out to the muscles of the body with disastrous effect.

Recalling brings forward a throughput from the distal end of the tape. A new copy is made, and the new copy becomes a new entry at the "recent" end of the tape. The throughput has been "exercised" and throughputs are retained in memory when they are exercised.

Whether a particular throughput stays in inventory or not is a qualitative matter and not a function of the chronological age of the entry. Setting aside whatever psychological factors that may influence remembering and forgetting, the raw mechanical factors are as follows:

1. The throughput will be exercised and retained if it is being requested by contemporary experience or if it can be exercised in

association with another throughput that is being exercised on a contemporary basis.

2. Throughout the wakeful day there are short spurts of reverie and longer intervals of day dreaming that will recall and re-enter throughputs on a random basis.

3. The cortex asleep re-randomizes inventory in both of its sleep modes (discussed elsewhere). Sleep activity serves several vital functions and one of them is rescuing fading throughputs, again, at random. Any factor that re-randomizes inventory (there may be additional randomizers) will tend to rescue fading throughputs, to nullify the straight-line-frequency-of-use parameter and to equalize the advantage recent entries have by virtue of their recency or redundant throughputs have by virtue of their redundancy.

4. The technical competence of the throughput statement is always the most important factor. I have a hunch those few cloying remembrances of our first few years are attributable to short intervals when the forming cortex was working especially well in a stable plateau of structural consistency sandwiched between bursts of growth. Incompetent throughputs are written by the forming cortex, one that has suffered trauma and one that has been damaged by booze and drugs. There are both transient and permanent versions of this problem. In any case, the fade process allows memory a means to get rid of its technically incompetent throughputs.

Since the memory molecule is recycled, it would be necessary to know the retention/fade ratio in order to estimate memory capacity. An elegant method for determining either the total capacity or the retention/fade ratio is not to be seen on the near horizon. None of this is amenable to experiment.

Subjective estimates of memory capacity or the retention/fade ratio are none too good either. Subjective estimates of the memory fade factor have a way of varying with the partisanship of the last person who appointed himself to make the representation. To one way of thinking, 90% of the information stored in memory, so much of it redundant, could disappear altogether and it would be good riddance. On the other hand, the "total recall" partisanship would insist every fleeting second of experience is indelibly embossed in memory.

The foregoing are the problems that will confront anyone who tries to estimate memory capacity. Taking both memory usage and the technical factors into account, we could probably safely reduce the technical estimate of storage capacity to much smaller proportions. As a guess, the memory molecule strand is probably around one foot long. Its total capacity is on the order of tens of millions of data events and with ten or more data events in each scenario, the number of discrete experiences that can be recalled is on the order of a million. The data rate on scan is tens of millions of events per second and the maximum pause time is less than one second.

Egotism tends to plead for a very high memory capacity. I think the "total recall" partisanship may have been misled by some experiments that were performed by electrically stimulating the cortex while it was exposed during surgery. Considering the elaborate and system wide provisions for neutralizing stray voltages (discussed later) the cortex has no tolerance for a foreign voltage. When the experimenter applies the external voltage, real-time cortical function immediately becomes incoherent, and, relieved of a real instruction, the cortical statement is written by the only function remaining coherent: the memory. During the experiment, memory free-scans and monopolizes the network.

The patient has vivid recollections of experience indigenous to the lobe under stimulation. When the auditory lobe is stimulated, the patient recalls sounds, or music, or phrases dredged from distant memory. Visual memory reconstructs a series of strong and distinct visual images when it is stimulated. The patient is surprised and impressed upon discovering this long forgotten information is still retained in memory. (One patient, a brick layer, recalled the individual bricks he had set in a wall twenty years earlier.)

The recall is so vivid, so pervasive so lifelike (so free of competitive images) the patient reports he seems to be reliving the experience. The recall of these images, thought to be long forgotten, is sometimes construed as an argument for "total recall". Topical as all of this may be, it tells us nothing quantitative about total memory capacity or the retention/fade

ratio. The exposed cortex is available for experimentation for
perhaps one half hour of the several hours of the surgery.
(Surgery is performed for clinical rather than experimental
objectives. One surgery, including electrical stimulation, lasted
17 hours.)

During the time available, the probe will induce a dozen,
possibly several dozen of these recollections. Since it would take
several months, running day and night, to "dump" the tape, there is
not enough time during the experiment to deliver a representative
sampling of the information contained in memory. The technique is
not useful in estimating the retention/fade ratio.

SHORT TERM MEMORY A POSSIBILITY

The real-time lobe of the visual cortex contains memory units and
meets the technical definition of being a short term memory. The
eye forages the visual image with a succession of quick jumps
followed by a short fixation on areas of interest in the image.
The visual acquisition is made during the fixation, the information
picked up while the eye was in rapid movement is not entered in
permanent memory. The short term memory in the real time lobe
stores these short bursts of visual experience for the length of
time it takes to make the acquisition. The time duration of the
burst varies from about one-fourth to one-half second.

The function of the real-time lobe more nearly resembles the
buffer memory in the digital computer than a short term memory as
such. In digital processors the buffer memory temporarily stores

the input until the central processing unit is available. The real-time memory of the cortex works a little differently, it organizes the visual scenario (i.e. the burst of visual images making up the visual scenario), and codes the rate of movement within the image.

A working short term memory should have a storage capacity exceeding the very brief storage of a technical or buffering memory. Real-time memory, structurally identical to permanent memory, is not used in a way that would qualify it as a short term memory.

Some theorists seem to be convinced the cortex incorporates provision for short term memory. In so far as this discussion of the cortex is concerned, I have no vested interest in the outcome of the argument.

Short term memory is an appealing idea because it seems like it ought to provide a mechanism for pre-fading throughputs before they are entered in permanent memory, a virtue that would expand total memory capacity. On the other hand, there is no need to expand memory capacity if the existing capacity is already more than adequate, and, if there is a need to fade throughputs, fading can be carried out in permanent memory about as well as it can be done in short term memory. I doubt the cortex has short term memory, other than the technical memory in the preceding paragraphs. It would complicate the system with extra apparatus to make and to

control the tricky transfer of data from short term to permanent
memory.

The persisting hunch that the cortex incorporates short term
memory is probably supported by certain oddities, real or imagined,
in cortical behavior.

There is one experiment the psychologists have run where the
subject is set at the task of memorizing a nonsense word list (an
enterprise notoriously spare of mnemonic landmarks to begin with).
Initially memorization will be consistent and predictable for a
short period of time. Memory seems to balk and further attempts at
memorization either fail or are not as efficient beyond this
initial interval. From this, the psychologists concludes there is
a short term memory and its storage capacity has been overrun when
the subject is no longer able to memorize the word list.

Functioning naturally, in an ambience of naturally occurring
experience, the cortex makes its first grasp of a new entry by the
reinforcement process. After the acquisition has been made, the
cortex "shifts gears" and slows down to think about the new entry.
"Thinking" about the new entry, in effect, re-enters the new
acquisition in memory, this time by forming associations with it.
A properly written entry is made by both processes. Bereft of
associations when there is no pause in the task for forming
associations, much of the mnemonic value is lost. Defeating the
associative process will balk the cortex and create the impression
a short term memory has either been overrun or has failed to make
the transfer of information to permanent memory. Here, the cortex
balks because the experimenter has clamped the subject in a

situation requiring uncharacteristic internal cortical strategies and information management.

The intelligent mechanism--with its fickle attention span and freedom of wit--is at the center of all cortical operations, it has a way of coming off second best when lashed to the Pavlovian confines and artifice of the psychologist's laboratory. With so many experiments of this kind, there is an ever present tendency to cold-deck the cortex with most abnormal performing situations imaginable and, from this, draft all sorts of inferences about the way the cortex is supposed to work normally.

The cortex behaves strangely following concussion and this behavior simulates the symptoms we would expect from a short term memory dysfunction.

Concussion (jarring, shaking violently) to the brain follows the blow to the head when the blow lands with sufficient force. The cortex, suspended, more or less afloat, in the cerebral fluids and protected by the bony skull and surrounding membranes, at times can withstand a remarkable amount of punishment to the head without being excessively disturbed. It is extremely vulnerable when the blow is strong enough to breach cortical protection.

The medical people do not entirely understand the pathophysiology of concussion. Concussion is the result of driving the cortex, albeit within its membranous coverings, against the hard surface of the skull. There is a transient insult to the brain accompanied by variable neurological symptoms. Loss of consciousness is not a necessary sequel to concussion and, where there is a loss of consciousness, it may not set in for minutes or days after the injury. The victim is pretty much out of it. Typically he is unresponsive, confused about time and place, sometimes stuporous and complaining about double vision and dizziness. In the least acute case, the victim may report a headache and unsteadiness the following day with no lasting effects.

With more severe concussions, the G forces near the brain and membranous tissue lacerate or bruise the cortex when it is slammed against the cranial bones and partitions. A bruised cortex, called a contusion, produces local areas of swollen tissue and capillary hemorrhage and, along with the hemorrhage, cerebral crisis. (The direction of the blow and the physics of deceleration may leave the cortical contusion on the side opposite to the impact. If the contusion underlies the point of impact it is called a "coup" injury and if it is on the far side, across from the point of impact: "contra coup" injury.

Hemorrhage infuses blood protein into the cerebral fluids so water must enter the cerebral space to equilibrate protein concentration. Normally there are no pressure differences between the organs of the body; whatever pressure differences there may be, they are very slight. When the cortex is bruised, cranial pressures rise and may threaten life. The cranium will not expand and the fluids cannot be compressed so pressures rise to a point where blood supply to the cortex is compromised and extruding pressure is applied to the nerves that penetrate the floor of the skull, including the vital spinal cord. Pressures can be relieved by drilling burr holes in the skull, sometimes on an emergency basis. With bad luck, the episode may be followed by brain damage syndrome: paralysis (usually to one side of the body), speech impairment and occasionally, protracted coma.

Amnesia (loss of memory) may accompany brain trauma, it is also found with senility, hysteria, epilepsy, alcoholism. Amnesia may be confined to a single lobe of the brain.

Memory loss for events subsequent to cortical trauma is called anterograde amnesia. Inability to recall stored experience prior to the injury is called retrograde amnesia. I think amnesia is a dysfunction of the real-time processes of the cortex and not a memory dysfunction as such.

With anterograde amnesia something like this may be happening: the cortex is presently writing incompetent entries because it has been injured, hence the difficulty with the recall of recent entries. With retrograde amnesia, the injured cortex is writing incompetent or incompatible retrieval instructions so memory has difficulty responding when interrogated for entries made prior to the injury. To me, difficulty with memory interrogation, a sequel of brain injury, is as significant in the amnesic picture as the loss of stored information per se.

There is one form of amnesia that goes along with concussion consistently. The victim is unable to recall the blow responsible for the concussion and the minute, or fraction of a minute, that immediately preceded the blow. It has been said the injury prevents the transfer of the just prior experience from a short term memory to permanent memory. Here the cortex makes the acquisition alright, an acquisition which it would have normally been followed by a period of time when it "thinks" about the acquisition just made. Both activities are necessary for a properly written entry and the concussion denied the cortex a chance to complete the entry by the associative process. Entered by the iterative process only, the entry is only fractionally written and does not survive in memory.

Amnesia is not found in neat packages of memory loss. The anterograde form is frequently accompanied by the retrograde form. Very early memories usually survive rather well. There are a number of odd amnesias, each with an odd interval of memory difficulty and each suggesting a short term memory of that particular interval. The hippocampal formation is a part of the cortical control system. There is an odd amnesia found with hippocampal dysfunction. The patient is unable to recall recent experience older than the most recent five minutes. He would be able to memorize a short grocery list, but would not be able to remember the things he wanted to buy if it took more than five minutes to get to the store. This dysfunction suggests a short term memory of five minutes capacity.

Some psychologists believe there is a tendency for memories to fade within a period of 48 hours after entry is made. There may be a fade, but I think it is the normal sleep mode equalization of the memory throughput ledger. Sleep is dealt with later.

ESTIMATING MEMORY CAPACITY

Proposals for short term memory in the cortex are never free of doubt. Most of the evidence for short term memory can be interpreted in more than one way. I do not think there is a need for short term memory in the system, but I am willing to listen to any reasonable proposal.

THE LATERAL TO THE AXIS RE ORGANIZATION OF THE DATA BUSES AND THE DATA THEY ARE CARRYING

Unreferenced data: information in isolation is not useable. There is a lateral re organization of the cortex out of respect for just such truisms.

A single symbol: "G", or an isolated burst of symbols: "ERGRE", will not convey useful information in isolation. The sense conveyed by the symbol will only become meaningful when referenced in some sort of context; "EVERGREEN". Information is encountered in one of its two aspects: "message" or "context". The "message" is the component in immediate traffic, the part we would expect to see at an instant of inspection. The "context" can be a lot of things: an expanded version of the message(s), a memory inventory of experience with similar messages, or even the fixed processing parameters of the computer. There is always "context" going along with the "message" somewhere; though, it may take a little hunting to find it. (Psychologists speak of "feature" and "surround" which are psychological variants of roughly the same referencing predicament.)

The "message" in the visual cortex is the statement standing in the active site at the moment. The "context" is a buildup of habits and prior constructions that make possible a useful disposition of the "message".

Suppose I pick up a photograph and take a look at it. My task is to identify the content of the image solely on the basis of the information given in the image. I am not allowed to make use of recalled information or resort to strategies other than interpreting the information as it is given in the image. It

flatly cannot be done. This is another way of saying there is no

such thing as instantaneous experience. Incoming experience is

only meaningful when it can be construed in a continuum and context

of similar and relatable experiences. A "message" is never an

orphan; it has to have relatives and ancestors somewhere.

The foundations of referencing begin with the single symbol, the

single data event, and, beginning with the single symbol, it may be

extrapolatable without limit but the single event is where it all

begins. Physically referencing the single data event in the cortex

is an operational variation of the referencing truisms.

In Fig. 25 the input modules are drawn in a three dimensional

lattice and this is a valid equivalent circuit of the cortex. In

situ, the network is folded in the middle and this lattice is a

"legal" topological manipulation of the folded network. Fig. 26

traces back through the steps that were taken to manipulate the "U"

shaped reentrant arrangement in order to end up with the lattice

equivalent. The equivalent circuit is justified because it is much

simpler to visualize the data flow in the lattice than it is in the

"U" shaped routing of the real cortex.

The bottom drawing does not quite tell the truth. The "fan in"

fiber, that is the fiber labeled "optic nerve" and the first cell

in the cortex ("ascending columnar") are the same cell. For

purposes of expository, nothing more, we will show it as two cells

because it makes the electronics easier to explain. Fig. 26 does

not show the cell body for the lateral cell. I think the long processes of the lateral cell are in the outermost cortical layer and the cell body is in the underlying layer.

These topological manipulations are neither grand nor farfetched. They are simple and as "safe" as it is possible to make them. Fig. 27 is a semi anatomical drawing of the real time (input) section of the cortical module. This is a sagittal section with the posterior to the left. The visual lobe is the rearmost and lowest lobe in the cortex. An electrical replica of the visual image originates at the retina (right), moves down the optic nerve to a crossover point in front of the thalamus, then around and under the thalamus and terminates in a couple of round protrusions at the posterior and underside of the thalamus. Reflex information is picked off at this point and the nerves that carry information to the visual lobe begin here. This is the fan in to the visual cortex, represented here by the lone fiber running from the thalamus to the cortex.

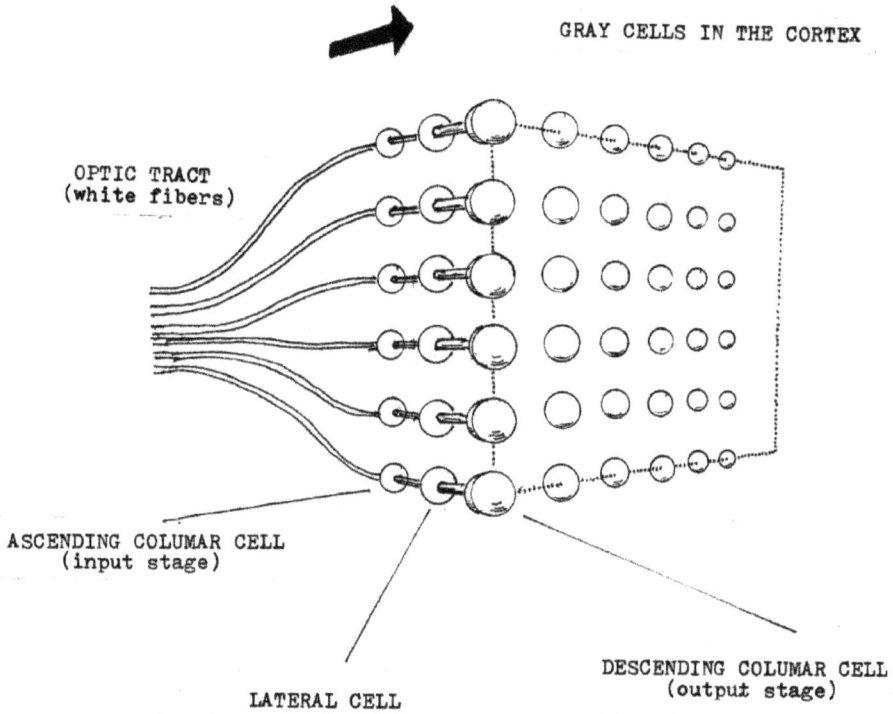

This is a "legal" lay-out of the cortical network. The network
is folded in the middle in situ. The lay-out in situ is a "legal"
topological manipulation of this lattice. Dotted line is the
physical plane of the exalted data stage.

Figure 25

STARTING WITH THE LATTICE,
WE WORK OUR WAY TO THE
LAYOUT IN THE CORTEX.

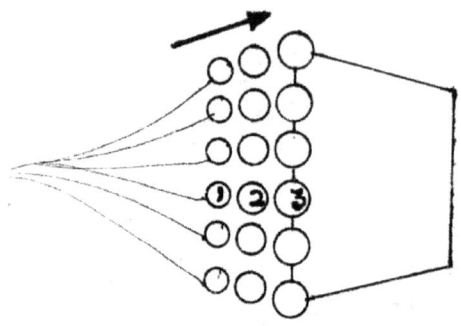

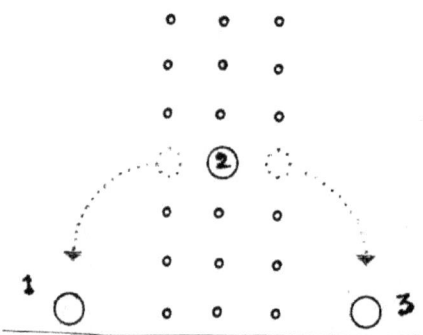

LOOKING AT THE SIDE OF THE
LATTICE, THE NUMBERED CELLS
LEAVE THEIR VERTICAL PLANE
IN THE LATTICE AND ARE RE-
TURNED TO THE PLANE THEY
OCCUPY IN THE CORTEX.

2   LATERAL

ASCENDING
COLUMAR

1   3

DESCENDING
COLUMAR

THE CELL BODIES ARE ELONGATED
TO PENETRATE THE LAYERS OF
THE CORTEX.

OPTIC NERVE
(See text)

Figure 26

We will say the white fiber delivers to the ascending columnar

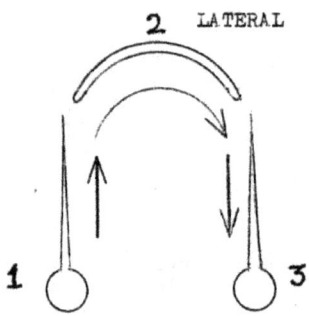

which carries the signal upward to the outer layers of the cortex.

(One fiber serves both the ascending and the fan in function.) The

lateral cell bends down a little to meet the ascending columnar which does not quite penetrate the outer layers. The lateral cell

picks up the ascending columnar signal and redistributes it

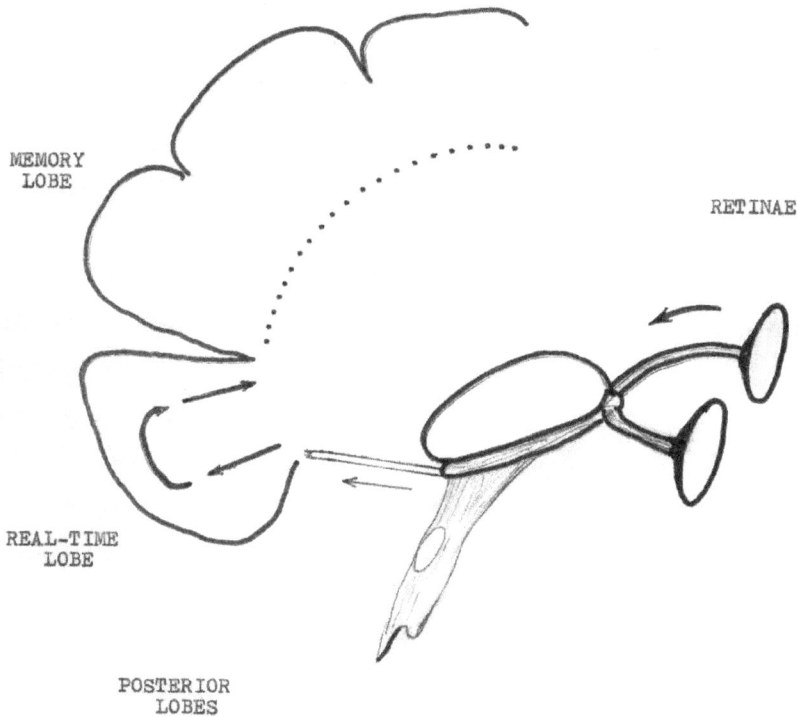

MEMORY
LOBE

RETINAE

REAL-TIME
LOBE

POSTERIOR
LOBES

FIG 25

to the descending columnar cel Figure 27 letes the "U" shaped

flow path in the input visual lobe.

The dotted line is the physical plane of the exalted data stage. The memory half of the module has an input face and an output face. The input and output faces terminate in their respective exalted data stages and these stages are laid out in the anatomy of the cortex with one slightly above the other to quiet cross talk. "Ascending" and "descending" indicate the direction of data flow and this may agree with the appearance of the cells in the microscope but I am not sure.

Fig. 28 looks at the lattice "end on" looking upstream and with the data flow toward the viewer. This is the output stage and contains the active sites.

We will say some sort of provision has been made to bring all of the sites in this stage into a collaborative operation except for the single data bus set out at the lower left. This is a data bus in isolations: an orphan. The data it carries is also in isolation. There are two problems here: 1. As far as "data" is concerned, the bus is carrying unreferenced data. The information on this bus is all "message" and no "context". Unreferenced, it is unusable. 2. As far as "process" is concerned, the network is divided lengthwise, along the upstream/downstream axis. It is divided into two, and operationally separate, pieces. Part of the visual image lands in one of the pieces and part in

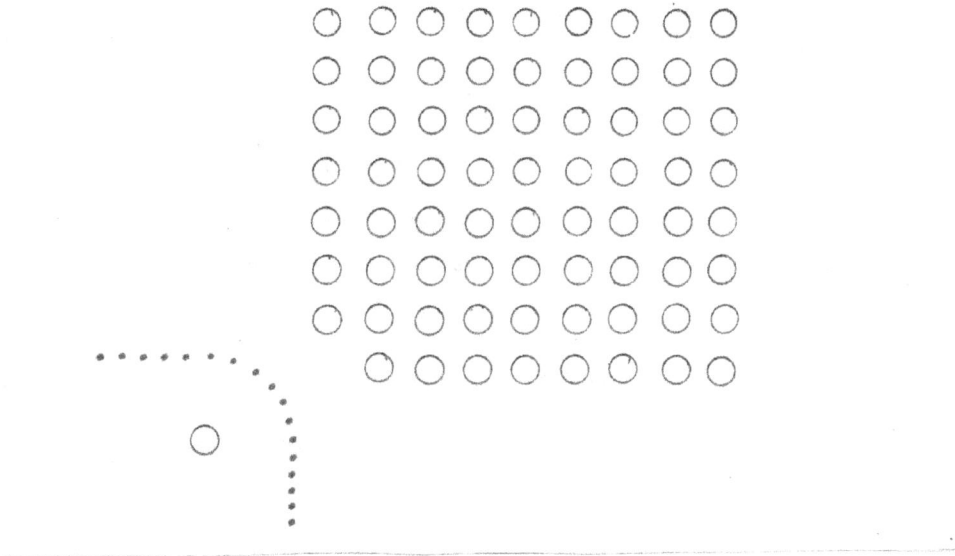

Fig.
28

the other. The system is "blind" to operations that depend on

collaborative processing of the two parts of the image. The

absence of collaborative processing leaves a processing artifact in

the image; the performance artifact is at the gap between the two

parts of the image (dotted line in Fig. 28). There is a lateral re organization of the cortical network to get rid of both the unreferenced data problem and the artifact problem. There is a relationship between referencing and artifact suppression--the more the referencing, the fewer artifacts in the throughput.

Ideally, each data bus would be referenced to all other data buses. If it only required one cell to bring about collaboration between two data buses, it would require one million to the million power data buses to produce collaboration between all of the data buses in the data plane. The 16 billion cells in the cortex are only the smallest fraction of the number of cells needed.

(Thirty years ago, theorists unerringly discovered this shortage of cortical cells. Their findings have never been taken to heart. This is a key issue, it sets extreme limitations on the degree of sophistication of process we can expect to find in the cortex. We will also show this as one of the "clincher" arguments which argue against the cortex having access to the subject matter of its throughput. If the cortex interpreted the visual image, a situation could arise where the information at the far edge of the retina could only be interpreted in conjunction with information arriving from a diametrically opposing area. There are not enough cortical cells to assure even a few of these relationships could be drawn.)

Fig. 29 is a (probable) physical data pick up schedule for the lateral re organization of the network. The ascending columnar delivers to the lateral cell. The lateral cell does not deliver to the "on axis" descending cell. The data bus and the data it is carrying is transposed and delivers to several descending columnar

cells with a lateral shift in the flow of data between input and
output cells. The lateral shift may be easier to see in the upper
drawing where the pickup is from one source. The bottom circuit is
the more probable arrangement. The data routing is "recursed"
which means the data appearing at a single input terminal will be
partially carried to the output terminals via, perhaps, hundreds of
recursive routings.

The lateral cell is a "summator". The cell accepts a D.C.
signal from many sources and adds the signal amplitudes
arithmetically.

The purpose of the lateral re-organization is to arithmetically
"add in" the referencing between the data buses and to "add out"
the artifact vulnerability. Upon completion of the arithmetical
addition, the information that would preserve the identity of the
data bus that was reporting has been composited (say, "buried") in
the lateral re organization of the network. The compositing
process has already begun at the retina and

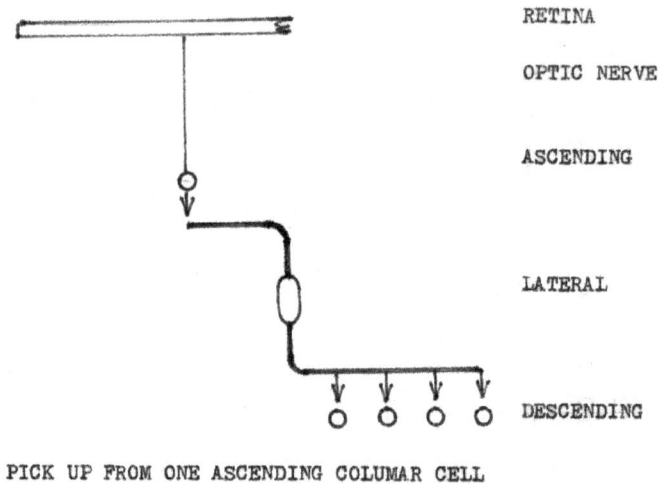

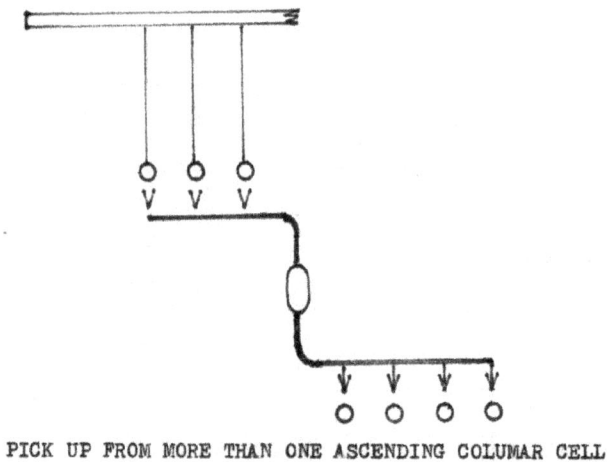

RETINA

OPTIC NERVE

ASCENDING

LATERAL

DESCENDING

PICK UP FROM ONE ASCENDING COLUMAR CELL

PICK UP FROM MORE THAN ONE ASCENDING COLUMAR CELL

Fig.27

Figure 29

the transpositions and summing   ortex are a continuation

of a process already in progress. Here again, the cortex cannot

have access to the subject matter of the throughput without

preserving the identity of the nerve fiber reporting.

THE LATERAL TO THE AXIS RE ORGANIZATION OF THE DATA BUSES AND THE DATA THEY ARE CARRYING

Here we have recursive routing through the cortex. In a recursive routing, an adjacent lateral cell picks up most of the information already being carried by the data bus it is recursing. In a stepwise fashion, each lateral cell adds a few new pickups and drops a few old ones, moving a few terminals laterally in the process.

Due to the "U" shaped folding of the network and the recursive data routings, it would take a very extensive lesion in the outer layers of the cortex before we had an assured severance of enough on axis data buses to create a problem.

The neurology people report the cortex has a remarkable ability to suffer this kind of damage without severe loss of faculty. A small lesion may have no noticeable effect. In the visual system, a lesion large enough to be damaging will produce a blind area in the image when it occurs in the real time lobe and the same lesion may have little or no effect when it occurs in the memory division of the lobe. Each lobe has its version of the damage problem.

Fig. 30 shows the confluent "U" shaped flow paths in the two halves of the module. The real time segments of the module make up the real time division of the lobe and memory segments make up the memory division of the lobe. The lobe of the cortex shown

MEMORY SEGMENT OF
THE CORTICAL MODULE

COMPARATOR SITE

REAL-TIME SEGMENT
OF THE
CORTICAL MODULE

Fan-in fiber is shown making a
connection with an ascending columar.

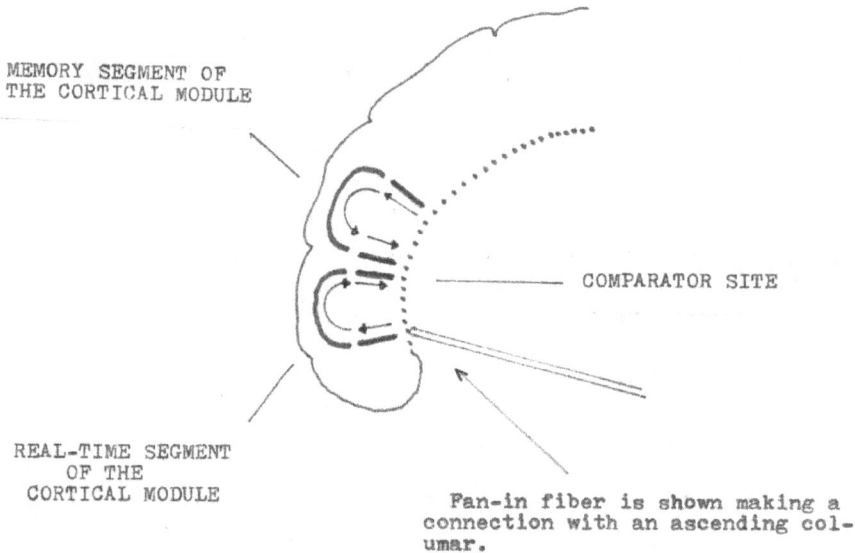

This is the physical arrangement of the
memory module and the direction of data flow
through the module. Columar cells contain
memory units and either originate or terminate in the exalted data stage. (dotted
line)

Figure 30

as the "associative" lobe in s͏͏͏͏͏͏͏   ' books is also the

memory division of the lobe.

In explaining the need for lateral reorganization of the network,

we have a million fan in fibers appearing at the input terminals to

the computer and each terminal is connected to a module, a

miniature computer; and we do not want one million separate
computers functioning independently of each other; we want one
computer with one million input terminals.

SUMMARY OF THE LATERAL RE-ORGANIZATION OF THE NETWORK

There is so much emphasis on brain "volume" or brain "mass" that
it could be misleading. Most of the mass of the brain is made up
of the white fibers at its center. The white fibers either carry
information to and from the cortex (radial fibers) or control
instructions between lobes (arcuate fibers). White fibers do
necessary work, to be sure, however, other than delivering data to
the right places, they contribute nothing to computation, or
intelligence--for that matter.

Only the gray and outer layer of cells do the computation, the
"smart" layer is about 1/8 inch thick and constitutes only 3% of
the brain mass, Fig. 31.

Discretion may be the better part of speculation, but never to
the point where it takes away all of the fun.

Only the gray cells in
the "bark" of the cortical
system are available for
computation.

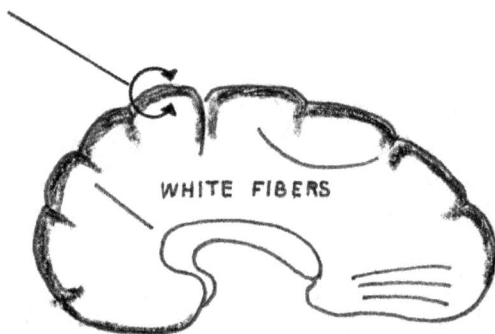

WHITE FIBERS

Fig. 31

The question is often posed about the way the hereditary code

dictates the complex connecting schedule for forming the trillions

of connections between cortical cells. It is thought the highly

site-specific nature of the connection about to be formed, along

with billions like it, would require a code of unimaginable

complication. Specificity, as such, is the problem. The thing to

142

do is to get rid of site critical specificity in the hereditary code, and the way to do this is to have the code dictate general routines for forming the cell and refer the specificity of the intercellular connection to some kind of gross histogenic formula. Part of this problem has already been attended to with the universal cortical module which will accept any optic nerve in the "fan-in" and does not require an instruction for connecting a specific nerve to a specific module.

An example I would choose for a gross histogenic formula would be the piezo-electric effect and its influence on bone growth. (The piezo-electric effect generates a voltage across, or at the surface of, a substance under mechanical stress.) Compressive stress in bone precipitates the deposition of calcium. The deposit is the thickest where the piezo-electric voltage is the greatest. The bone "grows under its load" becoming thicker and stronger where the compressive force is the greatest. The histogenic code for the formation and growth of bone is relieved of the extra work of specifying the thickness of bone versus stress.

The cortex begins as a widening and elaboration of the embryonic neural tube at its cephalic end. The precursor of the cortical cell forms on the inner wall of the tube and migrates to its final position in the cortex. It is not known if the cell is capable of self-propulsion or if is moved under the influence of a local chemical gradient. The direction of its movement is surely chemically guided. This kind of cell migration is called "chemotaxis".

The precursor cortical cell is called a neuroblast and is undifferentiated at its initial formation. When it reaches its permanent physical position in the cortex, it can differentiate into a supporting cell (called a glial cell, there are several kinds) or it can differentiate into a cortical nerve cell, one of many varieties. The mechanisms that position and differentiate the cell are not understood at the moment.

I think there is a gross histogenic formula for forming the synapses. The nerve fiber arborizes at its output end. At the end of these branches there bulbous terminals called synapses which form junctions with the next cell in the signal path.

The cell is almost always a summator. A cell is a summator when it performs additions and subtractions on the signals appearing at its input. A number of cells will form junctions with the summator. The contribution each cell makes to the summation is proportioned by the number of synapses allocated to each contributor.

Now we have the problem of forming the correct number of synapses for each contributor without encumbering the hereditary code with synapse-by-synapse specificity in the code. Suppose, shortly after the neuroblast differentiated into a cortical cell, its metabolic energy supply was hyper-active. At this stage of the cell's formation it is as small as it will ever be and the proportion of metabolic energy to cell volume is as great as it will ever be. A hyper-active cell is hyper-sensitive. A hyper-sensitive cell is prone to self-excited oscillation (in this case uncontrolled cell firings)

THE LATERAL TO THE AXIS RE ORGANIZATION OF THE DATA BUSES AND THE DATA THEY ARE CARRYING

The newly formed cell body arborizes and begins to form junctions with its neighbors. Suppose, as each new junction was formed, its formation tended to quiet the hyperactivity of the newly formed cell

An ascending columnar cell would seek out as many lateral cells as it could make contact with and continue to do this until it had quieted itself. If the formation of a junction between an ascending columnar and a lateral cell tended to further excite an already over-active lateral cell, the lateral cell would form as many junctions with descending cells as it could in order to quiet itself. When it ran out of nearby descending columnar cells, it would be forced to extend its branching to form junctions with descending cells at increasingly distant locations. I have a hunch the synaptic connections are formed by a gross histogenic formula such as this.

THE CODER ASPECT OF THE CODER/MULTIPLEXER

The sensory systems are known to be extremely sensitive and this
brings up another reality of the nervous system that needs to be
"taken to heart". An extremely sensitive "Automatic Sensitivity
Control" system must accompany these systems in order to control
their otherwise "run-away" sensitivity. We will keep the
discussion on automatic sensitivity control short and ASC is the
only abbreviation we use in the text. ASC, a relatively obvious
need, is the most neglected circuitry in the system.

Processes that overlay and collaborate with each other seem to
perfuse the nervous system. Automatic sensitivity control in the
visual system utilizes several ASC systems which overlay and
collaborate to reach an agreement on the sensitivity of the retina
under a given illumination.

The visual ASC systems are numbered in Fig. 32.

1. This is the straight-forward electro-mechanical system. A
sampling of light intensities is collected over the area of the
retina. Special fibers carrying this sample are separated from the
optic nerve. Iris control agrees on a consensus of light
intensities and this consensus is translated to the pupillary
reflex. A signal is sent to the muscles that control the aperture
of the iris based on overall average light value. The aperture is
reduced in proportion to the intensity of light stimulus falling on
the

THE CODER ASPECT OF THE CODER/MULTIPLEXER

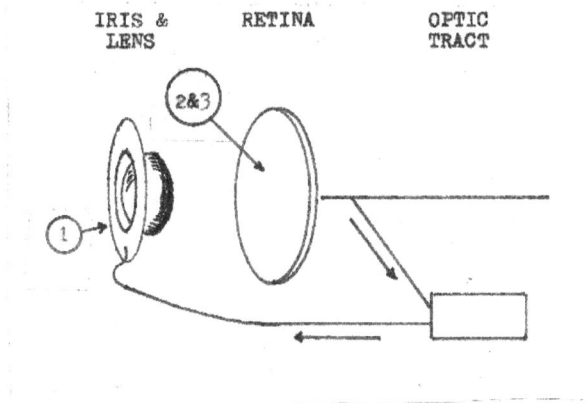

Figure 32

retina (not much different than automatic exposure control in a camera). This is a relatively slow acting system. (I have a hunch the special fiber extrication may be used for other purposes also, perhaps automatic focus control.)

2. Retinal "accommodation" is an optical-chemical ASC system. It is called "accommodation" in the visual system and "recruiting" in the hearing system; they are both parts of an "automatic sensitivity control" system. Accommodation and recruiting are the slowest acting of the ASC systems. In the visual system, the initial dark accommodation takes about one minute. Final accommodation trails off to the fifth minute after entering darkened surroundings. This is the slowest acting system.

Accommodation goes beyond controlling the iris aperture. There are 100 million photoreceptors and in full illumination the visual image should contain 100 million elements of visual definition. (Since the receptor will respond when its area is partially stimulated, the definition is greater than 100 million elements.) In the depths of dark accommodation, the individual receptors no longer function independently. As a part of the accommodation process, there is a reconfiguration of the way receptors function and a group of receptors, perhaps 100, will begin to report to the optic nerve as a single receptor in dark accommodation. A tradeoff is made wherein the system exchanges its ability to see detail for a gain in visual sensitivity when seeing in the dark. The definition is reduced from 100 million elements to near one million elements. This change in resolution from light seeing to dark seeing is a major artifact in the poorly illuminated visual image, yet it is so commonplace we scarcely notice

3. Photo-accommodation of the retina is thought to be a photochemical process. There is also a need for a fast acting system to protect the retina in the presence of a very bright light

with a fast attack, say the firing of a flash bulb. Rhodopsin, the light sensitive pigment in the rod cells, has been suggested for the fast acting light attenuator. One suggestion polarized the rhodopsin molecule at a right angle to the light path and another proposal sequestered the rhodopsin molecule in the membrane of the rod cell where it would move in and out to control the light excitation of the receptor. Neither of these ideas has been confirmed.

There is a voltage in immediate intimacy with the retina of about 40 millivolts. Theorists have suggested this voltage, or at least some of its component voltages (it is a composite voltage), is the fast acting ASC in the retina. I think this is the more likely case and the retinal voltage sets the retinal sensitivity.

The ASC voltage is probably generated by the photo-receptor and impressed on the surrounding retina. Each receptor makes a small contribution to the voltage. It is a D.C. voltage and varies as does the intensity of the illumination on the retina. I believe the voltage reduces the sensitivity of the receptor that generated it along with reducing the sensitivity of proximal receptors. All receptors contribute to, or respond to, the ASC voltage, so the process propagates through the span of the retina. The ASC voltage sets a fixed operating point for the sensitivity range of the photo receptor and the reference level is probably based on the average illumination of the retina. There is also another process, the coder process, where an illuminated receptor reduces the sensitivity of nearby receptors. The coder is a cell-specific process while the ASC voltage controls the span of the retina. The span wise process overlays and collaborates with the cell-specific processes of the coder. (The coder is a network of interconnected cells that accept the outputs of the photo-receptors.) Span wise ASC contributes a steady illumination reference signal to the coder arithmetic.

(There is a similar voltage in the duct containing the organ of Corti in the hearing system and it performs the same function. The voltage has been named the "cochlear microphonic". "Span wise automatic sensitivity control" would do for the retinal ASC signal. Maybe it should be shortened to "span wise automatic".)

There are five kinds of cells just behind the array of photo sensors. The first cells, more or less in layers, are <u>D.C.(only) cells</u> and they deliver their signal to ganglia of the optic nerve. This apparatus is the coder multiplexer and it is not as complicated as it may sound.

If we use the letter "E" as a symbol for the amplitude of the sensor output signal, we can set aside juggling voltages, membrane currents and chemical fluxes; all process the light signal passes through.

The arithmetic is simple addition or subtraction. E_{plus} is a positive contribution to the arithmetic and E_{minus} is negative.

Fig. 33 is the first step in the coder arithmetic. The visual image has been projected on the receptor array. The smallest element of details falls on the single receptor. (If the most minute element of detail is so small it does not entirely fill the end are of the receptor, it is useable anyway. The system normally functions at a resolution greater than single receptor resolution.

One experimenter working with a visual image with nothing more than a straight line with a break in it, reported resolution at 1/30 the receptor diameter.)

The element of detail is an analogue of the light stimulus on the receptor set, in turn, by the specific information in the visual image. It is immediately translated to an electrical equivalent signal at the receptor, this is the D.C. analogue of the signal and the "E" in the drawings.

The receptor in the middle of Fig. 33 (marked) has made this translation and the D.C. amplitude of the signal is started on its way toward the optic nerve. The receptor on the left makes a similar translation which is passed on to an inverter cell. The inverter cell changes positive signal amplitudes to negative signal amplitudes. A signal which started out as an amplitude increment at the receptor will be entered as a decrement in the arithmetic after it comes through the inverter routing. The D.C. (only) arithmetic of the coder now begins.

The signal arriving from the left, initially positive, is now negative because it is passed through the inverter; the sensor itself is the same as any other.

The receptor on the left, as a result of its signal inversion, is in E (minus) service as seen by the E (plus) channel. The signal output of the sensor on the left is positive, the same as any other sensor, and it is in its own "plus" service when its positive output is collected by its own "plus" routing.

The receptor in the middle of Fig. 33 will also be in its own "minus" service, delivering its signal to an inverter which makes a

"minus" contribution to a neighboring "plus" channel (not shown).
The sensors in Fig. 33 are separated by a microscopic distance.
The apparatus in Fig. 33 is on the left in Fig. 34.

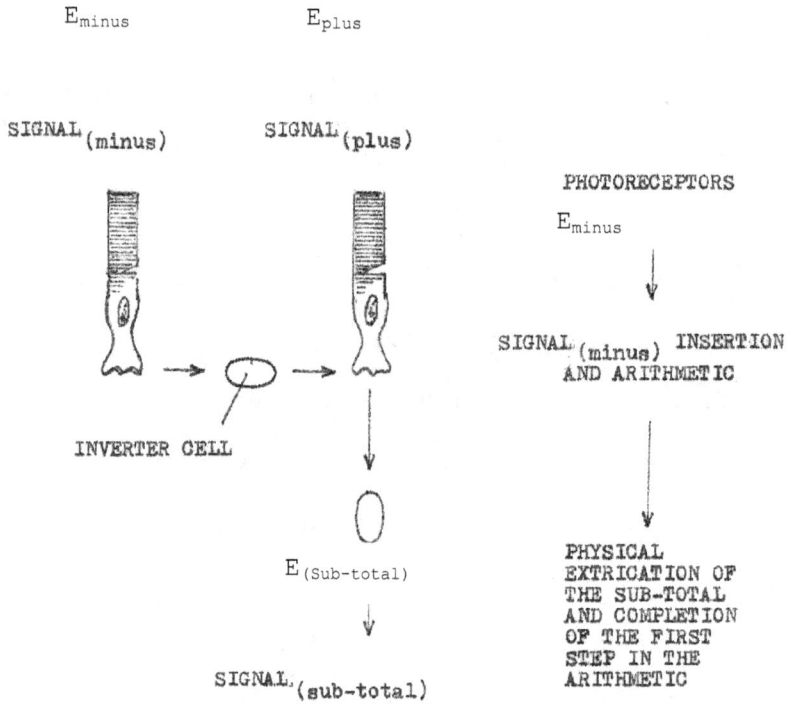

Figure 33

THE CODER ASPECT OF THE CODER/MULTIPLEXER

Another signal is collected from more outlying points on the retina, distances great enough to be called macroscopic--though barely. This larger sampling of the image is referenced to the microscopic detail of the adjacent

158

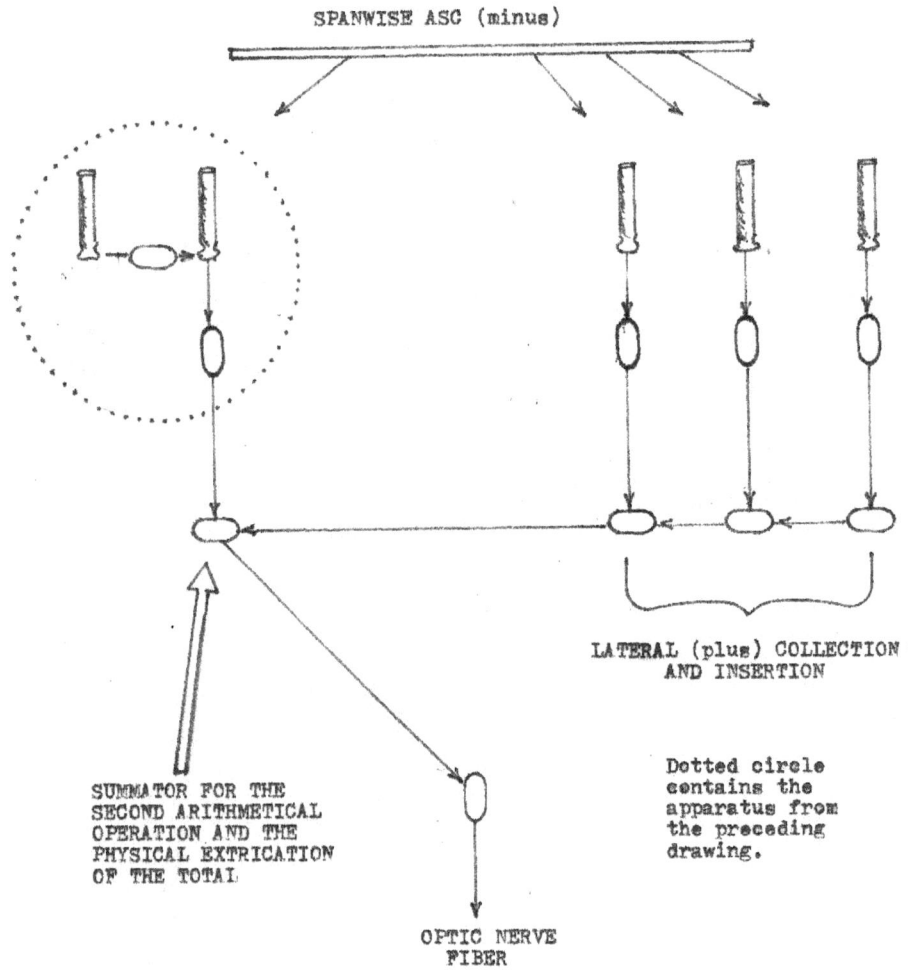

SPANWISE ASC (minus)

LATERAL (plus) COLLECTION
AND INSERTION

Dotted circle
contains the
apparatus from
the preceding
drawing.

SUMMATOR FOR THE
SECOND ARITHMETICAL
OPERATION AND THE
PHYSICAL EXTRICATION
OF THE TOTAL

OPTIC NERVE
FIBER

Figure 34

receptors. This is a positive signal. The separation between

positive pick-up points probably increases as the distance from the receptive field of a given optic nerve increases and the number of pick-up points decreases as the distance increases.

This lateral, somewhat span wise, positive contribution to the arithmetic is sensor specific, as contrasted with the gross ASC (minus) contribution. The lateral positive contribution is arithmetically added to the subtotal already computed and the total put on board the optic nerve.

The information that would identify and commemorate the specific receptor that was reporting has been arithmetically mixed (perhaps "homogenized" would be a better word) to the signals from all other receptors (about 100) in the receptive field of the optic nerve. (The receptors collected by a single optic nerve fiber are called the "receptive field" of the nerve. In dark accommodation, the receptive field functions as a single receptor.)

Traditional opinion of visual neural processing has held there are two components to the visual signal: one a "spatial" component and the other an "intensity" component. "Spatial" refers to the geometry of the visual image. If the coder was keeping track of the spatial component, it would write a statement that said, "Receptor number so-and-so is reporting with a signal of so many units of intensity". It does not do this, it simply adds intensities.

It might be argued the spatial component is somehow "implied" in the existing coder process. Implied or "real", it was clobbered when the intensity components and whatever it was that would have designated the spatial component were homogenized with all other signals in the immediate area. It can be looked at in several ways; the intensity components have been added to intensity components, the spatial identifiers have been added to spatial identifiers, the spatial components have been added to intensity components.

Once the signals have been compensated, the spatial component is not extractable from the intensity component downstream of the coder. This is a "clincher" argument for the cortex not having access to the subject matter of the throughput. For the cortex to have access to the subject matter of the image, it would require processing the spatial component and the intensity component in a separated format. (The cortex would need to know two things: (1) the amplitude excursion of the signal, (2) the physical receptor where the exclusion is taking place. It might be argued the cortex could somehow reconstruct the image in the separated format. The constants of the coder are set by the visual image itself, no such (central) information is available downstream of the coder to supervise the constants of the decoder.)

The coder erects an electrical replica of the visual image. The only requirement it has to meet is that it uniquely replicates the image. For every small intensity excursion in the visual image, there a corresponding signal excursion in the coder output. Nothing is lost or disregarded. The coder we have here meets this test.

Fig. 35 is a practical demonstration of coder arithmetic. A "minus" (or "inhibit") signal is flowing down the avenues between the squares toward the intersections. Since it is not opposed by an opposite signal gathered from the immediate surroundings, the minus signal darkens the intersections. I have worked out a gambit in the intersection at the lower right. Rather than shut off the lateral positive contribution altogether, the white circles restore enough of it to offset the effects of the minus (only) inflow to the intersection area.

Now we have a coder that uniquely replicates the visual image. For the time being we will settle for a "unique" replica, we will try for a coder output that is not only "unique", but "exclusive" in the next item on the multiplexer aspect of the coder multiplexer. The coder is a fine example of getting the most in performance out of a minimum of apparatus. Information about the spatial aspects of the image, shapes, sizes and positions, is "buried" in the coder arithmetic. The coder is not to be faulted for this quirk in its way of doing things. Here is a list of reasons for this extraordinary coder procedure:

1. The relative referencing of the data, an ongoing process in the cortex, has already begun at the coder. The coder

161

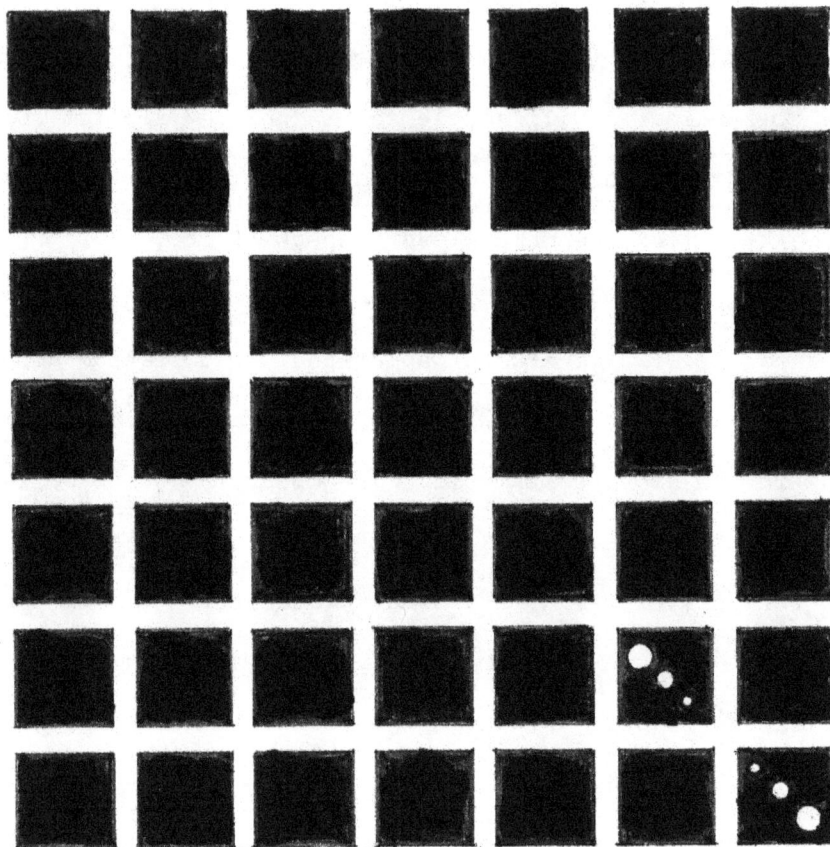

Figure 35

data format and the cortical format are compatible. The

microscopic areas of the retina are referenced to a more span wise

sampling of visual information. Intensities are referenced to everything it is possible to reference them to and most importantly; the average illumination of the retina is written in along with referencing specific light intensities on nearby receptors.

2. If the signal was not processed in the composited format, there is a possibility a naturally occurring visual image might "beat with" the physical geometry of the receptor mosaic (moiré effect) and produce an artifact in the visual image. The coder "adds out" the mosaic artifact.

3. The information from the 100 million receptors is conveyed to the cortex by the one million fibers of the optic nerve. The optic nerve flexes when the eye moves and this scheme greatly reduces the size of the nerve and improves the mobility of the eye.

4. If there was separate processing for the spatial and the intensity signals, it would forbid the re-organization of the sensitive areas of the retina under dark accommodation.

THE MULTIPLEXER ASPECT OF THE CODER/MULTIPLEXER

A multiplexer gathers information from a number of sources and squeezes the information, by one technique or another, so it can be carried on fewer channels than there are sources. There is "convergence" through a multiplexer. The convergence in the retina is 100 to 1: the information from 100 million receptors is converged so it can be carried on the million fibers of the optic nerve.

Fig. 36 is masterful for the way it takes liberties with the anatomy of the retina; the coder has been left out altogether to get across the gist of what happens when 100 channels are converged on one optic nerve fiber. Fig. 37 is more representative of the way multiplexing is done at the retina. Information from a given receptor is carried on more than one fiber. This is "recursive" multiplexing. The lower sketch makes the distinction between a "recursive" and the simpler "redundant" channel. A redundant channel carries exactly the same information already being carried by another channel: there are no redundant channels in the nervous system. The coder and D.C. multiplexing are inseparable: more like two ways at looking at the same mechanism than separate processes. The sketches leave out the coder and it is the coder that gathers the information from the receptors, converges it (as a part of coder arithmetic), and puts it on board the optic nerve.

Fig. 38 starts at the receptor and goes straight to the output, leaving out everything in between in order to see how the output behaves with respect to an element of detail in the visual image. The Greek letter "delta" (triangle) indicates there has been an excursion (say, a small increase in intensity) in the signal at the receptor. Due to the lateral reorganization of the network, the excursion will appear at several descending columnar cells in the cortex. For a given excursion at the receptor, there will be a unique and corresponding excursion of signal amplitude in several descending columnar cells. The absolute value of the excursion in the columnar cell will not be the same as the excursion at the receptor due to the proportioning in the inverter cell and the arithmetic entailed in the lateral reorganization of the network. Whatever arithmetic the element of detail has been through, however it has been scattered, it never gets lost, there is always consistent treatment of each element of detail. This is the only test we need apply to establish the "uniqueness" of the coder statement.

Establishing the "exclusiveness" of the coder will need a little more noodle work. I will sketch the terms of the problem. The coder is exclusive when we have assurance two,

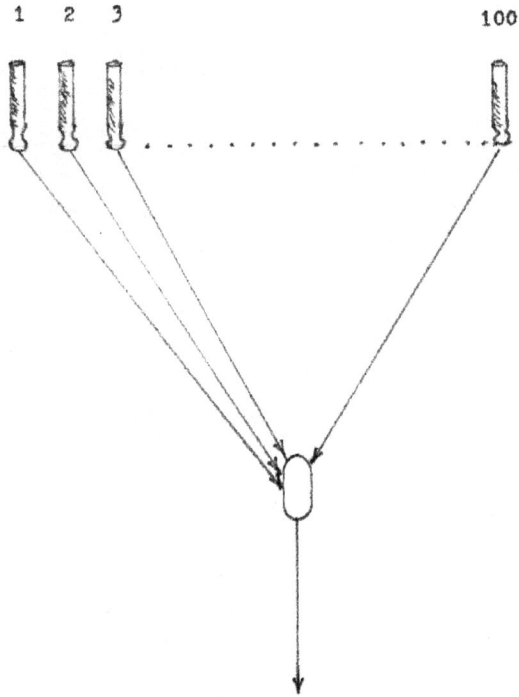

Figure 36

and different, visual images will never come out of the coder as
the same electrical statement. Exclusivity is achieved by a
scattering of techniques.

167

RECURSING MULTIPLEXER

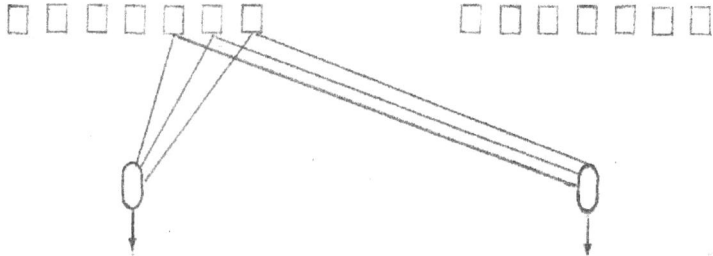

REDUNDANT SCHEME

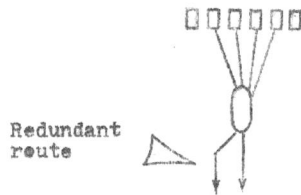

Redundant
route

FIG 35

Figure 37

163

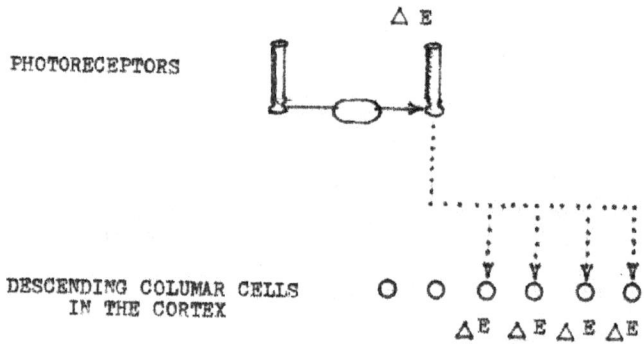

Figure 38

The simple circuit in Fig. 39 has a certain amount of

exclusiveness. The upper drawing has a 15 unit signal in the plus

channel and a minus 10 from the inverter. The subtotal is 5. It is true, another visual image could come along and produce this same subtotal at this site, (middle sketch). It is another visual image, however, and should have different signal values at most of the remaining photoreceptors in the retina. In any case, the span wise minus signal and the lateral positive signal will be different for different images, so it would take more than a few common subtotals to destroy the coder exclusiveness. I do not think is possible, but the coder would be ambiguous if the light signals falling on two receptors could be interchanged and still end up with the same subtotal (bottom sketch in Fig. 39).

There are a couple of ways the circuit in Fig. 39 can be made more exclusive:

1. If the receptor parameters follow some sort of curve, the minus contribution will be uniquely proportioned with respect to signal amplitude. This may not enforce exclusivity, but it does provide new dimensions to the ways the system can be exclusive.

2. The circuit layout will make a big difference with regard to exclusiveness. In Fig. 40, the minus signal from the receptor on the left will pass through and be entered in the arithmetic in four additional channels. The route on the right is the same as previous sketches (dotted channel). The receptor will report via its own positive channel with its unique arithmetic (middle channel). This same signal will make a specific positive entry in one or more positive totals, some going directly to the optic

170

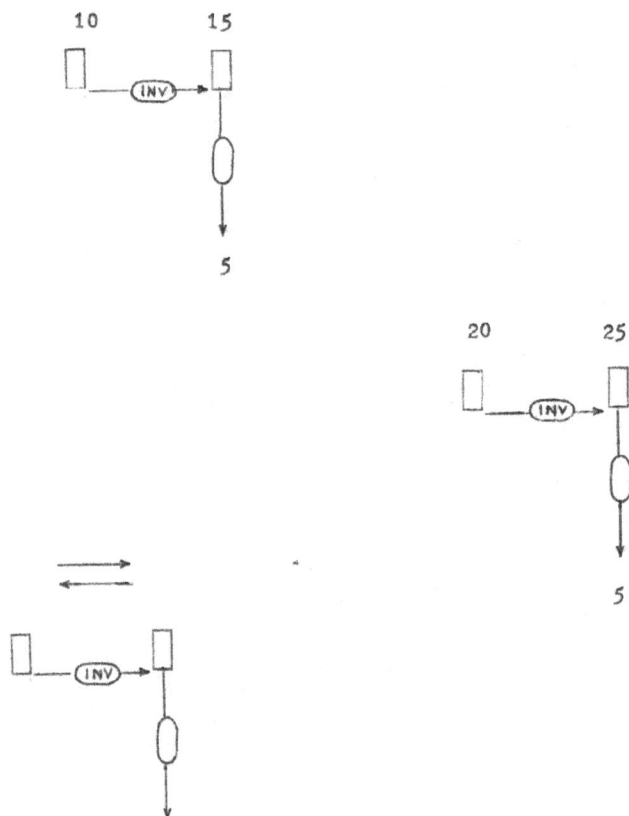

Fig 37

Figure 39

172

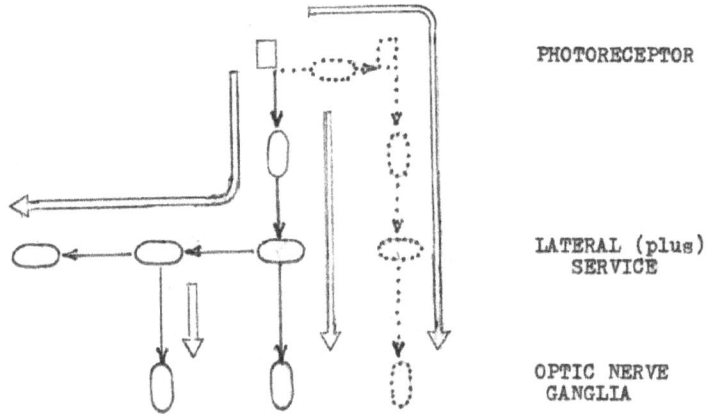

PHOTORECEPTOR

LATERAL (plus)
SERVICE

OPTIC NERVE
GANGLIA

Figure 40

nerve and some added to the lateral spread of the lateral "plus"

reference signal (just left of the middle channel). At greater

distances away from a given receptor, the lateral (plus) signal

becomes more of a referencing signal and counterpoises the span

167

wise ASC minus signal. A given receptor will contribute to both the lateral (plus) service and the span wise ASC minus.

It should not be possible to transpose the stimulus on two receptors, run the signal through all of these specially proportioned arithmetical summations, in four or more routings, and end up with the same totals at the same sites.

Not all of the artifacts and errors in the visual system are known. We have to allow for the possibility of an occasional practical failure of coder exclusivity as it processes a naturally occurring visual image. I doubt if much of this happens but it cannot be dogmatically ruled out.

Experimenters have tried experiments where the subject looked at a pattern of shaded bars. The image covered the retina and there were 100 graduations of shading in the pattern all of which the eye could resolve. At the moment, there is no elegant way to find out how many graduations of shading can be recognized by a single photoreceptor or by adjacent receptors. The contrast range of adjacent receptors would be pertinent here. Let us say the receptor is capable of responding to ten uniform increments in light stimulus. I would almost bet the system can do better than ten.

By virtue of the multiplexer convergence, the signals from 100 receptors, each of which can assume a value from zero to 10 units of amplitude, are to be impressed on a single optic nerve fiber. These small variations of signal amplitude can assume any combination so the optic nerve should be able to faithfully carry a signal that can be divided into 10 times 100, or 1000 small divisions. The experimenter tells us the receptor will respond if only a fraction of its area is illuminated. We will say it will respond if only half of its area is stimulated. We now have 2000 possible amplitudes.

This signal will be processed by a nerve cell and somewhere along the line the signal will be expressed as a membrane voltage. The useable signal excursion of the membrane is 50 millivolts. (A millivolt is 1/1000 volt) with 2000 amplitudes, the 50mv allowable excursion must be divisible into 2000 meaningful subdivisions, i.e. discrete amplitudes. In order to faithfully process this signal, the "resolution" of the cell must be one part in 2000. The resolution of the cell should exceed the bare requirements for processing the signal. A resolution of one part in 2500 would not be unreasonable. We will use the 1 part in 2500 estimate for openers, so to speak, because it is easy to defend. The actual resolution, if it is ever measured, may be somewhat higher. (One part in 4500 is probably in the ball park. Noise immunity problems come up if the estimate is made much higher.)

"Error" and "resolution" are not quite the same thing. Error refers to the ability of the system to process the signal without adding or subtracting anything extraneous to it, and the ability to do so repeatedly. In the case we have here, error should be less than 1 part in 2500 to preserve resolution. Error tends to accumulate as more stages are added. To produce error of less than 1 part in 2500 at the descending columnar stage, the upstream error would have to be much less that 1 part in 2500.

If the 50mv useable excursion is divided into 2500 meaningful divisions, each division will be 20 microvolts (a microvolt is one millionth of a volt). If the actual resolution turns out to be nearer 1 part in 5000, each division will be 10 microvolts. The very fine elements of image detail can be wiped out if a stray voltage became superimposed on the cell membrane. A 5 microvolt stray voltage would cancel useable information and a 10 microvolt unwanted signal would probably render the cell unusable.

Elsewhere I discuss the dire need for stray current, stray voltage and noise immunity measures in the nervous system. The tolerance a nerve cell has for stray voltages is on the order of one to several microvolts, ten at the most. My own view of the noise suppression measures are explained in the item on the nerve cell as the active element.

SUMMARY OF THE CODER/MULTIPLEXER

Fig. 41 is a sketch of a very badly managed experiment that has been a trifle misleading over the years. I mention it here because it appears in so many standard textbooks on the visual system.

Light is directed to a small area on the retina. This illuminated area can be thought of as the center of a bulls' eye. It is surrounded by an "inhibited" area, the first ring in the bulls' eye. A probe picks up the firing rate of the optic nerve fibers in this area and displays the firing rate on an oscilloscope.

THE MULTIPLEXER ASPECT OF THE CODER/MULTIPLEXER

When the light is on, the surrounding area is "inhibited" to the extent the nerve fails to fire at all. This refusal to fire is called a "refractory" interval. As far as I am concerned, excepting a half millisecond interval following the pulse, there are no legitimate "refractory" intervals in the normal operation of any nerve. The refractory interval we have here is attributable to over-stimulating the illuminated area. Over-illuminated, the surrounding area is "over-inhibited" by the outflow of the nearby minus signal and the affected retina ceases to function altogether.

This on-or-off, all-or-none, behavior of the retina was interpreted to be the basic nature of the retina and tended to argue against the system being an analogue system. (All-or-none systems are not analogue systems.)

We have here an experimenters error. It is said the photo receptor is capable of responding to a single photon of light.

177

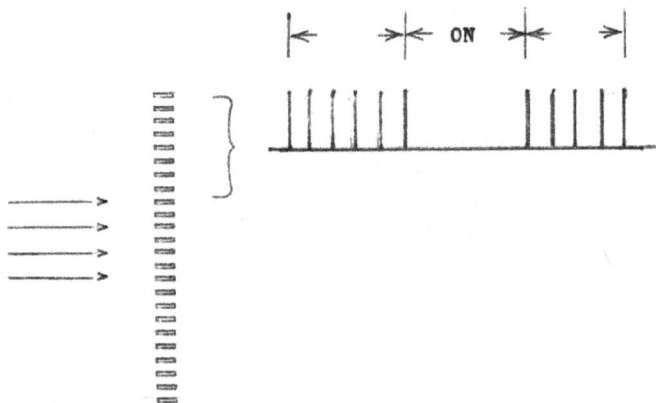

F16. 39

This extreme sensitivity (nay, incredible sensitivity) makes it

impossible to experiment with the mammalian retina. The light

source would have to be so weak, or using an attenuator, the attenuation so great that the noise in either the light source or the attenuator would be greater than the signal we are trying to measure.

The firing rate of a nerve is simply an analogue of the D.C. signal on the nerve. The experimenter should determine the linear operating range of the nerve first, and then set the constants for the experiment so they are well within the upper and lower limits of the nerve capability.

The mammalian retina should not be used in this sort of experiment. I have been working on this retinal theory for a number of years and do not think it is amenable to experiment. I did run across one experiment on the ommatidia of insects (the mosaic eye of insects). The experiment showed the D.C. arithmetic of the visual system to perfection, though it only demonstrated the E (minus) insertion and arithmetic. I have a hunch the E (plus) arithmetic is in there somewhere, perhaps closer to the bugs' brain than its eye, it just hasn't been located yet. The visual automatic sensitivity control program must be in the individual ommatidium, it would almost have to be for the experiment to work at all.

I see a certain amount of vindication for my coder theory in the D.C. arithmetic exposed by this experiment.

Fig. 42 brings home the consequences of multiplexing the spatial components of the visual image. In a practical seeing situation, data elements within the dotted circle on the left could be composited with elements from the circle on the right. This mixing of information can result from the coder process, or because the information is multiplexed, or it could happen in the lateral reorganization of the network. A lot would depend on the size of the image on the retina. Information from one subject matter: the shoe, has been scrambled with the information from another subject matter: the reclining letter. With the subject matter inseparably mixed this way, there is no way the cortex can have access to the subject matter. We will show the convergence through the coder as a bonus argument for the cortex not having access to the subject matter of its throughput.

The visual system does not interpret or classify the subject matter of the visual image. It can, and does, make phenomenal "separations" based on the phenomenology--not the subject matter-- of the visual image. It separately processes the following;

1. A luminance signal. This is the black and white high definition signal and conveys most of the specific data in the image. It is generated by the Rod cells in the retina.

2. There is a chrominance, or color, system subdivided into three systems, one for each color: red, green, and blue. (I am not sure how the chroma systems work. From experimenters reports and through intuition, I get the impression the color channels

180

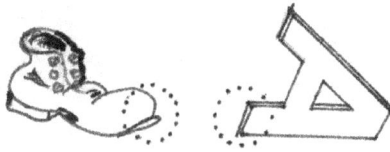

Fig 40

are "piggy back" systems, or as Ma Bell would say: "phantom circuits". Each color has a ph Figure 42 ensitive to the respective part of the spectrum and their outputs are arithmetically superimposed on the black and white signal.

175

I think these "phantom" signals are arithmetically extricated within the cortex. The anatomy of the visual lobe is strange. There is a clearly demarcated zone, a fatty insulator, that partly perfuse the lobe. The zone ends in a wedged shaped boundary and the rest of the lobe is normal. Only the visual lobe has a zone like this. I think this is the area where the color signal is extricated and the extra insulation is to electrically protect these extremely cross-talk sensitive "phantom" circuits.

3. There is a rate-of-change coder which codes movement in the visual image. This is an internal cortical efferent system and is discussed in a later item.

4. The cortical computer has a control system. The cingulate lobe controls the specific data cortex. It writes a control statement at the same time the visual system is writing the visual statement.

We now have all of the ways the image can be taken apart on a phenomenal basis. These phenomenal statements, or "separations", specify everything that needs to be specified in order to replicate the image on recall.

(As the cortex evolved, the color systems seem to be an add-on to the extant black and white system which had evolved much earlier. It would be a major histogenic disruption of the already established optic tract to introduce three additional optic tracts, one for each color. It would entail the physical insertion of three sets of dedicated nerves, each fiber surrounded by the several extant black and white fibers. Dedication would have to be preserved at both retina and cortex. The arithmetically superimposed "phantom" scheme is the only way color vision could

have evolved.)

COCHLEAR THEORY

The sound transducer translates sound vibrations in the air, in this case, the fluids of the inner ear into an electrical analogue of the sound. The sensor array in the hearing system is in a tapered spiraling tunnel in the petrous temporal bone. (Petrous, from Peter and the rock, the temporal bone is the hardest in the body, occasionally compared to marble.) A wax impression of the spiraling galleries in the tunnel resembles a snail (cochlea, snail). The micro-architecture of the cochlear system is both fascinating and complex. The hearing system has been a refractory area of study. The system has been studied by three generations of theorists and there is still no satisfactory account of the electromechanical translation that transpires at the organ of Corti (O.H.C and I.H.C. in Fig. 43, I.H.C. refers to the inner row of hair cells, O.H.C. to the outer.) The sound signal is impressed on the basilar membrane (B.M. of Fig. 43). The direction of motion is mechanically shifted 90 degrees and the movement is communicated to the hair cells in the organ of Corti. The organ of Corti writes a coded statement, an electrical replica of the physical sound disturbances of the sound image and puts it on board the acoustic nerve. Three cochlear theories have received the most attention. One theory treats the detector system as an assembly of resonant devices, something like an array of tuning forks. Another theory sees the cochlear membrane as a resonant line. A third theory is called the "volley" theory. The volley theory says a given

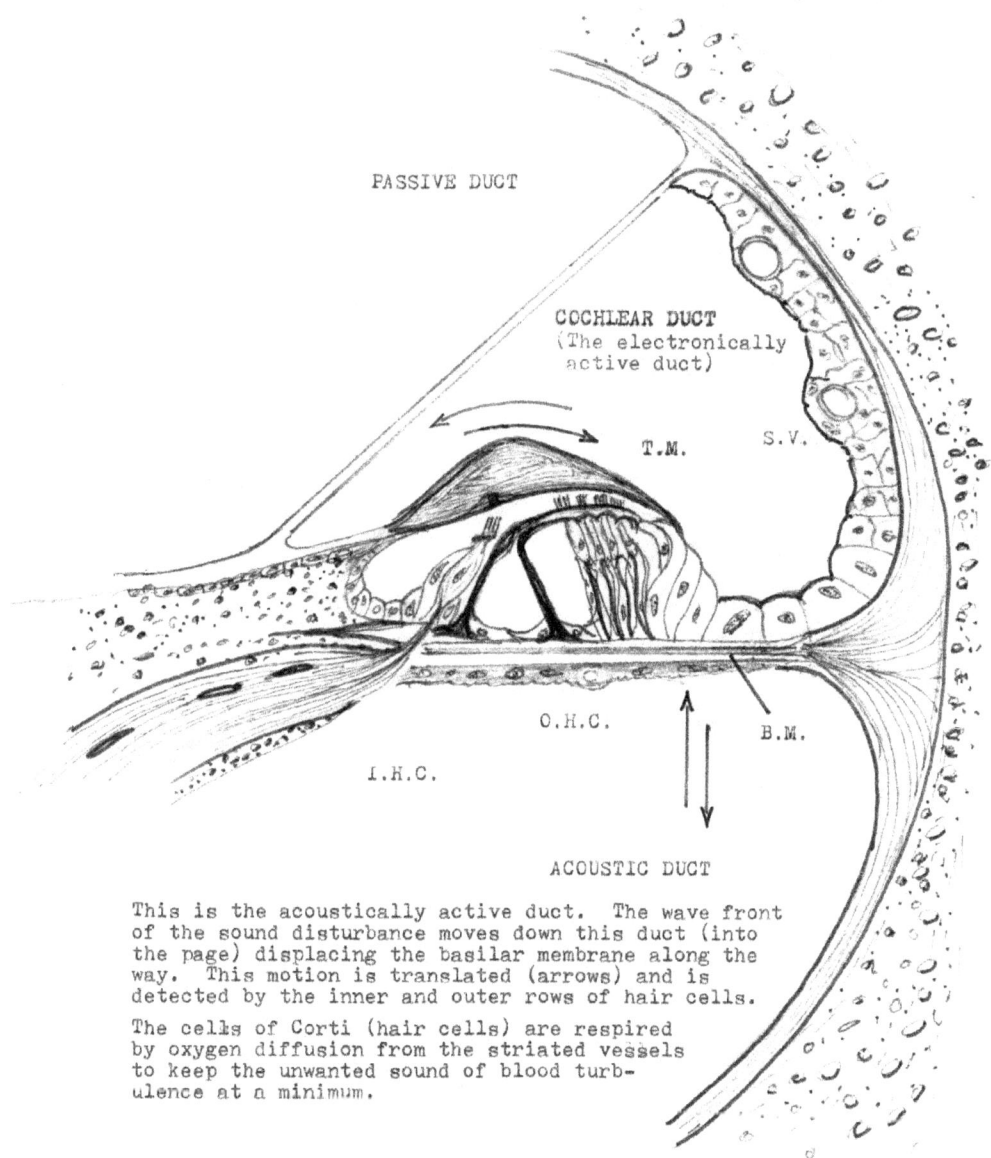

184

PASSIVE DUCT

COCHLEAR DUCT
(The electronically
active duct)

T.M.

S.V.

O.H.C.

B.M.

I.H.C.

ACOUSTIC DUCT

This is the acoustically active duct. The wave front
of the sound disturbance moves down this duct (into
the page) displacing the basilar membrane along the
way. This motion is translated (arrows) and is
detected by the inner and outer rows of hair cells.

The cells of Corti (hair cells) are respired
by oxygen diffusion from the striated vessels
to keep the unwanted sound of blood turbulence at a minimum.

Fig. 41

sound disturbance will produce a unique volley of firings in the

acoustic nerve--a point of view I roundly agree with; however, it

does not set out the de Figure 43 vay the coded statement is

written. We still need to explain how it is done.

I believe my circuit for the retinal coder multiplexer is essentially correct. Since I see no reason for the cochlear coder/multiplexer to be different than the one in the retina, I will take a shot at a cochlear theory. I don't think I can harm anything by doing so.

I enjoy studying this remarkable apparatus. Fig. 43 is a cross-section of the sound sensitive cochlear duct. The sound disturbance is impressed on the fluids in the lower duct and propagated down the tunnel, flowing into the page. The sound disturbance is a mechanical disturbance, perhaps "vibration" would be better, and it displaces the basilar membrane transmitting the disturbance to the hair cells in the organ of Corti. The motion is applied to the base of the hair cell. The upper end of the hair cell is denied movement by the tectoral membrane (tectum, roof, T.M. in the sketch). This is a fibrous membrane, but its consistency is almost a gel.

The hair cell is not rigidly affixed to the tectoral membrane; it is held in a firm, tight fit. The tectum is well developed in humans. In lesser developed hearing systems, amphibia for example, the inertia of the cochlear fluids in conjunction with elaborations of the upper end of the hair cell, constitute the upper anchorage of the hair cell.

The arrows show the relative movement between the base of the hair cell and the tectum. The hair cell is bent very slightly in the process.

The hair cell is an incredibly sensitive device and it is said to be able to generate an output when the distance it is flexed can be

measured in molecule diameters. (It has to be sensitive: the
attenuation of the system, measured from eardrum to hair cell is -
135db. If the eardrum is listening to the exhaust noise in a
missile silo at launch, the deflection of the hair cell would be
barely detectable under a microscope. Theorists do not believe
piezo-electric effect, as it is usually known, generates the output
of the hair cell.)

The two rows of hair cells are interesting. Perhaps the inner
row samples the total stimulus on the basilar membrane, averages
it, and computes an automatic sensitivity control signal based on
the average. The ASC signal would be expressed as a motor
instruction to a muscle called the "tensor tympani". The tensor
tympani is a muscle that controls the efficiency, hence the
attenuation, of the bony linkage between the eardrum and the window
to the inner ear. The mechanical attenuator is a part of the
automatic sensitivity control for the hearing system. (It could be
called the "automatic volume control", or AVC, I will use
"automatic sensitivity control" through the text.)

The upper and lower ducts are part of the lymphatic system and
the fluid they contain in about the same as cerebral/spinal fluid.
The fluid in the cochlear duct is a more exotic serum. It is
protein rich and the protein will condense into fibers under
certain conditions, perhaps aiding the maintenance of fluid
pressure in the duct.

The fluid in the cochlear duct is also electronically active. A
voltage generated by the hair cells is impressed on the fluid. The
voltage has several components and its crest value is superimposed

on its average value. The average value is a sample of sound intensity. The voltage is called the "cochlear microphonic" and it controls the sensitivity of the organ of Corti. This is the fast acting ASC system for the cochlea and the sensitivity of the hair cell is reduced in proportion to the average sound signal amplitude: the louder the sound, the less the sensitivity. This voltage is the cochlear equivalent of the retinal "span wise automation", it is also a reference signal in the coder arithmetic and its sense is "minus".

Most of the tissue cells of the body are never more than two cell diameters distant from capillary blood service. Oxygen support for the hair cell is provided by the striated blood vessels (S.V.) on the opposite wall of the cochlear duct. This arrangement immunizes the hair cell from the noisy turbulence of blood flowing in the capillaries. The hair cell depends on oxygen dissolved in the cochlear fluid for its only source. Oxygen concentration is so low in the vicinity of the hair cell it is remarkable it survives.

(Conspicuously, metabolites and oxygen must be available for the cell to survive. Metabolic pacing, per se, is also critically important. A precise metabolic rate is established to insure the vitality of the cell, for most tissue cells, this is the only rate needed. In excitable cells there is a precise increment in the metabolic rate, slightly over and above the cell vitality requirement, to supply energy for the extra work of signal processing. Some nerve cells depend on the signal to pace the metabolic rate and a few are so dependent they will die if there is a malfunction in an upstream cell, if it depends on the upstream cell for its excitation.

(Receptors are somewhat different and seem to possess a "keep-alive" metabolic rate which preserves vitality when the visual or sound stimulus is not present. There was a short paragraph in the February, 1977 issue of Skin Diver magazine about physicians at Nagoya Medical Center in Japan who used hyperbaric oxygen therapy to start hearing in patients who were born deaf. The patients breathed oxygen in a decompression chamber at a pressure of two atmospheres. Hearing was started in 33 of 39 attempts. I think something like this may be happening: the hair cell was in a state of metabolic repose, and the residual pacing was just adequate to preserve the vitality of the sensor. For unknown reasons, the incremental up-pacing required to initiate signal conduction failed to take place. The sensor, in all ways capable of functioning, began to function when assisted with a little extra oxygen, the metabolic rate became greater than the repose rate.)

The experts are not clear about the mechanics of the acoustic path within the hearing system. We will do the best we can with the acoustic path, it is not a critical matter in so far as the coder is concerned.

A sound is a vibrating disturbance of the air surrounding the sound source and it spreads out from the source like waves from a pebble in a pond. The air is alternately compressed and expanded with each vibration. The leading edge of the wave is the compression part of the cycle, followed by a half cycle of reduced pressure called rarefaction. The excursion of the eardrum, moving inward on compression, is communicated by a linkage of tiny bones to a membranous window, called the oval window, and is then impressed on the fluids of the inner ear.

The first bone in the linkage is the malleus (or hammer) and it moves with the eardrum and passes the motion on to the next bone in the linkage, the incus (or anvil). The contact between the two bones in by means of fretting surfaces: a "clutch", so to speak with warped but mating faces. The surfaces are inclined, a little "S" shaped and the curvatures are in addendal/dedendal opposition. The contraction of the tensor tympani modifies the relationship between the two bones (Fig. 44). The bony linkage is an impedance matching device and it matches the long-excursion/low-force movement of the eardrum to the short-excursion/high force movement of the oval window. The transformation ratio (or "mechanical advantage") is variable and controlled by the tensor tympani. The tensor Tympani is the slow acting element in the ASC (automatic sensitivity control) program for the hearing system. In Fig. 44, movement of the eardrum right is transmitted by boney levers to the stapes (stirrup) left. The bone is shaped like a stirrup and its oval footplate mates with the oval window which introduces the sound signal into the chambers of the inner ear. Mechanical advantage through the levers provides a signal gain of about 20db and almost compensates for the linkage loss (-24db).

Contraction of the tensor tympani applies both a mechanical bias (a residual inward force) and a pre-travel to the oval window. If not compensated for, the bias shifts the characteristics of the oval window and the pre-travel limits

190

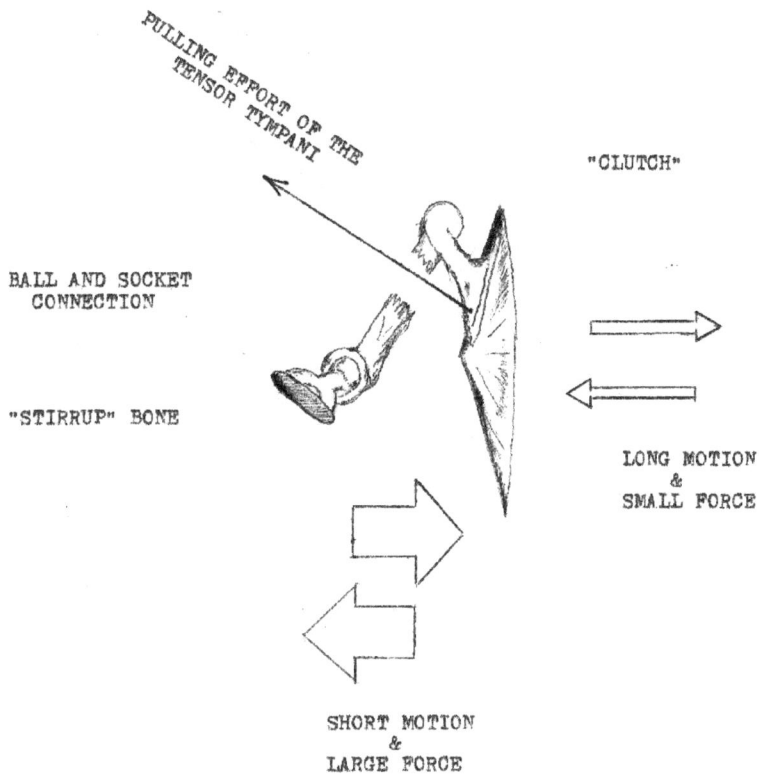

PULLING EFFORT OF THE
TENSOR TYMPANI

"CLUTCH"

BALL AND SOCKET
CONNECTION

"STIRRUP" BONE

LONG MOTION
&
SMALL FORCE

SHORT MOTION
&
LARGE FORCE

Fig42

Figure 44

the signal excursion range of   low. It also leaves

residual fluid pressure in the inner vestibules.

Fig. 45 is far from being anatomically accurate but it does

sketch, schematically, the action of a muscle called the

192

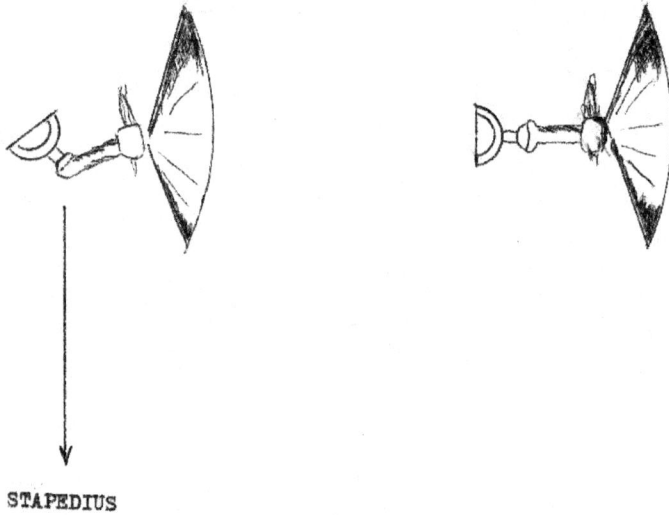

STAPEDIUS

Fig 43

"stapedius". Pulling is through a tendon and a sort of pulley; the

muscles proper is well away from the linkage. Both the pre-travel

and the mechanical bias of the tensor tympani is removed by

buckling the linkage with the pulling effort of the stapedius.
Tensing together, the tensor tympani and the stapedius muscles
cooperate with each other when the tensor tympani contracts in its
ASC function, the stapedius removes the resulting mechanical bias
and pre-travel. Pulling at a right angle to the acoustic path
avoids introducing the elasticity and the losses of the pulling
mechanism into the acoustic circuit.

A passerby, with a glance at the middle and inner ear, might
think inspection alone would tell us all we needed to know about
the acoustic path. This is not quite the way it is. Analyzing the
acoustic path through the boney linkage and the inner fluid routes
has been a study that has unraveled some of the best minds in the
business. The acoustic path is full of pitfalls.

To us, one of the pitfalls is the "clutch" at the junction of the
malleus and the incus. Apart from being controlled by the tensor
tympani, it may have additional special characteristics. On the
compression part of the cycle, and on inward movement of the
malleus, there is probably a hard, positive drive to the rest of
the linkage. On the rarefaction part of the cycle, accompanied by
relaxation of the linkage, I question whether the system is under
hard drive with outward movement of the malleus.

It is not essential for the fretting surfaces of the clutch to
physically bounce apart while transmitting the motion of the
malleus in order to have a difference of "hardness" of drive. If
there is a difference in the "hardness" of drive between the inward
motion and outward motion, the system becomes non-linear and there

is a possibility the junction between the malleus and incus may be acting as an acoustic rectifier.

Electrical rectifiers are a settled art. I have never seen anything written on acoustic rectifiers. I can only guess at the way an acoustic rectifier might work.

The upper half of Fig. 46 is the familiar electrical rectifier (small circuit) and its output wave form. It passes the signal on the positive half-cycle of the signal excursion and is nonconductive when the voltage reverses.

It would seem an acoustic rectifier, with "hard" drive in one direction and "soft" drive in the opposite direction, would conduct the signal on the positively directed segments of the wave form. In the absence of better knowledge, I will show it this way. The figure of merit for a rectifier is the "front-to-back" ratio. It is desirable to have forward resistance quite low and blocked conduction in the reverse direction if possible. Acoustic rectification in the linkage may have a small front-to-back ratio, it is a rectifier, nevertheless, and the front-to-back ratio can be improved by adding rectifiers in series. There may be other types of acoustic rectifiers in series with the acoustic path within

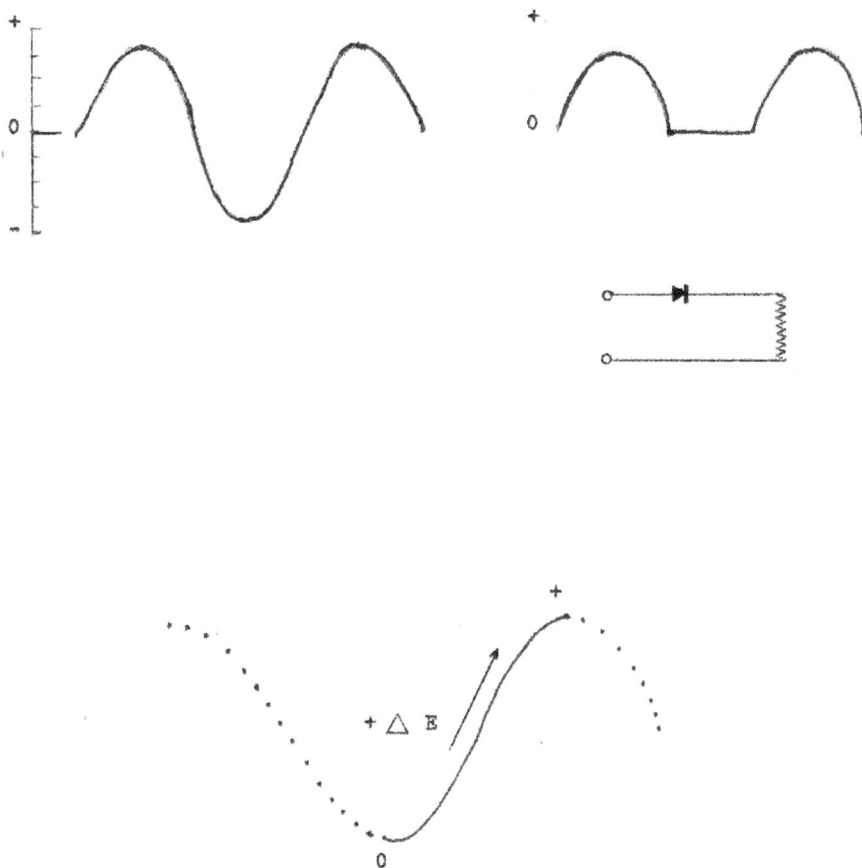

Figure 46

the inner systems. Any cochlear theory should tell us whether the

signal is rectified or not.

Two cochlear theories have failed. One theory regarded the organ

of Corti as a series of resonant devices with each device

responding to a particular frequency if it was present in the sound. This was to be a battery of mechanically resonant devices, somewhat like an array of tuning forks. When the appropriate frequency was present in the input, the device would resonate and the frequency would be selectively translated (or transduced) and a coded notation that the frequency was present was to be fed to the acoustic nerve.

The characteristic of merit for a resonant device is its "Q" factor and the higher the "Q", the more selective the device is at its resonant frequency. "Q" is the "flywheel effect" of a resonant circuit. (It is also the ratio of circulating energy in the device to the energy that excites it.) The "Q" of a tuning fork, a high "Q" device is about 600. The "Q" if the heavily damped organ of Corti is about 4. There are other problems with this theory and the flywheel effect is one of them. Once the resonant circuit has responded, it cannot be quickly damped and the resonance trails off in ever diminishing oscillations even after the original stimulus has been long quieted. There is a third major shortcoming of the resonant element theory. The rigidly selective resonant devices prohibit the interpolation of frequencies. There might be a provision for 400cps and another for 410cps, but the system is blind to, say, 403.2cps. Human hearing seems to have nearly unlimited interpolative capability. The resonant "site", or resonant device, theory has pretty much run its course and should drop out of circulation if it has not done so already.

At one time there was a resonant "line" theory which is a cousin to the resonant "device" theory. It will not work either.

According to this theory, the sound disturbance propagates down the basilar membrane until it reaches a point where the physical length of the excited segment will resonate with, or otherwise register, a particular frequency in the sound signal.

The physical dimensions of the basilar membrane argue against the "resonant line" theory or any other theory having a relationship between the length of the membrane and the frequency to be coded. The cochlea is so small it could be rested on a dime with room to spare. The uncoiled membrane is about an inch long and too short to span the smallest fraction of a wavelength at the sound frequencies it codes. To say it might be functioning on higher order harmonics, and it would be the tenth harmonic and higher, accomplishes nothing; the fundamental, the second and third are the important harmonics.

This theory has a lot of problems. The line (i.e. the basilar membrane) is restrained along its borders and consequently heavily damped. A resonant line should also be a high "Q" apparatus and here we have a damped, low "Q" device with no selectivity. The apical end of the basilar membrane is terminated in a special terminator section (right terminus of the membrane in Fig. 48). The terminator section terminates the membrane in its characteristic impedance which prevents standing waves and eliminates the prospect of using the reflected component of the wave.

The time has come to abandon the idea the hearing mechanism will extricate and selectively code each frequency in the sound image. The cochlea mechanism is not a frequency selective device; the "Q" is too low; the dimensions too small; and the problem of interpolating frequencies rules it out.

The osseous spiral labyrinth would look like Fig. 47 if someone excavated it from the temporal bone and sculpted the external surfaces in the sketch. The transition section between the vestibule and the spiral is slightly elongated and exaggerated to show the action of the round window.

The stirrup shaped stapes bone introduces the sound signal to the cochlear vestibule via the oval window. The fluids cannot be compressed and the bone will not yield, so the pressure excursion of the inward excursion of the inward movement of the oval window is relieved by the membranous round window. The round window is more or less in the "floor" of the vestibule, perhaps a little closer to the side than the drawing suggests. The vestibule tapers to meet the spiral ducts and the round window is at the place where the

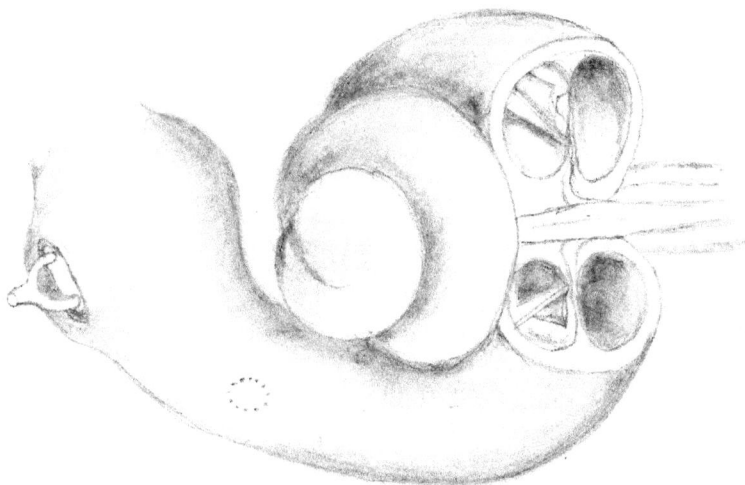

Figure 47

vestibule and the lower duct join. I call this adapter section:

the "nozzle". The nozzle is cle   r drawing.

The early theories had the cochlear system as a frequency

analyzer. Had this worked out, a second set of theories would be needed to account for it as an amplitude analyzer; and, perhaps, a third set of theories to explain how both the frequency and amplitude components were picked off the same sensitive membrane, sent down the same acoustic nerve together, yet maintained and processed separately at their destination.

According to my plan, the sound frequency and amplitude components are processed in a composited format. This format is reminiscent of the retinal coder and the way it codes the spatial and intensity components of the visual image in a mixed format. If we transplant the visual coder, making it the coder for the hearing system, the amplitude and frequency components of the sound signal will be composited at the coder when the coded statement is written. They cannot be separated later.

There are no internal sound amplitude or frequency standards, no filters or tuned devices, to confirm the presence of absence of a given frequency in the sound information presented to the cochlea. At an instant of inspection, there is both a scattering of frequencies and a scattering of amplitudes present in the sound image.

Each sound has a distinctive wave shape. One wave shape differs from another in the presence or absence and the relative amplitudes of its harmonic content. (The "fundamental" is the frequency we are listening to. The second, the third, the fourth "harmonics" are twice, three times, four times, and so on, the frequency of the fundamental.)

The wave shape in Fig. 46 before it is passed through the rectifier, is a "sine" wave, and it is the only known wave form that has no harmonic content. Since there is no devices in the inner ear that act as frequency standards, a given sound can only be registered in a framework of its own harmonics or other sounds present at the same time. Harmonics become all important in the case of the sine wave because, having no naturally occurring harmonics, it would be impossible, in principle, for the ear to hear and recognize a sine wave. The ear hears the sine wave as well as it does any other sound and it makes up for the lack of harmonics by distorting the signal. The cochlear system needs assured harmonics. Audio distortion is a magnificent generator of harmonics where none had heretofore existed and there is nothing quite like a rectifier for generating harmonics and distortion. This is the reason I raised the question about the incus and malleus being an acoustic rectifier. I think there are acoustic rectifiers elsewhere in the system.

(Sound distortion is not only permissible but desirable in the coding process. If a naturally occurring sound image tended to be spare of interesting and distinguishable features, distortion will scatter it all over the spectrum and give it degrees of uniqueness and recognizeability it could not possibly command in its original form.)

Sounds are meaningful with respect to other sounds. The ear tends to be ambiguous for monotones. A monotone is a single isolated frequency and presented monotones, hearing tends to confuse amplitude with frequency. This is one of a number of artifacts in the hearing process.

Another interesting hearing artifact has been incorporated in the design of the Pipe organ. The organ may have a stop marked "32 ft stop", but with no 32 ft pipe in the pipe loft. If I understand correctly, the stop couples the second harmonic, a 16 ft pipe and an octave higher, with a fifth above the octave and both are expressed together. The ear hears the 32 ft fundamental even though the sound is not physically present.)

The acoustic path within the cochlea is, and has been, a persistent pitfall. I will show an acoustic path that makes sense to me, though it may not agree with some that have been suggested. The spiral galleries have been uncoiled and the basilar membrane shown in plan view in Fig. 48. The hole in the membrane is the helicotrema. There is no anatomical barrier between the upper and lower ducts at either end of the cochlea. The helicotrema affords free communication

200

VESTIBULE

ELECTRONICALLY
ACTIVE DUCT

PASSIVE DUCT

ACOUSTIC DUCT

OVAL WINDOW

NOZZLE
SECTION

BASILAR MEMBRANE

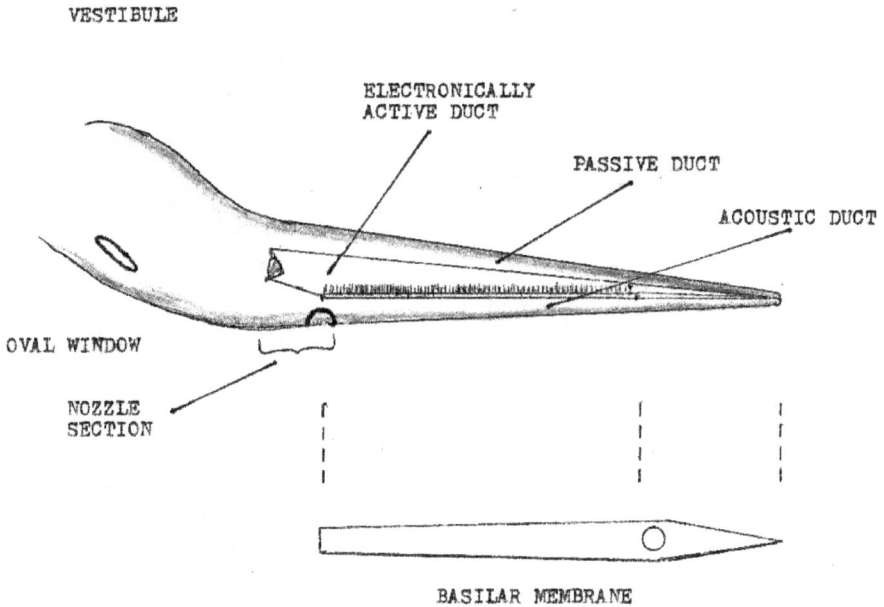

Called the helicotrema, the opening
in the membrane relieves pressure
differences between the passive and
acoustic dicts.

PRESSURE RELIEF WINDOW
Round window at the end
of the nozzle section.

FIG 46

between the ducts at the apical end and prevents pressure

differences between the ducts. If ; Figure 48   ue a pressure

difference, it would be attributable to the inertia of the fluids

and not absolute pressures. The apical end of the basilar membrane is on the right and the tapered section to the right of the helicotrema is the tapered terminator section which terminates the membrane in its characteristic impedance.

(The turbinate of the cochlea has three turns: basal, middle and apical. The third turn is not quite complete. The length of the duct varies so the turns vary from 2 1/2 to 2 3/4. The anatomist occasionally finds the apical turn or parts of the apical membrane missing, yet with no known ante mortem hearing impairment. Cochlear theories that critically depend on a membrane of precise length and damping may be embarrassed by findings such as this.)

There are two kinds of acoustic transducers. There are those that are pressure energy operated and another kind that responds to the kinetic energy of the sound stimulus. Analyzing the acoustic process within the cochlea is a job for the fluid dynamics expert. I may be doing this wrong, but will proceed with the idea. The pressure excursion from the oval window is translated to a kinetic disturbance and a wave front is erected and launched down the acoustic duct. In the upper drawing of Fig. 49 is a hypothetical kinetic energy version of the inner sound path. In the bottom drawing, the pressure disturbance from the inward movement of

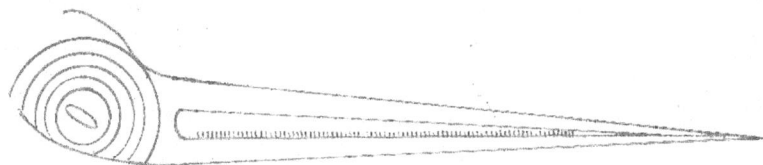

KINETIC ENERGY VERSION

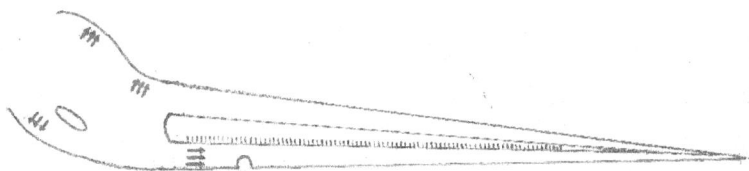

PRESSURE ENERGY VERSION

Figure 49

the oval window is uniformly and instantaneously (2 micro-seconds)

applied throughout the chamber. There is only one physical

location in the acoustic path where the pressure excursion could do

useful work and it is at the cross-section of the nozzle, just upstream of the relief window. Fig. 50 shows how the pressure wave is translated to a kinetic wave which is launched down the lower duct. The wave front propagates from the input end of the duct to its apex. The cochlear spiral is straightened out in Fig. 50 and the sensitive membrane is the "ceiling" of the lower duct. As the wave front passes, the sensitive membrane is displaced and the movement is transmitted to the sound sensitive hair cells. Energy is removed from the wave front by ablation as it moves down the duct until there is nothing left of it by the time it reaches the apical end of the duct.

I see the following virtues in the pressure wave to kinetic wave translation,

1. I do not think the acoustic sound, as it is introduced into the vestibule, is sufficiently energetic to stimulate the full length of the membrane, considering internal reflections and the generally inefficient look of the thing.

2. By translating the pressure wave to a kinetic wave, only the compression phase of the sound wave is used and the signal sent into the duct is unidirectional. We now have at least one more acoustic rectifier in series with the acoustic path, active only on the positively directed part of the signal excursion.

I doubt if there is, or that there could be, a backward moving wave, or echo, moving up the tunnel, apex to

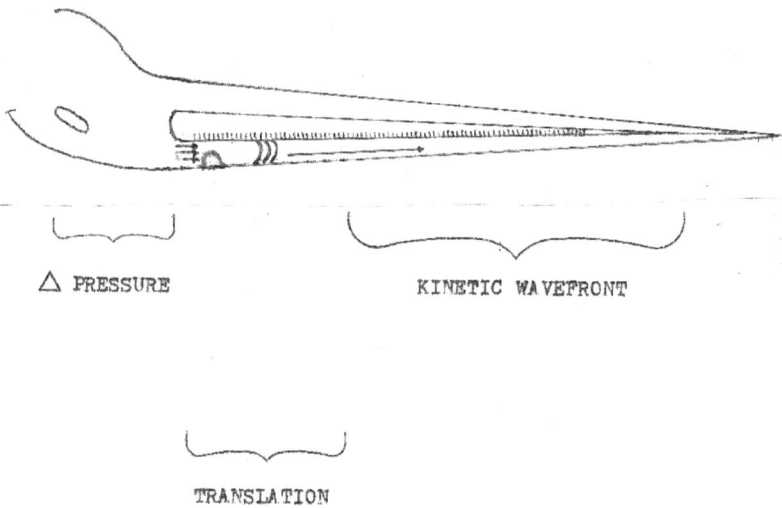

△ PRESSURE   KINETIC WAVEFRONT

TRANSLATION

Figure 50

vestibule. The cochlear tunnel probably has an exponential taper,

or nearly so, and an exponentially tapered acoustic column cancels

both standing and reflected waves. There is very little of the

right kind of apparatus to generate a signal capable of moving backward (apex to base) up the membrane. The removal of the backward moving wave is not strictly a third signal rectification, but it does improve the front to back ratio of the rectifiers we do have.

Fig. 51 is the archetype of the rectified sound signal envelope. The sound signal envelope is normally rich in ever changing detail. To make up for the lack of detail in Fig. 51; I have added a couple of marker blips to the signal envelope in Fig. 52. Whatever the acoustic path may have entailed, the waveform is put on board the sensitive membrane at its vestibular end. This is a traveling wave and the detailed waveform information in the sound signal envelope is translated into detailed local deformations of the sensitive membrane. The coder translates the detailed deformations of the membrane so they are replicated in the coded statement for the hearing system. The statement of this envelope detail is written "en passant", that is, while the waveform is still in motion down the membrane.

These displacements of the heavily damped membrane are too small to be seen with the microscope at normal and reasonable audio levels. The impression the signal envelope must be making on the membrane eludes imagining. A precise understanding of the physics and acoustic response in not urgently needed. All we need is certainty there is a unique relationship between the sound heard by the eardrum and the

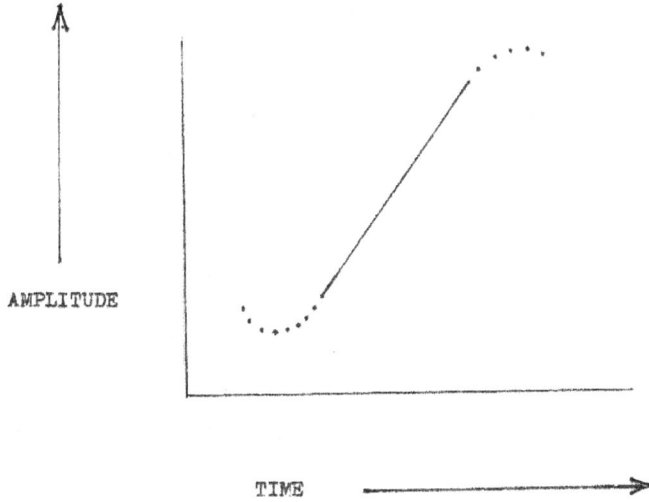

Figure 51

behavior of the membrane. I can think of no reason why this would

not be the probable case.

Without internal frequency standards in the system, sound

frequency, as such, cannot be coded. The signal envelope with

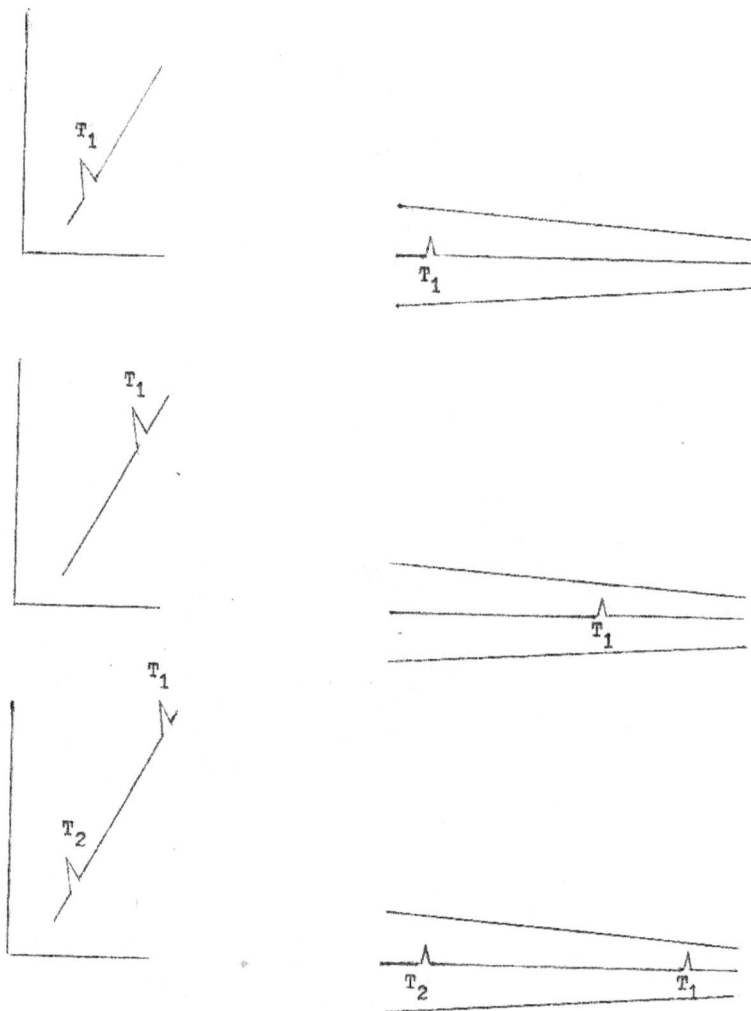

Fig 50

Figure 52

its ever changing rise rates, w ⎯ ⎯ 'sign" for the sound

signal without a complex analysis of the sound frequencies.

Overall, the coder does not code sound, it codes the behavior of the basilar membrane under sound stimulus. On the basis of the rise rate information impressed on the membrane, there is no way for the coder to determine if a sound event is producing a change in the amplitude or the frequency of the sound signal.

The chart in Fig. 53 shows a change in envelope rise rate can be caused by either a change in amplitude or frequency of the sound. Though an absolute analysis of the leading edge of the sound signal could be ambiguous, if we are assured the membrane will respond uniquely to a given sound, we have all of the information we need to write the coded statement.

(Be it an amplitude change or a frequency shift, the two are coded in a composited format. We will show the cochlear coder as a "clincher" argument which argues against the auditory cortex having access to the subject matter of the sound image. If the cortex is to have access to the subject matter, the frequency component and the amplitude component have to be available in separated formats. The cortex would have to be told a certain frequency was present in the sound image and (separately) this frequency was being expressed at this: particular and precise, amplitude. The membrane is an instantaneous translator and, using nothing more than the apparatus in the cochlea, it is not physically possible to

212

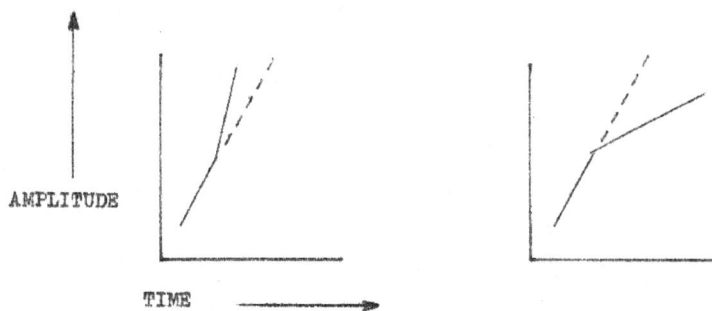

AMPLITUDE

TIME ⟶

ABRUPT INCREASE
IN RISE RATE

ABRUPT DECREASE
IN RISE RATE

1. There has been a change in the absolute amplitude of the signal to a higher amplitude	There has been a decrement in the absolute amplitude of the signal.
2. There has been a shift in a fundamental frequency to a higher frequency.	There has been a frequency shift to a lower frequency.
3. There has been a change in harmonic content, adding even harmonics, or there has been a shift in internal phase relationships toward leading phase.	There has been a change in harmonic content, adding odd harmonics, or there has internal phase shfts to a lagging phase.

Figure 53

separate the amplitude and frequency components in the sound.)

All of this does require a unique relationship between the sound

and the behavior of the membrane. Tapering the membrane will give

206

each millimeter of membrane a different set of responses so a given millimeter will respond to a given rise rate in one way and assure us the response will not be the same in the next millimeter.

Experimenters report the signal undergoes extreme phase shifting as it travels down the membrane--720 degrees toward leading phase. Phase shifting and other wise scattering the wave shape detail of the length of the membrane generates degrees of uniqueness and resolution the wave shape did not originally possess.

Anatomists do not always count the same number of hair cells in the organ of Corti. There are 6000 in the inner row-which I believe to be the sensors for the ASC system. The outer row is the coder and there are about 7000 (a low estimate) in it. Projecting the sound signal against the characteristics of the membrane provides an artificial, but helpful, exaggeration of the detail in the sound image. In addition to highlighting the detail in the signal, the coder is taking 17,000 samplings of the wave shape. The hair cell is an analogue translator and output of the hair cell is an analogue "vernier", further resolving the 17,000 sampled in more finely detailed elements of resolution. All of this makes the traveling wave more legible and adds to the number of significant elements of detail in the auditory statement. Though the hearing system is susceptible to a few acoustic illusions and confusions, it is fair to say both the "uniqueness" and the "exclusiveness" of the coder output are safe.

The basic coder/multiplexer is explained in the item on the coder/multiplexer. Allowing for a few special adaptations, the basic coder is probably incorporated in all of the perceptual systems. The cochlear coder, Fig. 54. resembles the retinal coder. The rectangles with the hairs sticking out of them in Fig. 54 are the sound sensors in the organ of Corti. The signal output of the hair cell is an analogue of the bending force on the hair cell. The sensor on the far left is in minus service as seen by the nearest positive cell. It is in positive service when it reports to its own acoustic nerve. The coder arithmetic is the same as it is in the retinal coder. Merely that the stimulus is moving along the coder array changes nothing with regard to the coder arithmetic: the retinal coder accepts a moving stimulus for that matter. The two coder techniques should be much the same.

When the flow of information is toward the cortex, it is "afferent" information. Information outbound from the cortex is "efferent" information, an instruction that "effects" a change of some kind, usually an instruction to muscles. There are efferent nerves in the acoustic tract.

The cells in the organ of Corti are arranged in a mosaic resembling paving tiles. The outer surface of the cell, the

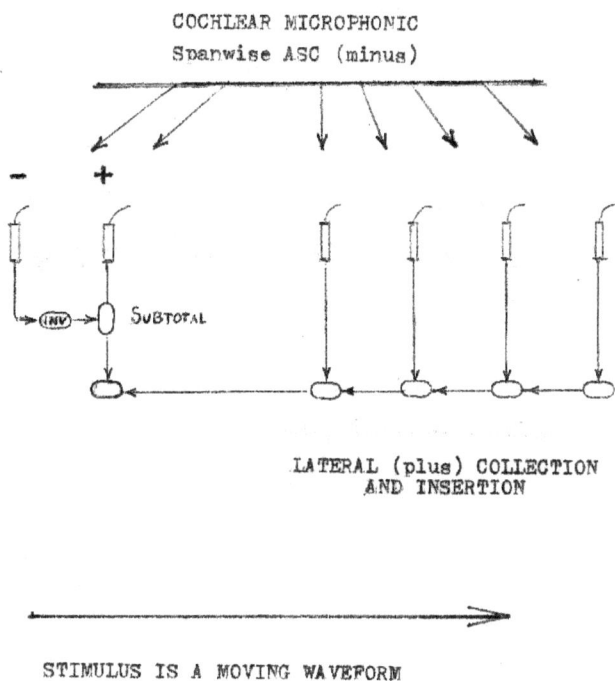

214

COCHLEAR MICROPHONIC
Spanwise ASC (minus)

− +

(INV) SUBTOTAL

LATERAL (plus) COLLECTION
AND INSERTION

STIMULUS IS A MOVING WAVEFORM

Figure 54

"tile", is a hard substance resembling insect hide. The sound

sensitive cell has a hair-like projection at its upper end and

there are "spacer" cells in between the sensitive cells. I think

the spacer cells accept an efferent instruction from the cortex and

either firm or loosen the bottom anchorage of the sensitive cells
in accordance with the cortical instruction. The cortex "figures
out", by trial and error, it can select a particular part of the
sound image it finds interesting by suppressing the remainder of
the image. It learns how to enhance the "feature" by suppressing
the "surround". The efferent instruction may even move along the
sensitive membrane in cadence with the sound waveform.

SUMMARY OF THE ITEM ON COCHLEAR THEORY

About twenty years ago I went to a telephone company exhibit
where a voice scrambler was demonstrated. Scrambling was achieved
by transposing the speech frequency spectrum, high frequency sounds
were converted to low frequency sounds and vice versa.

If you spoke the words "telephone company", into the microphone,
they came out of the speaker as "play-ah-feen creek-in-nole", If
you said "play-ah-feen creek-in-nole" into the mike, it came out:
"telephone company".

Naturally the visitors to the exhibit were saying all sorts of
things into the mike, I talked to the engineer who accompanied the
exhibit and he said he had been hearing so much of this chatter he
was becoming skilled at understanding what was being said at the
input by listening to the output of the scrambler.

If there were fixed interpretive structures in the cochlea (i.e.
fixed frequency or amplitude analyzers), surely this ability to
understand speech with the spectrum reversed would be forbidden.
In order for the auditory system to have access to the subject
matter of the sound image, it would need these interpretive

structures to segregate sound amplitude from sound frequency, if for no other reason. I see this ability of the engineer to understand the sound with the spectrum reversed as a "bonus" argument, arguing the auditory system does not have access to the subject matter of its throughput.

There is also a visual version of this same argument. An experiment has been performed where the subject wears spectacles fitted with prisms that invert the visual image, top to bottom. After three days of re-habituation, the subject becomes skilled at making use of the inverted image. The cortex is able to function with the inverted image and is still able to relate visual inputs to motor outputs and so on. If the visual image had to be projected through some sort of an interpretive standard, this experiment would be impossible because of the incompatibility between the image and the interpretive system. This experiment is a "bonus" argument, arguing the visual system does not have access to the subject matter of the throughput.

(Incidentally, the experiment will not work if the prisms reverse the image left to right. There is a fixed reflex structure in the lower brain and it requires the image to be in the proper left/right sense in order to instruct binocular aiming of the eyes. The left/right reversal experiment has been tried and its non-feasible instruction causes painful spasm of the rectus muscles of the eyes.)

THE NERVE CELL AS THE ACTIVE ELEMENT

Transistors are the active elements in factory made computers. The passive elements are the fixed resistors and the signal conducting path. The nerve cell is the active element in the nervous system; it is also, ipso facto, the passive signal path. In the light of the usual understanding of active elements in computers, a first impression of a nerve cell gets one to wondering how an improbably tissue cell--granted, it is a bio-chemical marvel in its function as a tissue cell--got around to passing itself off as an electronic device in the first place. Not all multicellular organisms need a nervous system. The jellyfish comes to mind. It seems to be a colony of polyps, each a specialized kind of tissue cell. There may be no need to control the separate parts of its anatomy, each may be capable of functioning self-sufficiently, or, if there is control, they may be coordinated by chemical signals. Without the evolution of the nerve cell, animal life on this planet would have been confined to polyps, diatoms and whatever marine animals that can supported in a passive symbiosis with the sea. I think the nerve cell evolved in three steps. It had to have its beginnings with the diversion to signal processing duty, of an extant tissue cell in a forerunner of a multi-celled organism. The concentration of ions, both within and without the cell, is a key factor in all living cell. Pertinent here, are the concentrations of potassium, sodium and chloride ions. For any living cell, there is a resting ion balance and preserving this balance is critical to the life or death of the cell. There are about 12 times as many sodium ions on the outside of the cell as there are in the inside.

The potassium ion concentration is the other way around with about 30 times as many potassium ions in the inside as there are on the outside. The concentration of chloride ions, along with whatever organic solutes there may be is such that there is a negative voltage inside the cell. The voltage is typically negative 60-70 millivolts, in cases -90 millivolts. I am using -70 millivolts for the typical nerve cell in this discussion. A millivolt is 1/1000 volt. Beginning with an extant tissue cell, the first step in the evolution of the nerve cell was the D.C. (only) cell. Is a D.C. (only) cell because it does not fire. I have never run across a study where this cell was written up quite the way I have it here. The only examples of pure D.C. cells I am sure of are the first three cells just downstream of the retina. The evolutionary adaptation of an extant tissue cell to an electronically active cell has to be done with the extent wherewithal, so of the ions available in extant cell, the potassium ion balance is allowed to depart from its normal cell vitality concentration under signal control and for signal processing purposes. Bones, muscles, blood flow and organs with high metabolic rates tend to be electrically noisy. I explain the importance of electrical noise and its counter measures later in this item.

The D.C. (only) nerve cell is sensitive to stray voltages in its surroundings and it will only be found in electrically sheltered parts of the anatomy where stray voltages and electrical noise can be controlled. The length of the D.C. cell is in millimeters and it does not extend beyond its protected surroundings. The first three cells in the retinal coder and, I believe, the first cells in the cochlear coder are D.C. (only) cells. It is not possible to be sure about the cochlea because the coder is housed in a small spiral slit in the temporal bone and not accessible to study. The cortical cell is a special type of D.C. (only) cell, it fires, but it is fired from an external source. Before the evolution of larger and more sophisticated animals was possible, the tiny cell body of the D.C. nerve cell had to be lengthened and the noise vulnerability of the cell had to be overcome so the longer cell axon could operate in an electrically hostile environment. Long nerve fibers are more susceptible to noise than short ones. The second step in the evolution of the nerve cell was a D.C. cell with a longer axon and yet noise immune. The axon is the tubular elongation of the cell body. In this case, noise immunity of the longer axon is improved by increasing its diameter. With a larger diameter, there is more membrane area and more ion current. Signal energy is a function of ion current flow through the cell membrane. Increasing the diameter of the axon, hence ion current favors the signal energy to noise energy ratio, or, simply: "signal to noise ratio".

Shell fish and squid, with their large diameter axons, are a favorite subject for experimenters because the large diameter of the axon makes the nerve fiber easier to work with. Some of their experiments produce waveforms that lead me to believe, with caution, this is a nerve cell arrested in its evolution halfway between a D.C. cell and a later kind of nerve that patterns its firings in a pulse rate code. This intermediate noise immunity plan may still survive in living shellfish. The large diameter nerve is an improvement over the much shorter D.C. (only) nerve, and it may be further protected from electrical noise in shellfish by routing it down the electrically quiet "core" of the animal avoiding the electrically noisy muscle and possibly the carapace which are toward the animal's periphery.

For any nerve cell, we must remember the signal controlled current flow is an inflow of ions that upsets the critical resting balances of the cell. The signal controlled activity of the cell amounts to a signal controlled leakage of potassium ions flowing through the cell membrane, outside to inside. The potassium ion is admitted to the inner cell as a charge carrier for the D.C. signal. There is an operational rule for this cell that requires at least one sodium ion to be sent outside the cell for each potassium ion admitted. (The working formula probably requires three sodium ions to be sent outside of the cell for two potassium ions admitted.) A drawback goes along with the increased ion current requirements of the large diameter and more energetic cell. The cell can be destroyed by the relative massive flow of potassium ions into the axoplasm of the cell. Then too, if nothing is done about the outflow of sodium ions, there will be a sodium ion imbalance that will threaten the cell. I may be wrong, but I think this type of D.C. nerve cell must take "time out" from its normal work of signal conduction to fire a short burst of pulses for the express purpose of restoring ion balances during the ion population inversion that accompanies cell firing. With this nerve, the firings serve no useful purpose as far as signal processing is concerned; they are nothing more than a necessary "house-keeping" procedure. Between

bursts the cell returns to its normal signal conduction and stays
in its D.C. mode until the accumulation of ion imbalances reach a
point where it is necessary to fire another burst of "equalizing
pulses".

The third and climatic step in the evolution of the nerve cell,
and the step that made vertebrate anatomy possible, probably
started with the large diameter shellfish nerve and ended with a
nerve fiber, much longer, and with a much smaller diameter. The
large diameter nerve was essentially a D.C. nerve that fired pulses
as a nuisance necessity. The longer and smaller vertebrate nerve
that replaced it incorporated the firings into a pulse rate code
which was superimposed over, and controlled by, the underlying D.C,
signal. The D.C. signal sets the firing rate.

The general purpose nerve in vertebrate anatomy is the long axon,
small diameter, nerve. It is usually called the myelinated nerve
because it is insulated with a myelin jacket. This remarkable
nerve resorts to a technique similar to FM radio to overcome the
noise in its surrounding. Without it there would have been no
vertebrate evolution at all.

The analogue signal receives one extra translation in the
myelinated nerve. To enhance the noise immunity of the nerve, _for
no other reason_, the signal is translated to a pattern of pulses
fired at a rate controlled by the analogue signal. The _rate_ of
firing is an analogue of the D.C. signal. A small amplitude
signal will fire the nerve about 40pps, a large amplitude signal
excursion about 450pps (pulses per second). There will be a firing
rate that corresponds to any and all signal conditions in between.

THE NERVE CELL AS THE ACTIVE ELEMENT

The pulse rate code is an accessory to the D.C. analogue activity already at work within the cell. As I see it, in cells that incorporate the pulse rate code, the two systems overlay and collaborate with other and the underlying D.C. analogue system controls the pulse rate system.

Fig. 55 is a D.C. analogue scheme. The D.C. signal starts at the receptor and is an analogue of the "haystack" excursion of lamp brightness. The lamp brightness was initially set at one-half brightness. The brightness was turned up to a new value then turned back down again. The analogue of the brightness excursion is the "haystack" profile in the graph. The haystack excursion is continuously translated from an analogue in one form to another as it moves from cell to cell until it reaches its destination.

The upper cell in Fig. 56 is the photo receptor and the next cell downstream is a bipolar cell ("bipolar" by reason of its shape, not its conducting direction.) The bipolar cell in the retina is the archetype of a D.C. (only) cell. Signal conduction within the cell is by D.C. processes exclusively and the signal is expressed as a D.C. analogue. The D.C. cell does not "fire".

There is a negative voltage on the inside of the cell membrane. At rest (no signal) the voltage is -70 millivolts. There is a reciprocal relationship between current and voltage. The -70 millivolts is the maximum voltage and minimum current value. It is fair enough to say the membrane itself is the active element. It is a current operated

217

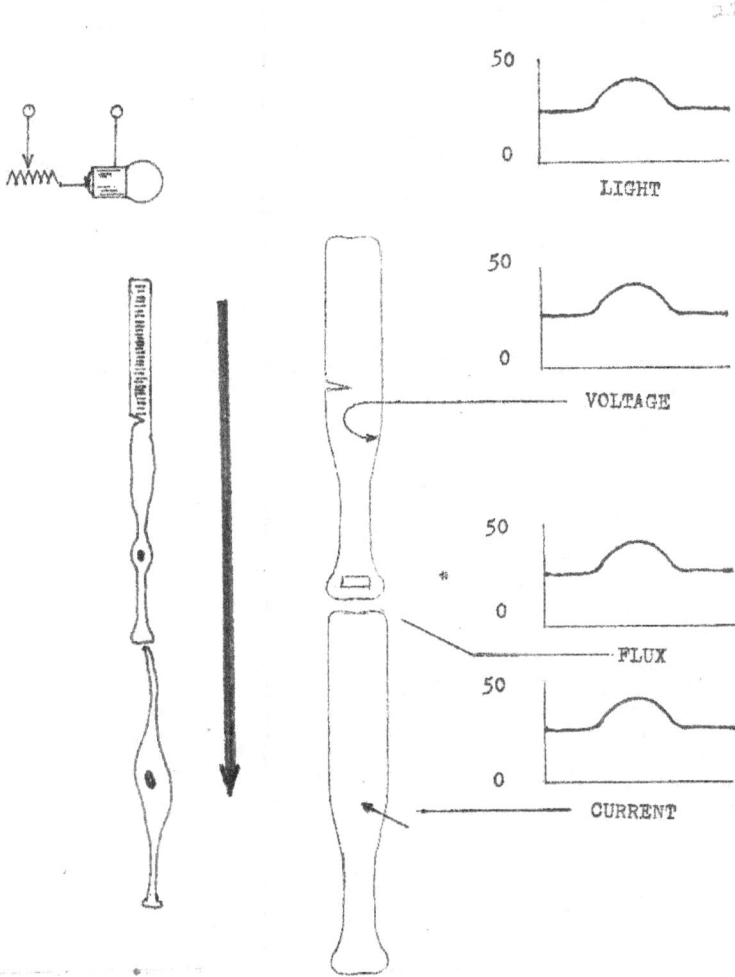

50

0

LIGHT

50

0

VOLTAGE

50

0

FLUX

50

0

CURRENT

*   The signal envelope for this D.C. junction between these
D.C. cells is a bit oversimplified. Let it suffice to say the
chemical flux within the junction will preserve the "sense" of
the signal so increased current in the upstream membrane will
appear as increased current in the downstream membrane in "normal"
or "non-inverting" cells.

Figure 55

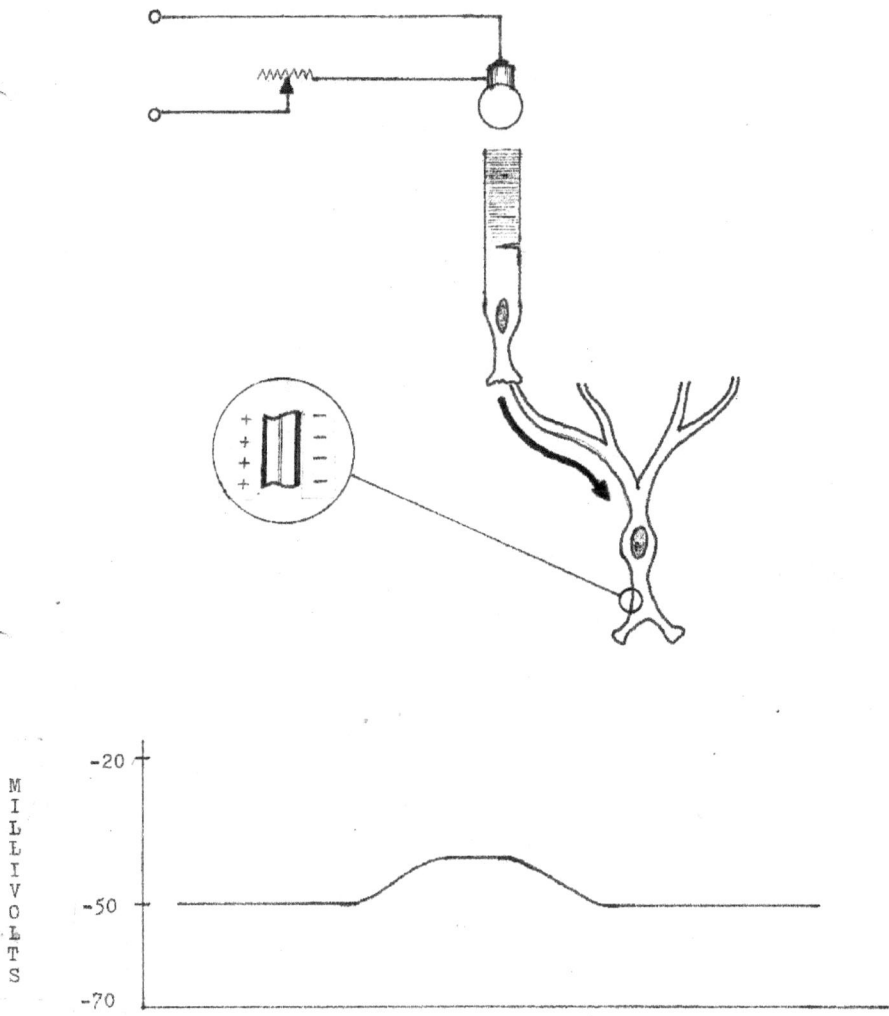

Figure 56

device and minimum current through the membrane corresponds to

minimum signal amplitude. When the signal is applied to the cell

membrane, the membrane will assume a voltage between -70mv and -

20mv depending on the signal amplitude. This is the operating range of the D.C. capability of the cell. According to me, nerve cells that "fire" the pulse rate code also have this underlying D.C. analogue capability. I explain this in this item.

The cells in Fig. 55 are D.C. (only) cells and the graphs, all analogues of the light signal, show the translations the analogue signal goes through as it moves down the data bus. To simplify the drawing, the signal amplitudes are arbitrarily shown between zero and 50 units of signal intensity and the absolute units of light intensity, voltage, chemical flux and ion current have been disregarded. Fig. 56 shows where the voltage is physically impressed and plots the absolute voltage on the graph.

In the series of cells in the drawing, the membrane voltage excursion controls the chemical flux at the synapse, and here the voltage excursion is translated to a chemical signal. Regardless of the signal translations that have taken place upstream of the synapse, the excursion in chemical current (or "flux") is still an analogue of the original excursion in light brightness. The chemical flux controls ion current in the membrane of the next cell just downstream of the synapse. The signal analogue is translated: voltage to flux, flux to ion current, current to voltage, followed by hundreds of repetitions of this same sequence from sensor to brain (Fig. 55).

The D.C. analogue plan is straight forward and the analogue is expressed as modulations of potassium current flowing radially through the membrane. The sodium ion outside and the chloride ion inside the membrane constitute the power supply for the D.C. system.

THE NERVE CELL AS THE ACTIVE ELEMENT

The nerve cell membrane conducts ion current in accordance with a set of parameters called the "cable properties" of the membrane. Potassium ion current sets the membrane voltage and this disturbance propagates down the axon as a result of the cable properties of the membrane. Signal processing by the D.C. characteristics of the membrane and its cable properties are all that is needed for a fully functional D.C. cell.

It seems to me, most of the time and money spent on nerve studies has been spent trying to find a "model" that will related the firing rate of pulsed nerves to the signal that controls it. At times, some of the studies of the fired nerve lose sight of the reasons for its existence. "PM" is "frequency modulation". Stray voltage and electrical noise degrade a desired signal by "amplitude modulating" it. The pulse rate nerve is a variation of FM signal processing and FM signals are not disturbed by AM noise. The pulse rate nerve, with its myelin jacket, is about as noise immune as the nature of nerve will permit. While a few odd pulses turn up in some experiments, they have to be accounted for in the light of the experiment. A strange experiment from time to time does not alter the integrity of the basic FM plan.

I will show my own model of the pulsed membrane. According to me, the membrane is "fired" by its metabolic power supply. Fig. 57 is an equivalent circuit. The apparatus on the left is the active element and we can look at as though it is a battery with an insulating separator between two electrodes. We will say the power supply is capable of delivering a voltage greater that the insulator can withstand. The power supply has a residual pacing

and it charges the battery over a short time. It charges for a
while, the voltage goes up, and, when the voltage reaches the
breakdown voltage of the insulator, there is a strike through.
Ions pour through when the membrane is breached and this discharges
the battery. The power supply charges it again; there is a uniform
amount of time needed for charging between each of the "firing"
cycles. The residual pacing of the power supply sets the residual
firing rate. The firing rate can be increased if the power supply
is up-paced. The firing rate can be made a function of the D.C.
signal if the D.C. signal is allowed to control the power supply
pacing.

The resistor in the drawing (zig-zag line) merely makes the
drawing "legal" as an electronic circuit, it prevents the active
element from shorting the power supply. In the model of the real
membrane, the trick is to remove the resistor and

228

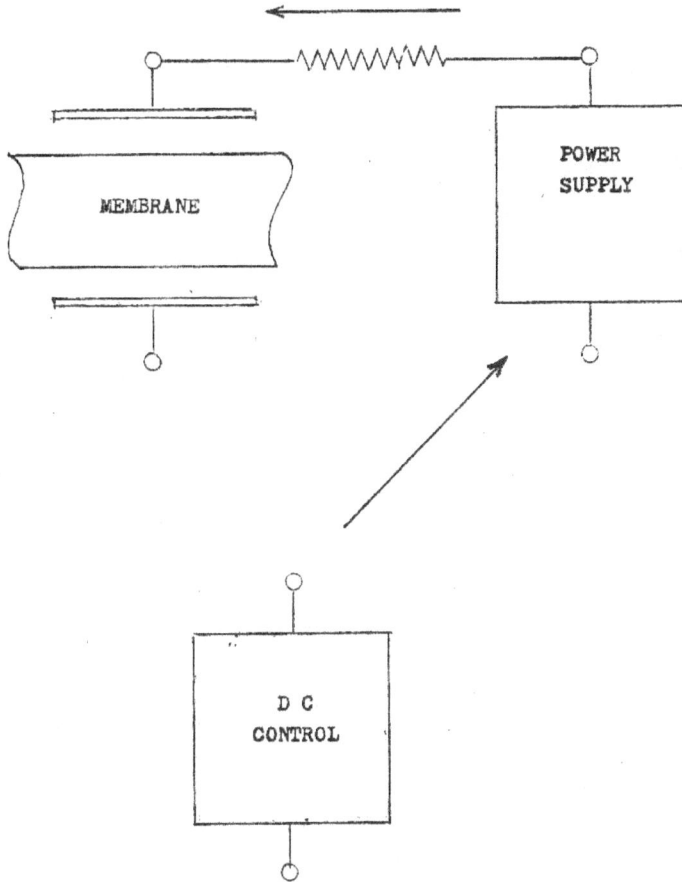

Figure
57

overlay all three circuit elements in the drawing, using the same

input and output terminals.

The fired nerve is still a D.C. nerve. It has a pulse rate system superimposed and the firing rate controlled by the underlying D.C. system. The D.C. system uses the membrane parameters as a "current" operated device and the pulse rate system uses the same membrane as a "voltage" operated device.

The sequence begins in the upper sketch in Fig. 58. A chemical neuro-transmitter has been delivered from the synapse of an upstream cell. The flux (quantity) of neuro-transmitter is signal controlled and the chemical has the property of changing the ion conductivity of the membrane. As conductivity increases, membrane resistance goes down, ion current goes up, all under signal control.

The mechanism responsible for the inflow of potassium ions (K^+, in the drawing) is not clear. The D.C. analogue signal is expressed as a potassium ion current through the membrane. Of the cellular ions, the potassium ion is the most mobile in the pores of the membrane. There is a negative voltage on the inside of the membrane and, as I see it, the potassium ions are "falling" down the voltage gradient. This would be the view that makes sense electronically. The potassium ion is also falling uphill against the ion concentration gradient, so it is thought the inflow of potassium ions is assisted by an enzyme pumping action to bring them into the cell against the concentration gradient. If this is the case, the potassium ion "pump" would be the complement of the sodium ion pump in the sketch. (The enzymes and the chemical steps in the pumping action are not known, indicated by the

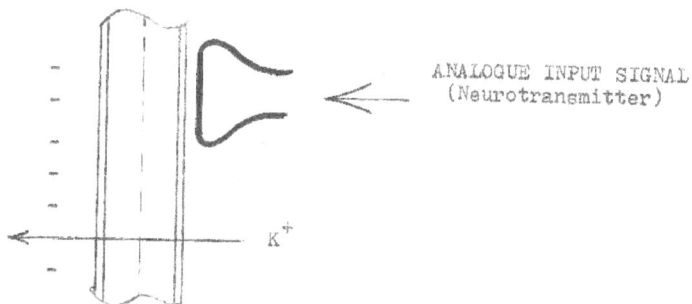

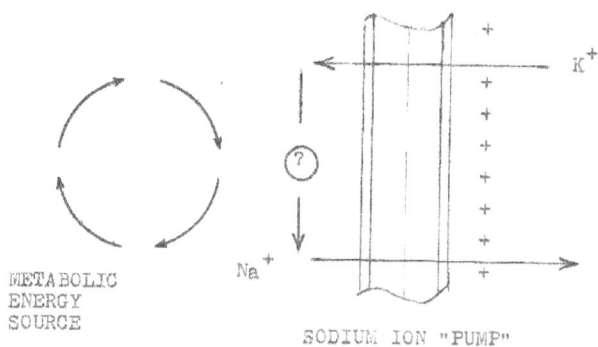

ANALOGUE INPUT SIGNAL
(Neurotransmitter)

K^+

METABOLIC
ENERGY
SOURCE

Na^+

K^+

SODIUM ION "PUMP"

Fig 35

question mark in the lower sketch. Ions are said to be "pumped"

across the cell membrane by a n Figure 58 p".)

To me, bringing the <u>potassium</u> ion into the cell sets the <u>sodium</u>

pumping action in motion and paces its rate. If one sodium ion is pumped out for each potassium admitted, the membrane voltage is equilibrated. If more than one sodium ion is sent out for each potassium ion admitted, there is a possibility for a "gain" in power supply delivery capability, and the ionic "battery" will gain charge. The sodium ions on the outside of membrane are the power supply for the potassium ion "current" operated system.

If the sodium pump is able to "gain" on potassium ion influx, its output must exceed the pumping energy needed for, maintaining cell vitality ion balances, equilibrating the signal controlled potassium ion influx and compensating for all leakages. The slight power supply "gain" will make the membrane parameters increasingly sensitive as the signal amplitude increases. The signal amplitude increases and the membrane parameters become hyper-sensitive. It is easier to trigger a firing when the power supply is hyper paced. This is true of any bi-stable electronic device. Later drawings will show the pulsed firings of the membrane separated by a serration which is the D.C. analogue signal. The increased power supply delivery capability does not raise membrane voltage immediately because the voltage increase has been off-set by increased potassium ion current in the serration. As the signal amplitude increases, the serration are shortened and the firing rate increased.

I will pass along a dubious but interesting idea that occurred to me (Fig. 59). Usual caution is recommended with this idea. The drawing is the nerve cell membrane. The water soluble heads of the lipid molecules that make up the membrane form the interstitial (outer) and axoplasmlc (inner) surfaces of the membrane. (The open

226

circles are the water soluble ends of the lipid molecules.) The water repellent tails point inward to the midline of the membrane. A voltage across the membrane implies a bombardment of ions from both sides: the greater the voltage, the more intense the bombardment. If the ion bombardment compressed these fairly long lipidic molecules, the diameters of the pores in the membrane will be reduced, restricting the permeability of the membrane for potassium ions. The ion conductivity would then become a function of the voltage across the membrane.

The height of the vertical lines suggests the membrane voltage at positions along the membrane. The voltage is greater at the point where the membrane is compressed. The zig-zag line suggests the Brownian (random) movement of an ion looking for a pore that will accommodate its diameter.

Experiments show the membrane has special electrical characteristics. An increase in ion current will reduce membrane voltage, which decreases resistance, followed, in turn, by an increase in current and so on. A reduction in current has the opposite effect, voltage rises, rising

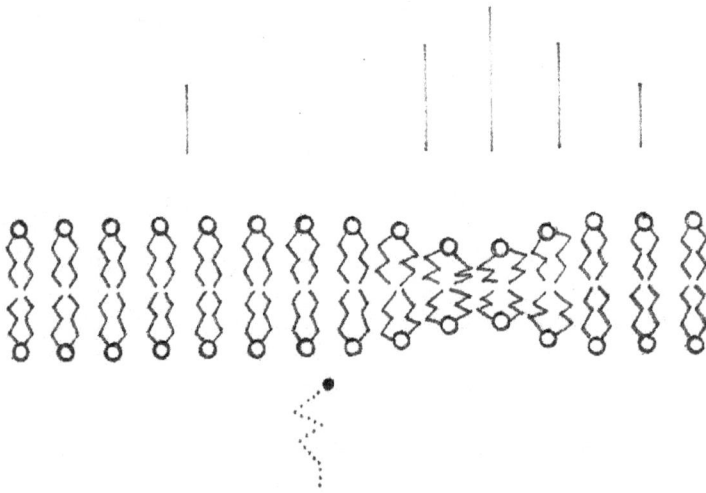

Fig 56

voltage increases membrane resis— — — — reduces current, and

Figure 59

membrane voltage goes up in a se— — ng, increase-begets-

increase, parameter. Be it higher or lower, the membrane voltage
makes an uninterruptable, all-or-nothing plunge.

The hyper-energetic power supply sets conditions so the small
increment in voltage attributable to "shot effect" is all that is
needed to trigger a shift from the equilibrated D.C. analogue state
in the serration to the all-or-nothing parameter of the membrane.
(Power supply pacing, controlled by the D.C. analogue sets the
firing rate. The instantaneous decision to disturb a resting
equilibrium and to initiate one cycle of firing is made by
extremely tiny bursts of thermally excited charge carriers--the
always present "shot effect".)

The membrane functions in both a "current" mode and a "voltage"
mode, the "voltage" mode is the firing activity. Once the shift
has been made from the current to the voltage mode, the membrane is
committed to complete its "one-shot" (though repeating) firing.

The rise rate, or fall rate, is quite abrupt (less than a
millisecond) and, because of the steep rise rate, at any one point
along the axon the pulse is clearly being generated locally, at the
point where the experimenters probe finds it.

This all-or-nothing parameter of the membrane is called the
"ancillary" parameter. It could also be called the "voltage
dependent resistor" or "VDR" parameter of the membrane. This same
membrane will also function in a stable D.C. analogue mode.
Oscillating devices, "one-shot" or otherwise, have a point in their
operating cycle where currents, voltages and parameters are in a
carefully balanced equilibrium. When the VDR parameter is at an
equilibrium point, voltage neither rises nor falls and potassium

ion current and power energy are in equilibrium. This equilibrium endures in the serration between firings.

Fig. 60 traces the events that come into play in order for the D.C. analogue to set the firing rate. Fig. 60 is a "busy" drawing because there are so many operations involved. The heavy line in the drawing plots membrane voltage, the waveform is shown the same way it would appear if it was seen on an oscilloscope.

1. This is the serration between pulses. During this interval, the signal is expressed as a D.C. analogue and the system is functioning in the "current" mode. The D.C. analogue is expressed as a potassium ion current. The voltage follows the current inversely and the voltage plot in Fig. 60 works out rather well if we note an upward movement of the voltage profile corresponds to an increase in signal current. During the serration, while the membrane is in the "current" mode, the power supply has been up-paced by potassium ion influx. While it tries to raise membrane voltage, it's up-paced output just compensates for the lowering of membrane voltage attributable to increased ion current. An equilibrium is reached which is a function of

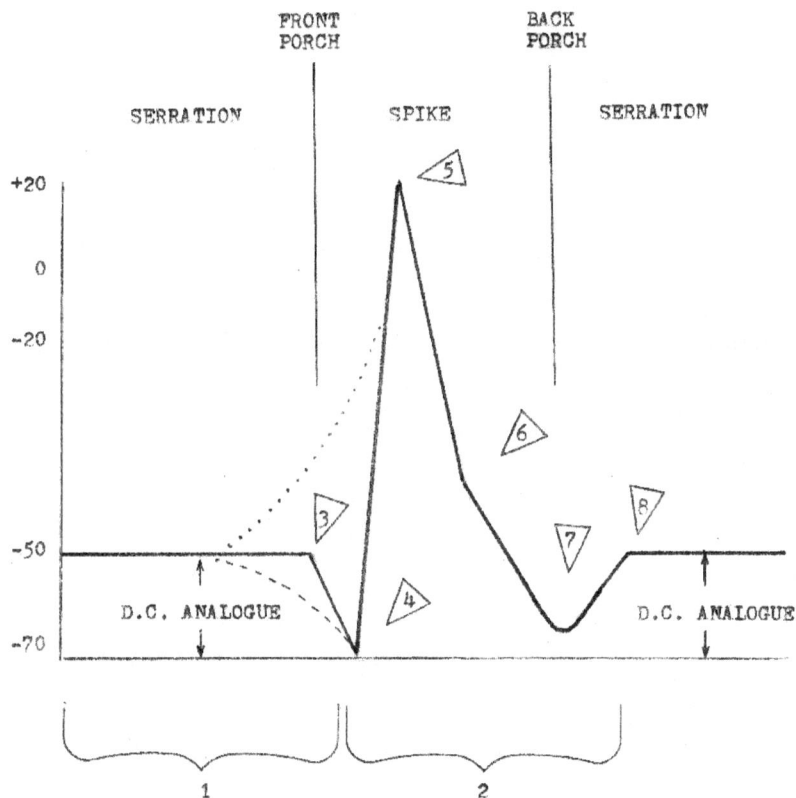

FIG 57

Figure 60

the D.C. signal. The power s .s: probably slightly

"hyper," otherwise it would equilibrate indefinitely.

  2. During this interval the cell is firing. The membrane

executes one cycle of a bi-stable oscillation. The firing rate is up-paced from its residual 40pps rate by up-pacing the sodium ion power supply. While power supply output has increased--it was re-paced by the analogue signal in the preceding serration--there will be no visible evidence of this in the scope trace, save we assume the higher firing rate to be evidence of the up-pacing. I have to assume this, there is no way to experimentally look into the power supply pacing.

The pulse has a front porch (3 to 4), a spike (4 to 5), and a back porch. The time required for the spike is one millisecond, each porch takes about .5 milliseconds.

(500 pulses per second is the absolute upper limit of the firing rate because there has to be some sort of serration if only to clear the front and back porches. I am wary of experiments reporting firing rates near 500 PPS. The experimenter maybe irritating the nerve and this may not be a naturally occurring firing rate.)

The drawing is my version of the wave shape. The straight edges and sharp corners will not be seen on the oscilloscope due to both series and shunt capacitance in the probe connection. The downward sloping line, from 3 to 4, may not be visible unless the signal is put on board naturally, that is, through a synaptic junction.

There is a difference between "avalanching" and "firing". In an experimental set up, where membrane voltage is influenced by an external source, the membrane will avalanche on the ancillary parameter. An "avalanche" is an all-out dumping of ions through the membrane resulting from a loss of membrane resistance. The foreign voltage reduces membrane resistance without a compensatory up-pacing of the power supply. The membrane immediately goes into its population inversion without firing. ("Avalanching", an experimenter's artifact, would follow the upward slanting dotted line in the drawing.)

3. Arrow 3 is the "mode shift" point where the membrane switches from the "current" (and analogue) mode to the "voltage" (and pulse rate) mode. The sodium ion power supply is the common link between the analogue system and the pulsed system. Increased potassium ion current (the signal current) has up-paced the power supply which increases the system sensitivity. The sensitivity is right (hyper), the stage is set, and a small, always present disturbance will shift the voltage slightly and the membrane shifts from equilibrated stability of the analogue mode to a fast and furious firing of the membrane. (The thermal disturbance is far too small to be plotted on this graph.) At the mode shift point, the slightest increment in voltage is enough to produce a slight increment in membrane resistance and the extension of these mutually regenerative processes is displayed in the very fast rise in voltage between 3 and 4. (While the curve slopes downward, the voltage is nevertheless rising.) Here, the pumping action and the VDR characteristics of the membrane are working together to enforce this abruptly rising voltage. The actual mode shift point probably lies somewhere between the acute angle at "3" and the dashed line. The dashed line is the probable trace on the scope.

4. Once the membrane has been committed to make the mode shift, the voltage will irreversibly go to its maximum limit about -70 millivolts. At -70mv, the membrane has reached the limits of its

dielectric strength (its strength as an insulator) and ions puncture through the membrane. A voltage on the order of 70mv may not seem like it is great enough to breach the insulating properties of the membrane but it amounts to 100,000 volts per inch, enough to strike through almost any insulator.

Ions flow through the breach and the ion current and the VDR parameter take over. The current lowers resistance which increases current and we have the same mutually regenerative parameters in reverse. This time the VDR parameter is enforcing a minimum resistance/maximum current and least voltage excursion in the parameters. The steep leading edge of the spike, 4 to 5, is caused by the ion population inversion, a sequel to the firing, in conjunction with the VDR parameter.

From the time the membrane voltage goes through the -20mv point of the leading edge of the pulse until it goes back through the -20mv point on the trailing edge, the membrane is not an effective barrier to ions. When the membrane voltage is less than -20mv, the membrane cannot be used in the D.C. analogue mode. This sets the upper and lower limits on the D.C. analogue signal excursion. The signal excursion limits are -70mv to -20mv. A total of 50mv is available for the D.C. analogue excursion.

In the nerve cell, ions are borrowed from the cell vitality ion balances to process the signal. The ion debt has to be repaid and this done during the ion population inversion that is a part of the firing process.

5. Point 5 is the positive overshoot of the membrane voltage. The experts are not sure of the reasons for the overshoot.

6. The VDR parameter is turned around again. The rapid voltage increase between 5 and 6 is caused by the pumping action working in conjunction with the VDR parameter. At point 6 there is a short-fall in the pumping action <u>rate</u>. Energy has been removed from the system to generate the pulse. The voltage increase between 6 and 7 is still brought about by the pumping action working in conjunction with the VDR parameter but the rise rate is not as steep between 6 and 7 because of the flagging contribution of the pumping action. (It may seem odd, but downward is a rising voltage.)

7. Position 7 is the <u>absolute</u> short-fall in pumping action energy. With a short-fall in sodium ion pumping, there is a short-fall in membrane voltage. At point 7 the membrane voltage is not quite high enough to restrike a voltage break-through of the membrane. The back porch of the spike is also the "absolute" refractory interval of the nerve. (The "refractory" interval is a refusal to fire. The back porch refractory interval serves nicely to prevent the pulse from moving backward along the nerve. As far as I am concerned, this .5 millisecond refractory interval is the only "legal" refractory interval. When experimenters show refractory nerve experiments, the nerve refuses to fire because it is fatigued.)

8. At position 8, the membrane has reset to the D.C. analogue mode and it will stay in this mode for the duration of the upcoming serration. During the serration the analogue signal will proportionately up-pace the power supply and another pulse will be fired with its rate set by the D.C. analogue current. The

foregoing is my version of the firing event, it should be regarded with caution.

The pulse rate system is an adjunct to an already adequate D.C. signal process within the cell. It is a strategy which compensates for the problem of routing an unshielded, and unshieldable, nerve through an environment hostile with stray voltages, stray currents and cross-talk between nerve fibers. Here we have a complicated pulse system, almost a FM system, serving no useful purpose other than making up for the basic vulnerability of the nerve to electrical noise in its ambience. Nothing like the pulse rate code would ever be used in a factory made electronic processor. Their signal conductor would be protected by shields and ground buses and there would be no need for the FM scheme.

(The capacitance of a long nerve sets the "high frequency roll-off" of the nerve. The "haystack" transient in some of the sketches is a case in point, if its rise rate was on the order of 1/100 second, there is a good chance it would be attenuated by capacity effects before it reached the end of the nerve. With an auspicious selection of modulation constants, there is a possibility the pulse rate code may assist in extending the high frequency response of the nerve.)

A look at a nerve in its tissue surroundings can be deceptive in that it tells us nothing about the drastic measures needed to shelter the sensitive nerve from the electrical crudities of its tissue matrix. Those crudities are; stray voltage, stray current and an unwanted coupling between nerves called "cross-talk".

THE NERVE CELL AS THE ACTIVE ELEMENT

I think most writers and theorists do not clearly see the signal versus noise problem. I have thought about this for many years. I am fairly confident I understand the, less than conspicuous, noise immunity measures of the nervous system.

The problem has its beginnings in the resolution of the nerve cell as the active element. Resolution refers to the ability to carry the precision signal from its input to its output without adding electrical errors. In so far as I know, no one has tried to estimate the resolution of the nerve so I will try to make the estimate myself. In the item on the coder, I show where a minimum resolution of one part in 2500 is easily required and the practical resolution is probably nearer one part in 5000. The D.C. analogue signal has a total excursion of 50mv. For a resolution of one part in 2500, it will be necessary to be able to divide the 50mv excursion and express the signal in one of 2500 small excursions. One meaningful division will be no more than 20 microvolts (millionths of a volt). If the resolution is one part in 5000, the nerve fiber must be so carefully protected from electrical noise in its surroundings that a stray voltage impressed on the membrane will never exceed 10 microvolts. It is probably protected down to one, perhaps several, microvolts.

There are two additional noise immunity measures, so potent they almost eliminate the noise problem, yet heretofore neither has been properly understood as a noise immunity device. They are the "node of Ranvier" (Rahn-vee-ay) and the electrotonic synapse.

The lipidic (fatty) jacket, perhaps: "tubular insulator" would be better, surrounding the myelinated nerve fiber is an end to end

237

arrangement of Schwann cells. This is a flat cell, rolled up like a carpet and it forms fatty insulating layers in a concentric spiral (upper part of Fig. 61). The myelinated nerve has the appearance of linked sausages under magnification. The cleft between the links is the node of Ranvier. The nerve axon is at the center of the Schwann cells.

Our man in the sketch has an ulnar nerve that is not only well insulated with Schwann cells but well-grounded at the nodes between the Schwann cells. The zig-zag lines are the resistive connections between the nerve environment and the excitable membrane of the axon. The small voltages we would find on a member of the body, as measured through the horny layer of skin would not create much of a stray voltage problem. Bones, muscle and organs deeper in the body, especially organs with high metabolic rates, surround the nerve with a more hostile environment by impressing stray voltages and currents in the nerve surround.

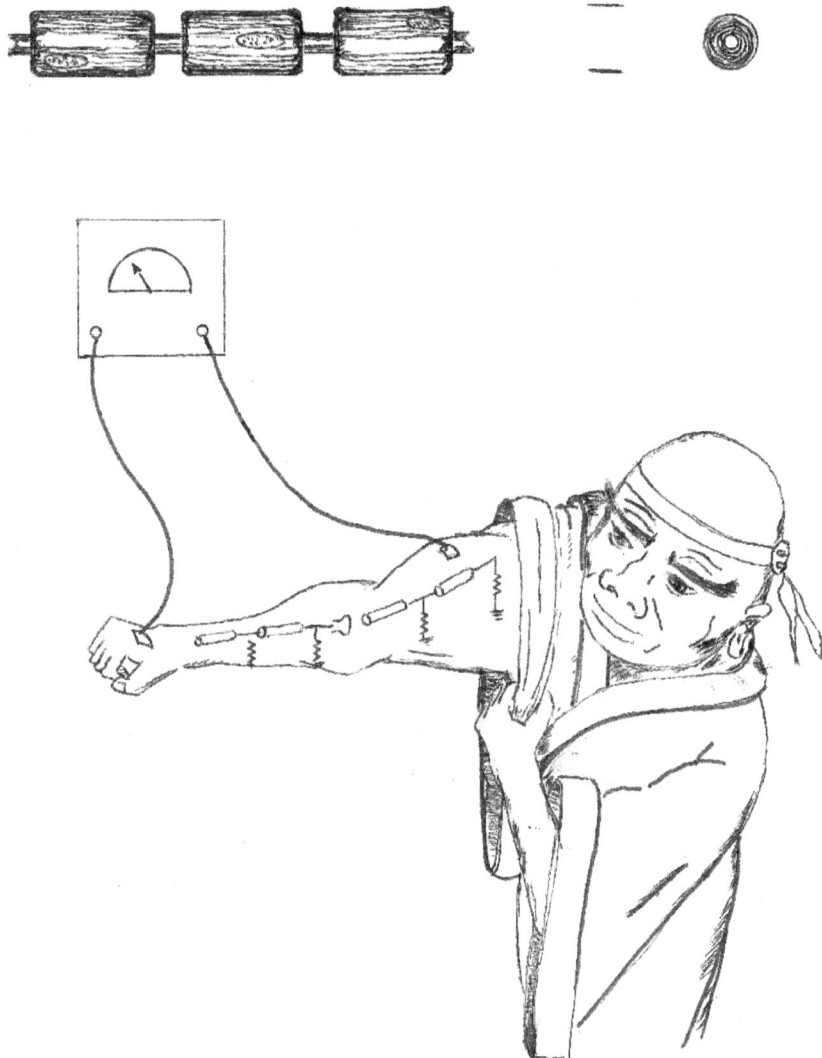

Figure 61

If the full length of the axon was enclosed in an uninterrupted

insulating tube, the insulator itself would bring new problems into

the picture. Stray voltages and currents would concentrate at the

arborization of the nerve at one of its ends and the cell body at the other.   If the tubular insulator was uninterrupted, there would

be a longitudinal voltage on the axoplasm.   In order to produce

this longitudinal voltage, there has to be a radial current

somewhere.   The stray voltage or stray current would then be

superimposed on the coherent signal.

The stray voltage, or the voltage drop produced by a stray

current, must be kept under the ten (or less) microvolt limit.   The

very accurate resolution of the nerve will tolerate no more.   The

node of Ranvier is a minute gap in the insulation and provides a

restricted path for a small current between the axoplasm and the

extracellular fluids.   These resistive pathways at the nodes (the

zig-zag lines at the nodes in Fig. 62) will permit each unit length

of axon to assume the voltage existing at each unit length of the

voltage gradient in the surrounding tissue.   Stray voltages are

divided up into small pieces and "bled" off before they reach

concentrated values that would destroy the calibration of the

nerve.   The layout of resistors in Fig. 62 is an equivalent

circuit.   The membrane is the active element, and it is sandwiched

in the bleed paths which is just where it should be to remove stray

voltages.

Some texts refer to the "salutatory" (jumping) behavior of the

pulses. the pulse is said to "jump" from one node to the next.

The jumping business is just an opinion, though it dates back years

and years, and the opinion may be based on trying to find a useful purpose for the odd looking node of Ranvier.

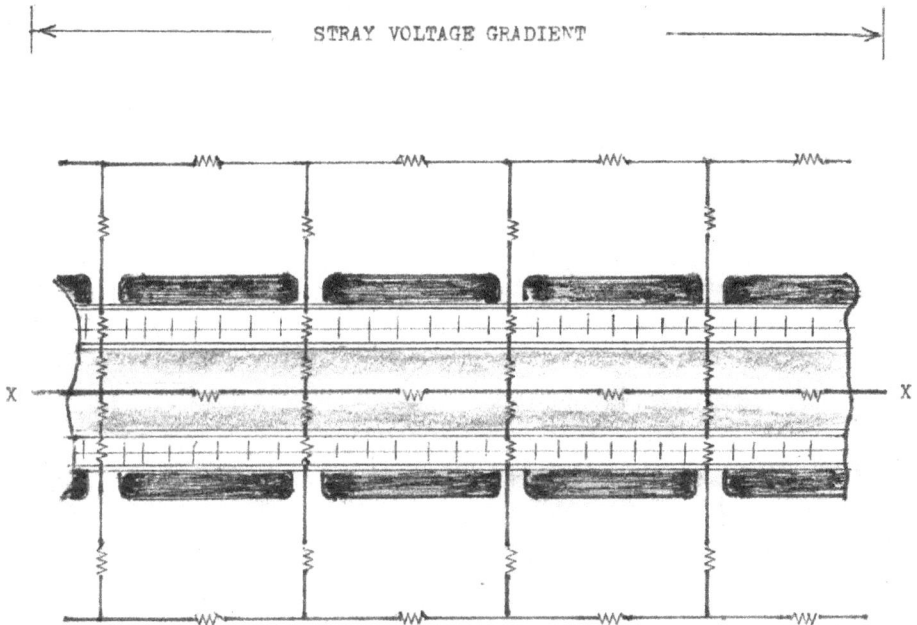

STRAY VOLTAGE GRADIENT

Figure 62

According to me, the pulse d from point to point along the nerve, it moves at a dignified, unvarying rate starting at the cell body and on out to the end of the nerve. A pulse that jumps from node to node has not been confirmed experimentally.

I view the node of Ranvier as an element in an extensive stray voltage, stray current, noise immunity program that perfuses the nervous system. Let me put it this way: if the node of Ranvier doesn't work the way I say it does--it ought to.

The signal is passed from an upstream cell to a downstream cell through a bulbous expansion of the end branch of the nerve axon: the button synapse. The upper drawing in Fig. 63 is the "electrotonic synapse". I think the state of the art has a view of the electrotonic synapse that is dead wrong. According to me, the electronic junction does not, and cannot, process the signal as has been thought. I will explain this prohibition in the summary of this item.

The electronic junction is a continuation of the stray voltage immunity scheme. Fig. 63 explains the difference between an active, signal processing junction, and the electrotonic synapse. Signal processing junctions contain a vesicular apparatus and the presence of vesicles should be taken as a landmark for distinguishing between signal-active and signal-inactive junctions. The apparatus consists of a honeycomb framework which supports and confines the bubble like vesicles. This mechanism releases precisely

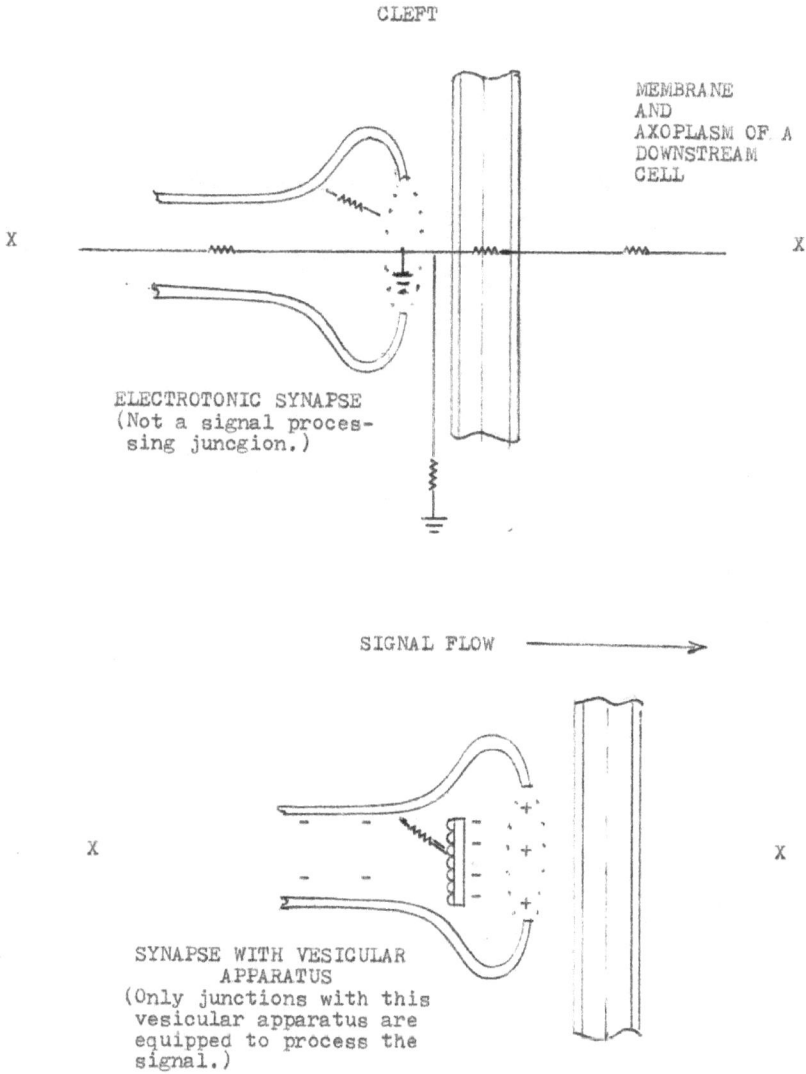

CLEFT

MEMBRANE
AND
AXOPLASM OF A
DOWNSTREAM
CELL

X   X

ELECTROTONIC SYNAPSE
(Not a signal proces-
sing junction.)

SIGNAL FLOW ⟶

X   X

SYNAPSE WITH VESICULAR
APPARATUS
(Only junctions with this
vesicular apparatus are
equipped to process the
signal.)

Fig 60

controlled quantities of chemicals called neuro-transmitters.

Experts believe the control is Figure 63 , possible controlled

to molecular quantities.

The vesicular structure is one pole of an electrophoretic apparatus. The grounded area (elliptical dotted line in the bottom drawing) is the other pole. Two poles (electrodes) are needed for an electrophoretic device, one positive and the other negative. Molecules of neuro-transmitter migrate from the negative to the positive pole (from vesicles to cleft in the drawing) under the influence of the voltage gradient between the poles. The voltage gradient is controlled by the signal voltage on the membrane which is coupled to the vesicular apparatus via the resistor (with arrowheads) in the bottom drawing.

Stray voltages cannot be impressed on signal junctions, axoplasm-to-axoplasm ("X" to "X", in the bottom drawing), because the stray voltage would also be superimposed in the voltage gradient in the electrophoretic apparatus, destroying its precise calibration. Stray voltage between the axoplasm of the upstream synapse and the axoplasm of the downstream cell must be neutralized. The problem is worse at junctions between segments of long nerves that transverse several environments and with different voltages at the ends of the nerve segment.

The upper part of Fig. 64 is the electrotonic synapse. Again there are resistive paths to either bleed off stray

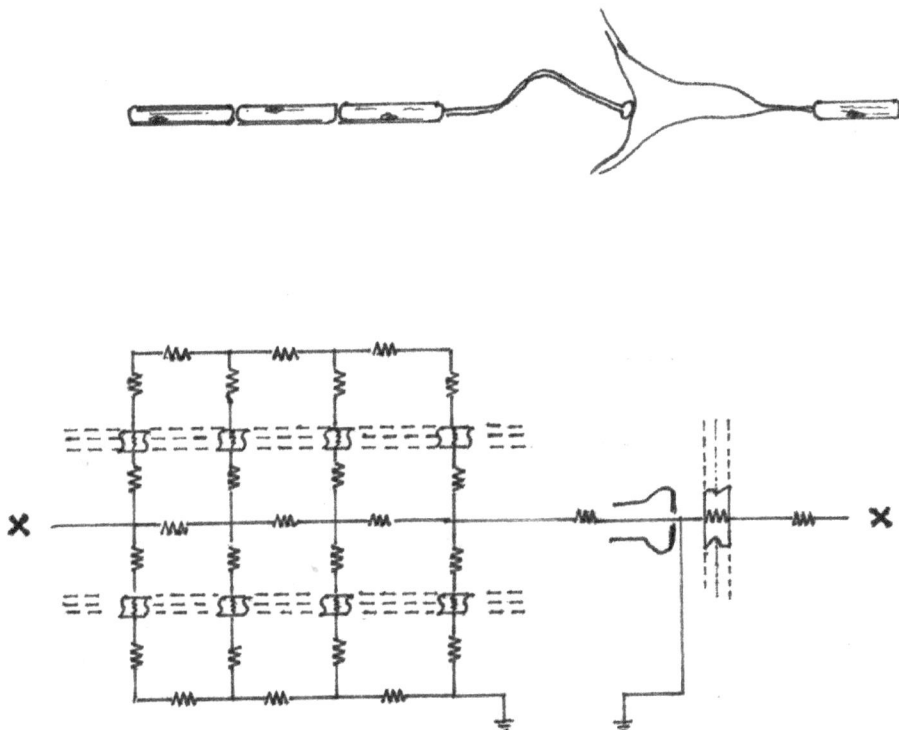

Fig. 64

voltages or to provide an axoplasm-to-axoplasm "shunt" resistance

between the two nerve cells. The shunt is between "X" and "X" and

stray voltage is kept to manageable levels rather than allow

unrestrained stray voltage to appear across the precise

electrophoretic gradient in the cell's active signal processing junctions. The cleft is electrically "grounded" to the world outside the cleft, serving the two fold function of acting as an additional node of Ranvier and providing an anode in the signal processing junctions.

The bulbous shape provides a high resistance path between the membrane and the cleft. A straight termination would eliminate the resistance (resistor with arrows, top sketch) and shunt the signal directly to the cleft.

The short lines cutting the membrane are speculative and suggest there may be a discontinuity in the characteristics of the membrane near the synapse. The central section of the membrane facing the cleft is probably not excitable membrane.

Fig. 64 puts the node of Ranvier and the electrotonic junction together in a working noise immunity layout. The pulse rate code is also a part of the noise immunity plan. Ingenious as it is, the entire noise immunizing scheme does nothing more than compensate for the lack of shielded signal conductors. Discarding the electrotonic junction as a signal processing junction is my idea, so the usual cautions are in order.

Any nerve cell is a signal "conductor" or a signal "repeater". The signal is put on board at one end and delivered at the other. Chemical neuro-transmitter is stored in the synapse and released in measured amounts to control the conductance of the downstream membrane. The neuro-transmitter is "excitory" if it increases firing rate of the downstream cell and "inhibitory" if it is reduced. Fig. 65 shows a cell in "inverter" service (middle cell, right data bus). The nature of the neuro-transmitter determines whether the cell is an inverter or not. The "excitory" neuro-transmitter is a "plus" contribution to the downstream arithmetic and the "inhibitory" neuro-transmitter is a "minus", or inverted, contribution. The rules of arithmetic are the same for both D.C. cells and the pulse rate kind. Fig. 65 shows the way the "haystack" transient is treated by the inverter cell.

Inverter service is simple enough application of a nerve cell but a couple of cautions must be kept in mind;

1. The inverted signal is negative in the downstream arithmetic and enough positive inputs must be added to establish a positive reference bias and to furthermore assure the negative signal will not drive the downstream membrane into potassium ion cut-off (signal cut-off). (Ion current cut-off is deliberately incorporated in the comparator arithmetic.)

2. Nerve cells do not have mixed outputs. If a cell has one positive terminal, then all other outputs from the cell are positive. All outputs from an inverter cell are inverted outputs. (Again, the rule for uniformity of synapses: for a given cell, they must be all of one kind. If one synapse has a memory unit in it, then all synapses must have them.)

256

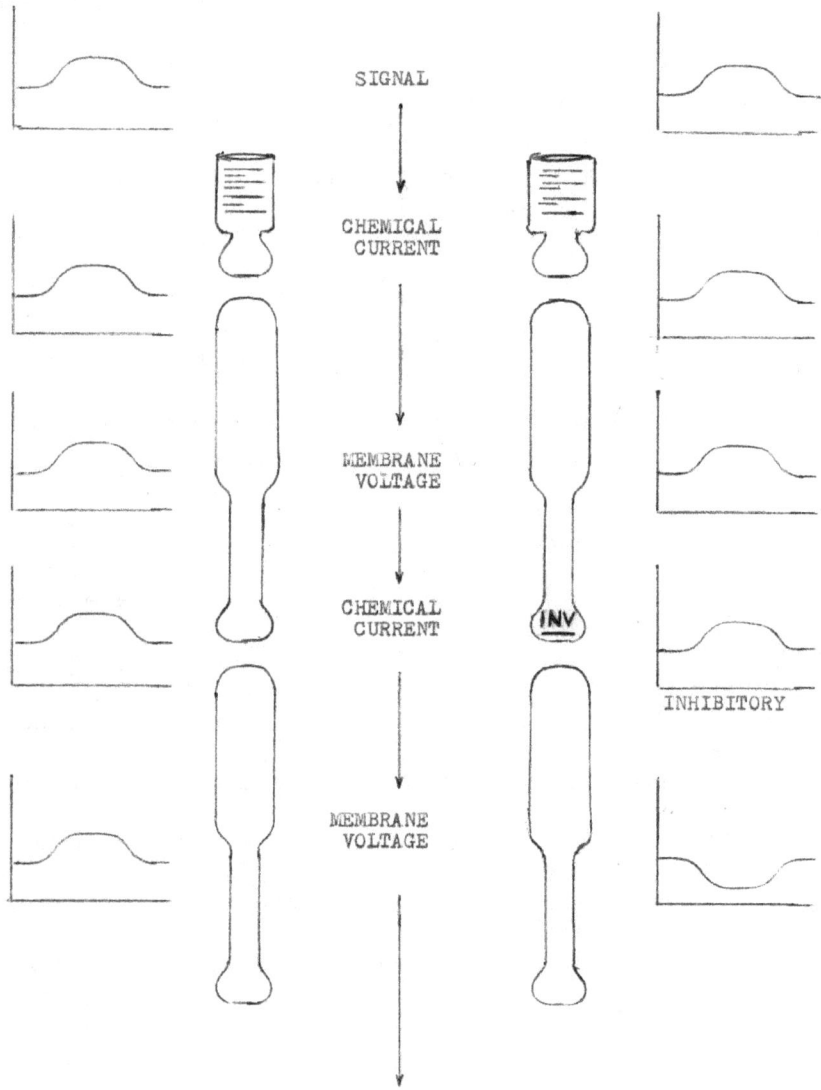

SIGNAL

CHEMICAL
CURRENT

MEMBRANE
VOLTAGE

CHEMICAL
CURRENT

INV

INHIBITORY

MEMBRANE
VOLTAGE

Fig 62

The nerve cell is always a "repeater" an Figure 65 r is usually a

"summator". A summator is a repeater witn more tnan one input.

Fig. 66 is a section of a cell in "summator" service. More than one discrete junction is needed to form an operational input junction. Under the microscope the cell body is covered with thousands of synapses but, after allowing for electrotonic junctions which carry no signal, and the multiple synapse requirement for single operating junctions, there are fewer inputs to the cell than a count of junctions would indicate.

The conductivity of the downstream membrane for potassium ions is controlled by the neuro-transmitter from the synapse. The number of discrete junctions allocated to a given input terminal will set the proportionality the input contributes to the summator arithmetic. One input is "advantaged" over another if it has more discrete synapses making up its terminal.

The downstream cell is a summator in Fig. 66. If the input from the upper group of five junctions is positive, with a total of nine junctions, the positive contribution will be proportioned by a factor of 5/9. Let us say the positive input is carrying a signal of 25 units of signal intensity and the negative, 20 units. The arithmetic goes like this:

+(25) times 5/9 = 125

-(20) times 4/9 = -80/45

The "advantaging" of the positive contribution cannot be so great it drives the membrane voltage to the -20mv zone, where

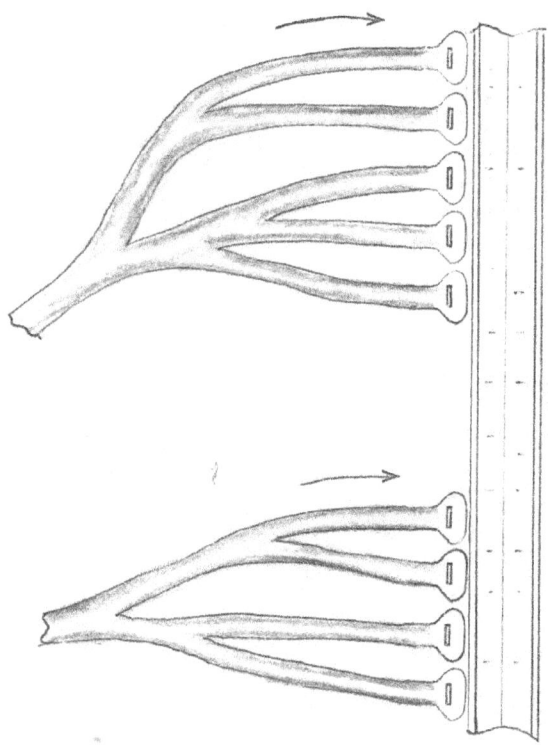

MEMBRANE OF THE
DOWNSTREAM CELL

Figure 66

the membrane is non-linear, and the negative contribution cannot

drive the membrane to cut-off.

Fig. 67 in an arrangement of summators and inverters to perform

an operation called "comparating". The signal

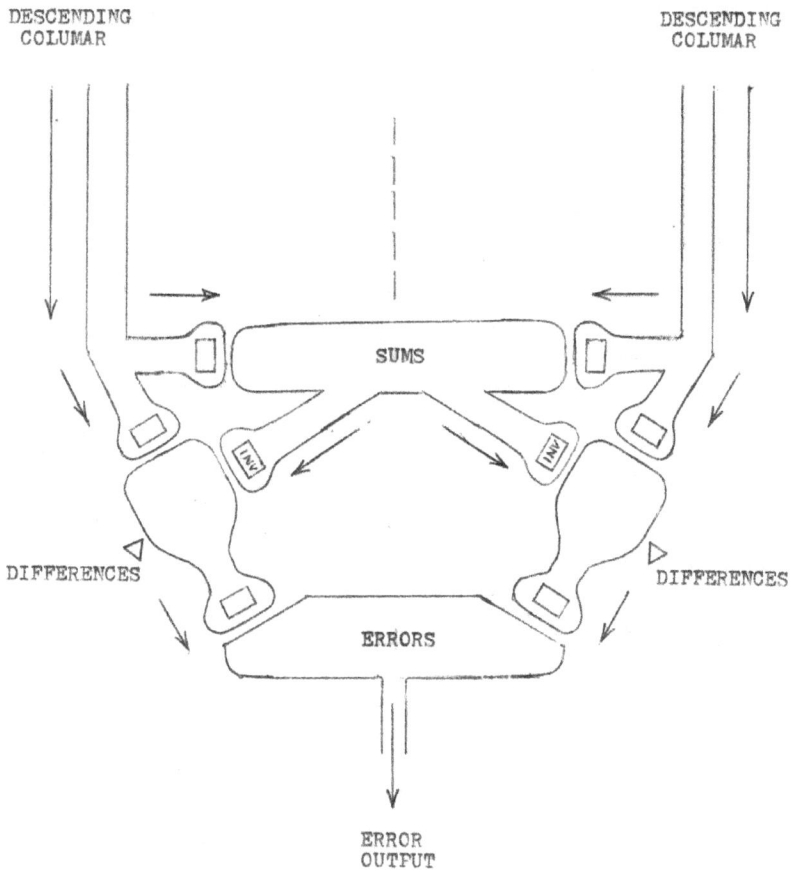

DESCENDING
COLUMAR

DESCENDING
COLUMAR

SUMS

INV

INV

DIFFERENCES

DIFFERENCES

ERRORS

ERROR
OUTPUT

Figure
67

descending from the columnar cell on the left moves toward the

center of the comparator where it will be compared with an opposing signal from the descending cell on the right. The vertical dashed line is the common interface at the midline of the comparator.

(In order to comply with the rule of uniform synapses: if one synapse has a memory unit, then all synapses in that cell must have them. There could be terminals in the comparator with memory units that are not strictly needed. The "differences" cell, which does not need memory units, is a case in point. If there are unneeded memory units, they do no harm because there is only one signal, regardless of its source, and it is uniformly distributed over the inner surface of the membrane. Within a given cell, the additional memory units raise the "Q" factor--flywheel effect-- of the memory system and help preserve synchronization of all memory units.)

This may not be the only comparator circuit possible in the living cortex because the circuit may double up on cell function which would require fewer cells. For purposes of expository, I will show the minimum number of cells necessary to get the job done step by step. Doubling cell functions makes the circuit harder to explain.

The signal coming from the left is compared to the signal on the right and, if they are of equal amplitude, the error output is zero. If there is an inequality, the error cell delivers an output which is a <u>function of the inequality</u>.

Fig. 68 is the same circuit as the previous sketch. Values for the signal amplitudes have been added at the input terminals and the comparator arithmetic is not complicated. The upper drawing shows no error output when the two inputs are equal. With unequal inputs, one of the "differences" cells will be driven to cut-off by the inverter and a difference, equal to the amplitude <u>difference</u> <u>between the two signals, will appear at the output</u>. <u>The error</u> <u>value is the difference between two signals</u>; <u>only the error is</u> <u>expressed at the comparator output: matched signals cancel and</u> <u>report no error</u>.

The apparatus in Fig. 68 and a couple of additional control cells make up the exalted data stage. The retrieval instruction and the memory response are presented "vis-a-vis" and, in effect, at the dashed line. With the vis-a-vis finesse, the fast and precise memory signals can be terminated in this stage and only the error signal needs to be sent to other parts of the cortex. The fast and precise signals delivered by memory will degrade if they are conveyed over great distances. The comparator circuit fits in with the several finesses of the exalted data stage.

The nerve tissue preparation has been mechanically sliced, vacuum dehydrated, metal plated or infused before the electron beam in the microscope gets a shot at it. The micro-architecture of the synapse is not easy to study; about

15 UNITS   EQUAL INPUTS   15 UNITS

+15   +15

$$\frac{15}{2} + \frac{15}{2}$$

+15   -15   -15   +15

0   0   0   0

0

9   19

+9   +19

$$\frac{9}{2} \qquad \frac{19}{2}$$

+9   -14   -14   +19

0   0   5   5

5

NEGATIVE BIAS EXCEEDS
POSITIVE BIAS AT THIS
CELL SO THIS CELL IS
CUTOFF

ARITHMETIC FOR THIS
CELL GOES:

$$\frac{19}{2} - \frac{14}{2} \times 2 = 5$$

THE ERROR OUTPUT
SIGNAL IS 5 UNITS

Figure
6̶0̶

all that can be seen is the wreckage of the synapse. In spite of

this problem, a good general understanding of the synaptic

mechanism has accumulated over the years.

THE NERVE CELL AS THE ACTIVE ELEMENT

Fig. 69 is a signal processing junction with its vesicles and supporting structure. The vesicles, collectively, are the emitter and the synaptic cleft is the anode. The plasma in the cleft is at grid voltage in this positive ground system. This is the electrical anode of the synaptic apparatus.

The physical structure of the anode has escaped the sight and wit of the microscopist. It could be a stiffened annular ring with most of the synapse opened to the cleft, or it could be a grid with generous openings in it. Cortical synapses contain memory units. About all the microscope will ever tell us is the suspected memory junction contains more wreckage than other synapses, if that much.

The anode and the emitter must be rigid enough so they will not distort or pull together under the influence of the electric field in the electrophoretic gradient. Microtubules are always found in the synaptic bulb and I show them in the drawing of the micro-architecture of the memory device used as spacers to fix the spacing between the structures in the synapse

The synaptic mechanism is a simple, dutiful servant and does several jobs at the same time. It has many facets and one of them is its function as a "buffer". In fired nerves, there is a translation from the pulse rate code to a chemical analogue at the synapse. For D.C. nerves, there is a voltage

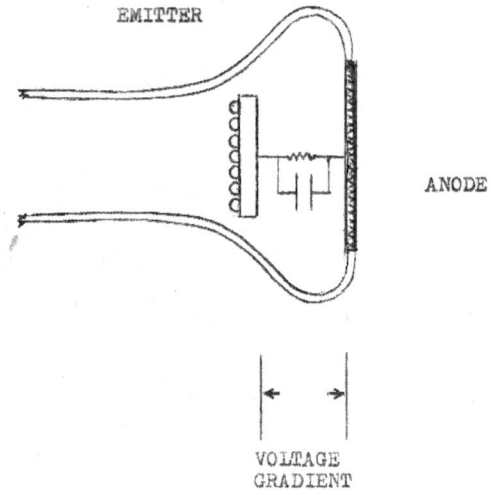

EMITTER

ANODE

VOLTAGE
GRADIENT

Figure 69

to current translation, and the emitter acts as an "emitter

follower" and prevents "blast-through" of pulses from an upstream

synapse so they do not penetrate the junction and add noise to the downstream nerve. It serves as a buffer for pulsed nerves too and prevents blast-through while it is translating the pulsed code back to the analogue format at the junction.

The capacitor (between arrows) in Fig. 70 is not a structure but an electrical equivalent of the emitter acting as one plate of a capacitor. The pulse code is translated back to a chemical current by the integrator capacitor within the junction. The chemical current is an analogue of the pulse rate. Everything to the left of the dashed line is in the pulsed format and, to the right of the line, in the D.C. chemical current format as the signal moves from left to right.

When the pulse train is impressed across the integrator capacitor, the capacitor charges to the amplitude of the pulse. There are resistors in the circuit and the resistor-capacitor time constant is so large the capacitor is unable to fully discharge during the serration, leaving a net charge on the capacitor. Alternating charge build-up during the serration and charge loss through the surrounding resistance paths will average the D.C. value which is always present at the integrator capacitor. The chemical current will be function of the D.C. voltage. The voltage, in turn, is a function of the pulse rate.

The D.C. values are shown opposite the pulse train in Fig. 71. The upper plot is a very slow pulse rate with the output

267

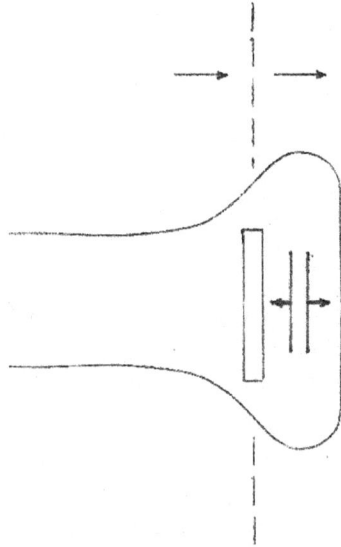

PULSE RATE CODE   D.C CHEMICAL CURRENT

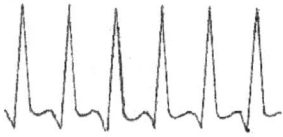

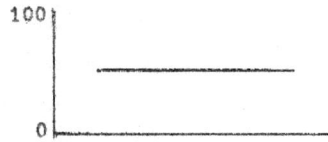

Figure
70

correspondingly small. The output graph shows "ripple". The

ripple is a remnant of the pulsed wave shape and is greatly

exaggerated in the drawing. The combination of high

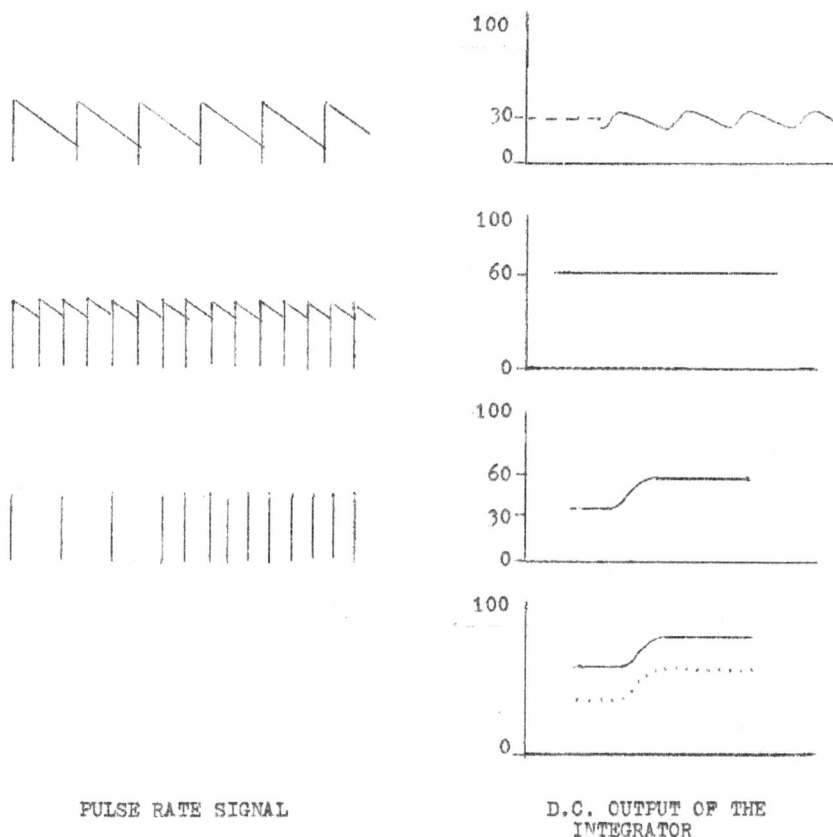

Figure 71

frequency pulses and the large integrator capacities tend to keep ripple at a minimum; it is probably not measureable.

The middle plot is a pulse train at a higher pulse rate and the output is plotted as a steady D.C. output. The lower wave train

259

starts at a low frequency and shifts to a higher firing rate; this is just what the wave train would look like if the leading edge of the "haystack" transient signal was passing through the junction. The D.C. voltage from the membrane is also superimposed on the integrator output. If the dotted line in the lower plot was the integrator output, the solid line above it would be the combined signal with the gradient D.C. superimposed. In this final translation, the pulse firing rate is translated to a chemical current and the signal, now in an analogue format, leaves the cell.

The item: "Estimating Memory Capacity" explained the need to have the memory device in the synapse. In Fig. 72, the middle element in the electrophoretic gradient is the memory device.

This element may be a perforated grid, or mask, with a memory molecule spanning each opening in the mask. Physically it may be closer to either the emitter or the anode, probably the anode, I will have it in the center of the gap, pending better knowledge. It too, must be held rigidly to prevent movement with variations in voltage. The memory grid will assume its voltage via the voltage divider resistors in the sketch. The plasma in the gradient provides the resistors.

There is an extra 20mv across the electrophoretic gradient that is not used for signal processing. The useable membrane

270

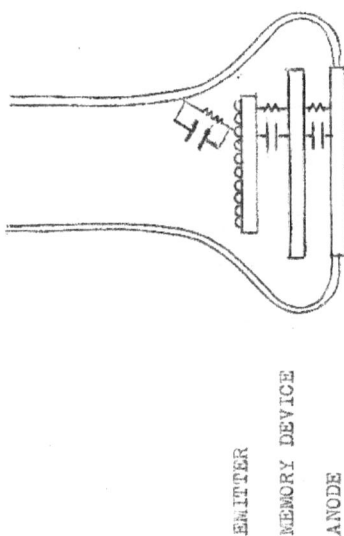

EMITTER

MEMORY DEVICE

ANODE

Figure 72

voltage is -70mv to -20mv. The voltage across the electrophoretic

gradient is -70mv to 0mv. The extra voltage may be used to assure

a pedestal current in the current path and a resting bias on the

memory mask.

Fig. 73 is the micro-architecture of the proposed memory device. The unkempt memory molecule strands are probably organized in an annular repository of some kind. Fig. 74 is a rung of forming memory molecule standing astride its opening in the perforated mask. The electric field, perhaps the extra 20mv, holds the molecule in position until the entry has been made and the control system orders the molecule to move the distance of one rung into the vault.

The data event is stored as a piezo-electric stress across the rung on the memory molecule. On delivery, the data event moves backward down the stationary molecule toward the entry position. The piezo-electric field of the data event controls the chemical current through the respective opening in the mask. If the electric field of the data event, working alone, is able to control the current through the opening, and I think it is, no external energy supply is needed to supply the memory system. If this is the case, we have a "non-destructive read-out". Digital computers often erase the data event on read-out and make up for the loss by re-entering it immediately after it was read-out.

The signal voltage excursion is translated to a chemical current and the current is fractionated into 3000, or so, smaller currents which are entered on the respective memory molecules in "parallel".

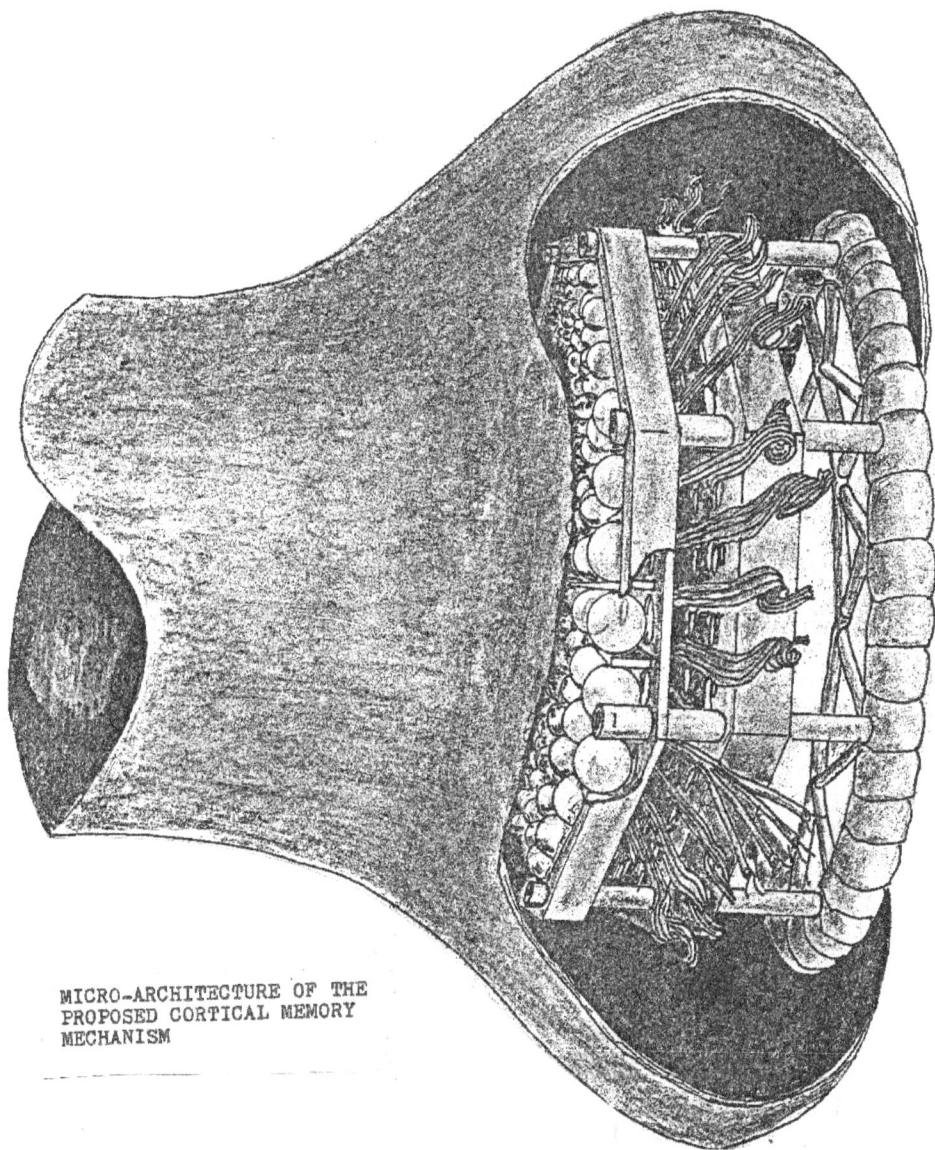

MICRO-ARCHITECTURE OF THE
PROPOSED CORTICAL MEMORY
MECHANISM

Figure
73

(I keep looking for some prints   n micro-photography that

would indicate the number of vesicles in the vesicular apparatus.

I found one which looked like two or

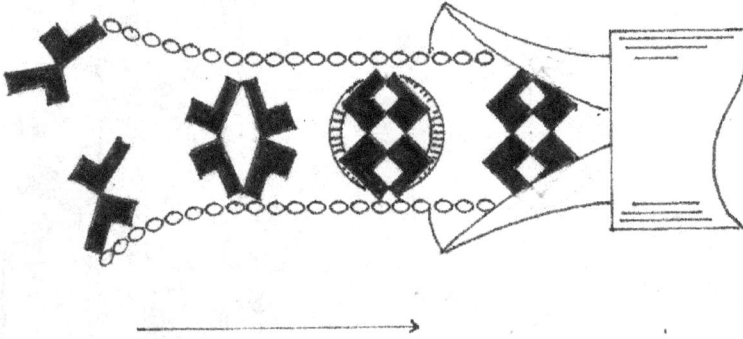

Figure

three wedged shaped pieces of pie left on the plate after most of

the pie had been eaten. I am not able to tell if there were 6 or 8

wedges to begin with. There could have been 3000 vesicles at a minimum and a possible 4800 at the most. With 3000-5000 vesicles,

it is a precision apparatus and there are as many strands of memory

molecule as there are vesicles. There also seems to be a type of

synapse with several hundred vesicles.)

On the memory "deliver" command, memory delivery is initiated at

the same instant for all memory molecule strands. The time

required to move the data event one position, or a given number, of

positions, on memory delivery, though quite short, is uniform and

invariant. All memory units in the cell will be delivering the

same element in the same data plane because they all initiate

delivery at the same instant. The "Q" factor, or "fly-wheel"

factor, preserves synchrony of the scattered memory units

throughout the memory delivery cycle.

Now we have the problem of controlling the memory molecule.

There is no "handle", no special terminal on the cell that goes

directly to the memory device and is capable of controlling it.

The cortical cell is a special type of D.C. (only) cell. It does

fire, but the firing mode is externally controlled and used in a

separate and distinctly different process that supervises the

enter/deliver cycle of the memory device.

(Here again, a special operation must be brought off with only

the extant characteristics of the nerve cell to do it with. The

membrane of the cortical cell may be slightly thicker than most

excitable cells, giving it a larger usable D.C. signal excursion.

The intrinsic firing rate may be less than 10 firings per second.

The cell is normally fired from an external source. If the

external commands fail to pace the cell, it will exercise itself at its residual rate. If all the cells in the lobe fire at the residual rate, it is the "alpha" exercise of the lobe. The alpha exercise is discussed later.)

The external memory control signal (firings) must be superimposed on the D.C. (analogue) signal. There are no alternatives to this way of doing things. The memory unit, isolated in the micro-universe of the synapse, cannot be broached by any other means.

The memory unit is to be found in one of three states:

1. In its inactive state, the memory unit is "following" the ups and downs of the D.C. analogue signal. As the chemical current flows through the opening in the mask, the piezo-electric stress at the rung follows the signal modulations of current flow.

2. The traditional view of the electrotonic junction was based on the idea the pulse from an upstream cell was to "blast through" the junction and become a factor in downstream firings. This idea is dealt a final blow in the summary of this item. Now, the thing to do is to reinvent the idea as it should properly be done.

I think there is an "avalanching" synapse of the vesiculated kind, rather than the electrotonic synapse with no vesicles. It probably contains fewer, but larger, vesicles than the precision synapse. The sync pulse is forced on the cortical cell via the avalanching synapse and the pulse sense is positive or "excitatory". Potassium ion current in the accepting cell is also avalanched (driven to saturation) and its membrane is immediately forced into "mode shift" and the membrane fires.

The memory unit has been "following" the D.C. signal up to the instant of forced firing. The D.C. signal amplitude has been continuously impressed on the memory unit and signal amplitude at the instant of firing is the amplitude permanently fixed on the memory molecule. An instantaneous sampling of the D.C. amplitude has been "chopped" from the normally continuous D.C. signal, fixed and entered in memory in the D.C. "event" format. All that is needed to "fix" the memory entry is a rapid advancement of the memory molecule(s) during the front porch of the firing.

The minute sequence of events at the grid can only be guessed at. When the mask is positive with respect to the emitter, the voltage between the emitter and the mask could hold the memory molecule in position over the opening in the mask. The capacity effect of the mask will not permit the mask to assume a new voltage rapidly (during the .5 millisecond front porch). A sudden positive swing of the emitter voltage will temporarily reverse the emitter to mask voltage. For a very short interval, the emitter will be positive with respect to the mask. The negative voltage which holds the memory molecule over the opening is removed and the memory molecule advances one position.

3. On memory delivery, the memory molecule "dumps the tape" while it is scanning for a data plane that will match the retrieval instruction. When the data plane is reached and the match is confirmed, the cell fires and the data event is entered in memory. The control signal that controls memory delivery must also be superimposed on the D.C. analogue processing function of the cortical cell. Here we have another avalanching synapse to control memory delivery. The physical synapse is probably the same as the "fire" synapse, only this time the neuro-transmitter chemical is

inhibitory. A microscopic flood of this neuro-transmitter cuts off potassium ion current through the membrane and the membrane voltage goes to -70mv, nullifying the D.C. analogue voltage. The potassium ion is not present inside the membrane, the pumping action does not up-pace and the cell does not fire. At maximum current, the rung over the opening is stressed in such a way that the remaining rungs will relieve their own piezo-electric stress by passing it along the memory molecule delivering it to the unformed rung over the opening in the mask. The piezo-electric voltage appears across the rung in the opening and the voltage modulates the steady and otherwise un-modulated flow of chemical neuro-transmitter.

In order to self-reinforce entries, there has to be a reciprocity between the voltage and the formation of the rung in the opening. This time, the about-to-be-formed rung is "following" the voltage delivered by the memory molecule, and, at the instant of firing (dictated by external command) the stress in the rung is fixed and the memory molecule advances one position, removing the molecule from the opening and closing out the formative process. The data event or the data plane just delivered is reentered in memory.

The memory molecule is the most speculative component in the system, if we need to be reminded. If it functions the way I have it here, it should have a tremendous delivery rate. We can concede the memory delivery rate is on the order of a billion data events per second. A more accurate estimate requires a tradeoff between the three factors involved: the total amount of data in storage, the rate it is delivered and the length of time the cortex can be paused for scanning.

THE NERVE CELL AS THE ACTIVE ELEMENT

Fig. 75 is the "enter" command from the control system. It is superimposed on the D.C. analogue signal. Only the front porch, and the leading edge of the front porch at that, is pertinent here. The rise rate is so fast, and is immediately

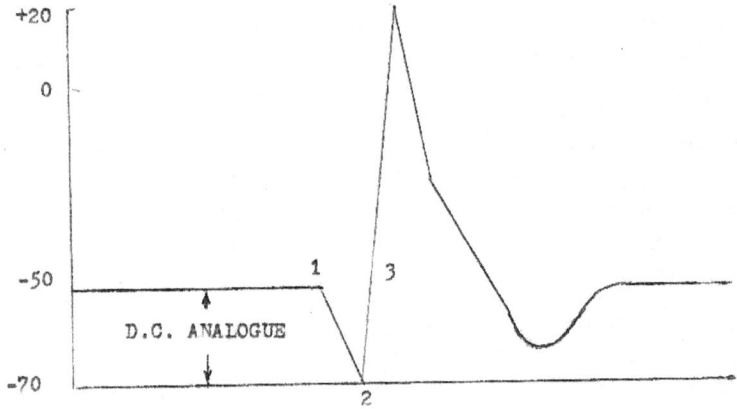

Figure 75

followed by a rise rate in the opposite direction, that it does not

add or subtract anything from the D.C. analogue. The reverse is

also true: the D.C. signal cannot precipitate a memory entry. It doesn't because it would require the D.C. system to convey a signal well beyond its high frequency roll off.

Fig. 76 is the memory "deliver" command from the control system. There is no interference between the D.C. analogue and the control signal because the membrane is cut off during the command to scan and because the signal amplitude excursion limits prevent the D.C. analogue signal initiating "deliver" command.

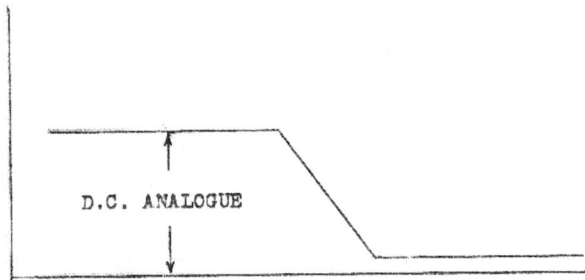

Figure 76

THE NERVE CELL AS THE ACTIVE ELEMENT

SUMMARY OF THE ITEM ON THE NERVE CELL AS THE ACTIVE ELEMENT

1. The real and practical aspects of acupuncture, more modest than sometimes claimed, derive from the very real and practical aspects of the Automatic Sensitivity Control systems that overlay the perceptual systems. We will take a quick look at automatic sensitivity control first, followed by acupuncture.

In addition to the on-axis movement and processing of the specific data in the throughput, nerve cells are also found in control and supervisory service. In general, supervisory cells are structurally the same as specific data cells, varying only in the specialization of their assignments. There may be exceptions, the control cell with the avalanching terminals is a case in point.

Automatic sensitivity control (ASC) is one of these special assignments. Light, sound, tactile stimulus ranges in intensity from barely perceptible to nearly unbearable. The problem of making the perceptual systems linear, given the wide range of signal amplitudes, is managed with transducers of extreme sensitivity (for weak stimuli) combined with a massive automatic sensitivity control program to reduce sensitivity when the sensor is exposed to intense excitation.

The ASC signal, the signal which turns down the system sensitivity, is a function of the amplitude of the raw excitation and it matches the amplitude to, and within, the amplitude handling capability of the downstream cell.

The sensor is at the front end of the data bus and ASC is applied as close to the front end as possible, <u>at</u> the sensor or even <u>ahead</u> of the sensor array in systems incorporating mechanical ASC. (As the item on the coder explains, mechanical, chemical and electronic ASC schemes can be overlaid. The thing to do with automatic sensitivity control is to "get it over with", up front, at the input, where it will be most effective. This applies to off the shelf electronic equipment as well as the nervous system.)

ASC circuits are fairly simple but there is a pitfall we must be alerted to. In Fig. 77, we have a closed loop with all of the cells delivering outputs in the "positive" or "excitory" sense. This circuit is a forbidden circuit (it is a "delta" circuit because it resembles the greek letter). In this sort of loop, the smallest disturbance in one cell is passed on to the next cell and so on around the loop. The loop will now generate a self excited oscillation and is, as a matter of fact, a "ring oscillator". No such circuits exist in the nervous system and anti-oscillation measures perfuse the nervous system about as much as anti-noise measures. (Some texts refer to "reverberating" circuits. There is nothing like this in the nervous system.) A circuit with three legs forming a triangle is permitted in the nervous

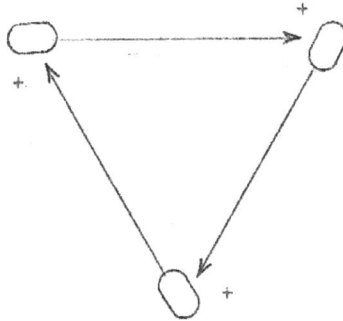

FORBIDDEN "DELTA" CIRCUIT

Figure 77

system only if one of the legs is negative--nullifying the oscillation problem.

Fig. 78 is the classis ASC layout. It is a delta circuit but one of the legs is negative so it does not oscillate.

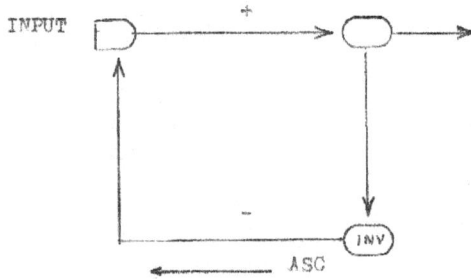

Figure 78

This circuit is represented in the nervous system by the mechanical ASC systems: the iris and the tensor tympani. It is more typical of manufactured electronic gear.

THE NERVE CELL AS THE ACTIVE ELEMENT

In Fig. 78, the input signal begins its stage by stage movement down the data bus. Somewhere downstream of the input, a sampling of the signal amplitude is picked off, inverted, and fed back to control the sensitivity of the input. This is "all electronic" ASC and, while it is a feasible use of nerve cells, it is not used in the nervous system because there is a much better way to do this job.

Fig. 79 expresses the belief the array for cutaneous sensors is processed through a coder about the same as any other coder. The bottom half of the drawing is the familiar and perhaps "standard" coder we found in the rest of the perceptual systems. This coder erects an electrical replica of the tactile "image". There is probably more than one coder somatesthetic perception and at least one coder will process cutaneous pain signals. The upper half of Fig. 79 is a special overlaying ASC circuit with its own receptors for sampling the intensity of stimulus and its own paths to control the sensitivity of the coder (dashed lines). The intensity of the stimulus is sampled and a consensus is agreed on with regard to adjusting sensitivity on a local basis.

The drawing has the ASC control signal impressed on the extant inverter cells in the coder. The chances are, the ASC network

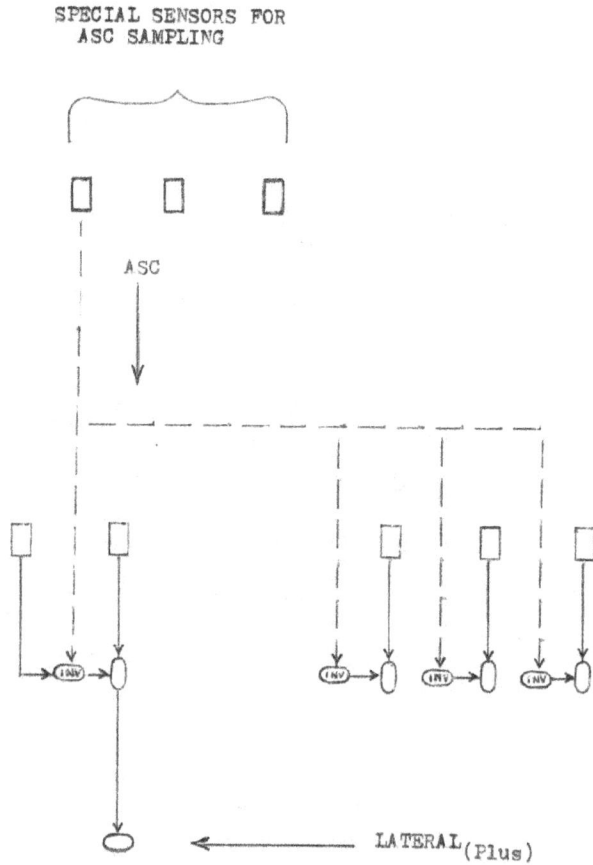

SPECIAL SENSORS FOR
ASC SAMPLING

ASC

LATERAL$_{(Plus)}$

Figure 79

incorporates its own inverter cells in a lateral elaboration of the

network. Configured this way, the ASC system functions as an

operational equivalent to the "span wise" automatic sensitivity control we found in other coders. Local ASC is a consensus of local stimulus and enters in the arithmetic as a reference signal.

ASC can have its own inverter cells or it can use extant inverters, or both, ASC synapses probably have "advantaged" proportioning so sensitivity is reduced at a slightly faster rate than the intensity of the stimulus increases.

Working through inverters, or through ASC cells with inverter output terminals, the ASC network is always in keeping with "delta" circuit rules. The scope and incisiveness of ASC authority can be greatly enhanced if the distal insertion in Fig. 79 is also allowed to penetrate deeper parts of the network, perhaps as deep as the spinal ganglia level. This can be done anywhere along the data buses and still be in keeping with delta circuit rules.

Further downstream insertions expand ASC control over the dermatome and expand local referencing to the level of the dermatome. (A dermatome is the area of skin innervated by the fiber bundles from one segment of the spinal nerve. Typically, for torso innervation, it is a band about three inches wide, coursing around the torso more or less like a belt. It originates at the spine and terminates in front at the midline of the body where it meets an identical band from the other half of the body. The "fan-in" the segment of the spinal nerve is one or two vertebrae higher than the dermatome.)

The tactile systems are not easy to study and the experimenters and tissue studies people have yet to answer a number of questions. To make things worse, there are two kinds of circuits in these systems: specific data circuits and control (ASC) circuits contra-

invested in the same nerve embedments all over the body. The study of pain sensing in the skin seems to produce more questions than it does answers. There is always the question of how much raw percepta contributes to our appreciation of pain and how much of it is based on habit and expectation.

(There have been surgeries for people who suffer from chronic intense pain. Fibers running from the lower brain to the cortex are severed: I don't know the site of the cut. After surgery, the patient reports the pain is still there, however, it no longer bothers him. He no longer pays attention to it.)

Also in connection with "subjective" versus "real" tactile sensing, some textbooks mention a "phasic" aspect to somaesthetic perception. A "phasic" activity has an onset, a plateau and a decay, and contrasts with a "cyclic" activity which is repetitive. We put on a wrist watch and, for a while, we are aware of it touching our skin. A little time passes, and our awareness of the watch seems to fade away. Some texts believe this is a "phasic" desensitization of the cutaneous tactile receptors.

This is a wrong opinion as far as I am concerned. The de-sensitization is much too distal from the cortex for safety. I think the desensitization is a cortical "feature extrication" or "feature suppression" strategy, The cortex becomes saturated with the repetitive stimulus and the parietal lobe tries to find more interesting things to feel.

A sensor, clearly a pain sensor, has not been located in the skin. I will take it upon myself to recommend the extant dedicated receptors, each dedicated to its own assignment, will become pain receptors when uncommon excitation (or over-excitation) drives it into a higher signal level operating regimen. With normal excitation, we subjectively appreciate the output of the receptor as its indigenous output: touch, temperature and so on. When driven into an unusually intense and infrequently occurring operating regimen, we habitually appreciate the output as pain, pain which has been "signed" with the indigenous character of the receptor. I see the pain detector system as a doubled usage of the already extant skin receptor system(s).

Acupuncture does suppress pain and the only equipment needed to account for this is the "feed forward" and "advantaged" ASC system and the mechano-receptor in the skin. (The classis ASC scheme in Fig. 78 is a "feedback" system.)

The horny layer of skin is an electrical, thermal, chemical and mechanical insulator between the nerve endings just beneath the skin and the crudities of the outside world. The horny layer is a massive signal attenuator permanently interposed between the stimulus on the outside and the transducers within. The microscopic mechano-receptor is suspended in this fairly rigid semi-plastic matrix. When the skin in mechanically disturbed, the receptor must deform slightly in order to translate the disturbance into its electrical analogue. Without breaking the skin or concentrating stresses in the skin by extraordinary means, this is a sort of mechanical improbability, something like deforming an apple seed by squeezing the outside of the apple. The mechano-receptor almost has to be an extremely sensitive transducer if it generates its output from outside disturbances that are so loosely coupled and so severely attenuated to begin with.

When the acupuncture stylus penetrates the outer layer of skin, the attenuator is bypassed and the microscopic domain of the sensor invaded by this now efficiently coupled and relatively enormous disturbance. Both the pain sensors and the ASC sensors are over-excited. The over-excited ASC system turns down the sensitivity of the pain system it is controlling. Sensitivity is reduced almost to the point of cut off and {minimally) the skin in the vicinity of the stylus is insensitive to further stimulus, even if it is quite intense.

Acupuncture comes to its maximum pain deadening effectiveness about ten minutes after its initial application and pain continues to be deadened for 20 minutes after the removal of the stylus. Evidently acupuncture involves two pain suppression processes: one fast enough to act in real time and an overlying and lingering process about which nothing is known. Some theorists think the delayed process is attributable to a chemical which is released in response to the pain stimulus and which requires a certain amount of time to have its fullest effect. As an alternative to this, I think the cutaneous receptors, and possibly downstream nerves, are driven into saturation conduction and held at maximum signal level for a period of time so long the cell's metabolic power supply cannot keep up with the extra demand for sustained operation at this unusually intense signal level.

The key to acupuncture is an overdriven ASC system and, artfully used, it should be an effective pain deadener. Given time and a willingness to develop the art, acupuncture may someday become the anesthesia of choice in surgical procedures where it is applicable. Acupuncture has no demonstrated therapeutic value and if it ever does it will be in connection with a nerve related dysfunction.

The smallest possible stylus should be used and the stylus insertion should be intradermal, between and parallel to the layers of skin. I have no idea what the straight-in stylus is supposed to accomplish. A pulsed voltage makes the technique more effective. Several styli can be used and they should be positioned so the nerve tracts between the styli and the spinal ganglia are not severed when the incision is made.

Whatever value acupuncture may have as a home remedy can be realized by digging the thumbnail into the skin, avoiding a bleeding and infection hazard. Pressing to the point of pain, a thumbnail dug into the web of skin between the thumb and forefinger will end light transient headache.

CONTINUING THE SUMMARY OF THE NERVE CELL AS THE ACTIVE ELEMENT

Here are the things I see as the main bottlenecks to understanding the nerve cell as the active electronic element.

1. The excitable membrane is a mechanism with a half dozen key parameters to be reconciled with sustaining cell vitality on the one hand and with the membrane as an active electronic element on the other. A resounding declaration of the signal format, a clear and emphatic view of the signal being expressed as an analogue, is, somehow, always just around the corner. There has been a

proliferation of models and still a problem of accounting for the parameters that compel the pulse rate to follow the analogue signal. (I am showing my own model where the sodium ion power supply is the common element coupling the D.C. analogue to the pulse rate code.)

2. The experimenters probe irritates the nerve, rendering it hyper-sensitive. The hyper-sensitive nerve has a way of sprinkling the text books with all sorts of exotic wave forms, some of which are in fact exotic and others a matter of probe artifact. We have to be able to sort out the wit and craft of the experimenters' laboratory and separate it from a few of the experimenters gaucheries and indiscretions.

3. Contributions from the electronic experts have been grand in concept but lacked a lot in practicality. The tendency is to dabbling and, for something that needs hard study, no one is willing to set down and dig in. There are a few things the tissue studies people cannot do, at least not very well. The seasoned electronics specialist should have studied the nerve mechanism to the extent needed to point out the system is an analogue system and the pulse rate code, the biggest and most unnecessary bottleneck of them all, is strictly an ancillary issue. It takes study, but a lot of the circuit can be worked out without knowing all of the parameters of membrane firing. The noise immunity procedure I discussed earlier should have been worked out. The electrotonic junction has been a conceptual obstruction for far too many years and long overdue for removal. A little wisdom, a little conviction should have alerted someone to the implausibility of the

electrotonic junction as a data processing terminal. Fig. 80
explains the reasoning.

The electrotonic junction in Fig. 80 is thought to be a "brute
force" synapse where a pulse from an up stream nerve "blasts"
through the junction and lands in the midst of the pulses being
generated in the downstream cell.

The instant of landing would have to be carefully controlled. If
the outlander pulse landed in the serration between pulses, it
would appear in the downstream arithmetic. If it landed on another
pulse or during the refractory interval following the pulse,
Nothing would happen. The instant of landing is not, and cannot,
be controlled.

I think ions, in Brownian motion, bombard the nerve membrane and
the compressive force squeezes it, reducing its porosity and
increasing its resistance. This would account for the "ancillary"
parameter where current is a function of resistance, which in turn
is a function of voltage. The idea appeals to me: though it needs
careful scrutiny. The compressible membrane may account for a few
experimenters artifacts in addition to its normal behavior as the
active element.

There is a type of probe made from a glass tube which has been
heated and stretched to a very slim diameter (about 50

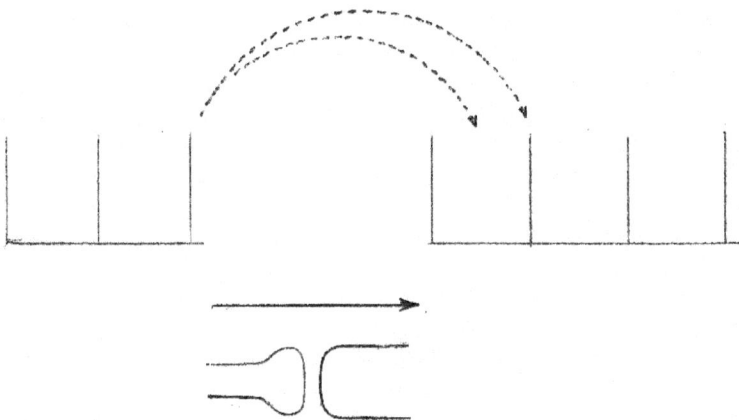

Figure 80

microns). The center conductor within the probe is externally

supplied electrolyte. The probe is pushed up the axon and it unavoidably deforms the membrane mechanically. Any deformation can only stretch the membrane.

The nerve cell membrane is the active element and it must perform with constant precision and invariant parameters. In experiments where the probe stretches the membrane, stretching makes it thinner which changes its resistance and it becomes more permeable to ions. The precise calibration of the membrane has been destroyed.

The bottom of Fig. 81 is a wave train that turns up in a few text books. The probe has lowered membrane resistance and there is an uncontrolled invasion of potassium ions. The abnormal concentration of potassium ions will surely trigger a run-away up-pacing of the sodium ion power supply and the nerve becomes (electronically) hyper-sensitive. Instead of generating a precisely controlled train of pulses, the nerve breaks into self-excited oscillation. The membrane is a low "Q" device. It does not oscillate at a single frequency but oscillates through an arpeggio of the frequencies it is capable of generating. This is called "squegging". ("Squegging" is correctly spelled and rhymes with wedging. If this wave train was amplified by a sound system, it would sound like cricket chirps.)

Fig. 82 is the worst version of the same problem. Initially the amplitude of the pulsed firing is normal but the firing rate is so high when it is squegging, the metabolic power supply fails to supply the energy needed to sustain oscillation. After a burst of squegging, the

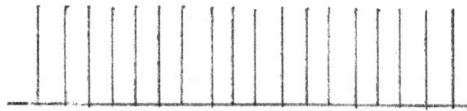

NORMAL

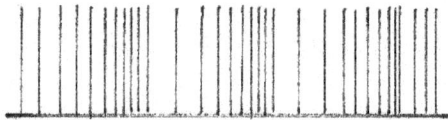

SQUEGGING

Figure 81

membrane ceases to fire. This paused firing of the membrane is

sometimes erroneously referred to as a "refractory interval". This

is not a natural refractory interval; it is an artifact of probe interference.   I think there is only one

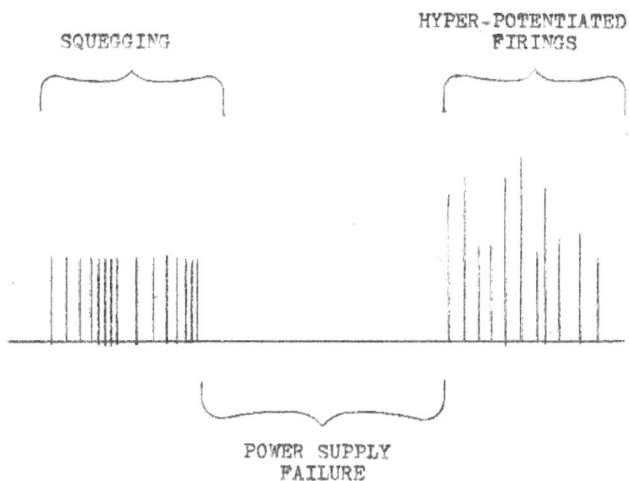

Figure 82

"legal" refractory interval, the back porch of the pulse.   (The

membrane cannot be fired for about .5 millisecond after the spike.

If there are additional "natural" refractory intervals in

vertebrate nervous systems, they have to be explained
individually.)

During the power supply failure, the power supply was unable to
supply the energy needed to equilibrate the surplus of potassium
ions and, at the same time, raise voltages enough to fire the leaky
membrane in the system to provide a reference which will assure the
system will stay in calibration. A calibrated energy source, long
term is necessary because all of the parameters are interdependent
and the calibrated power supply will calibrate sensitivity and the
rest of the parameters will fall into place as needed. (The
precision membrane will not tolerate mechanical distortion,
chemical invaders that change the resistance of the membrane, or
paused intervals. All of the forgoing, defeat the always needed,
always constant, calibration of the system.)

Keeping the cell vital, keeping it paced and calibrated is
probably something of an art in itself. Signal processing keeps
the cell paced, without it the cell will languish and certain types
of cells will die. The photo-receptor and the hair cell in the
organ of Corti would seem to be special cases of this problem. The
photoreceptor has to be able to survive the pause from closing the
eyes and remain calibrated and the hair cell in the organ of Corti
has its variation of the same problem. Perhaps these cells have a
"repose", or "keep alive", pacing that preserves calibration during
the time interval they are un-stimulated. (It may be the
hyperbaric therapy for deafness up-paces the "keep alive" pacing to
a higher pacing capable of supplying the slight surplus of energy
for signal processing.)

THE NERVE CELL AS THE ACTIVE ELEMENT

The cortical cell has special calibration problems due to a couple of odd factors in the way it is used;

1. The cell is fired externally and by brute force without regard for the cells' indigenous and dedicated calibration. The control system selects the time of firing and firing is independent of the ongoing D.C. potassium ion current parameters and their attendant energy requirements.

2. The firing rate of the cortical cell is quite slow, say, 10 to 40 firings per second with an average in between. Primary metabolic pacing is complicated by the need to fire the cell hear its high speed rate for some time, say, a substantial fraction of a second. Following this burst of high speed running, the cell may be abruptly switched to running at, or near, its slowest rate and for a period of time that cannot be predicted in advance. Primary pacing cannot down-pace during slow speed running because the cell may be called upon to instantly jump from slow speed running to high speed without time delay or provision to recalibrate metabolic pacing for the transition. Having jumped to high speed, metabolic pacing must be fully prepared to sustain the higher firing rate, again for an unpredictable period of time.

The cortical cell is not down-paced for slow speed running. Metabolic pacing is paced for high speed running regardless of the running speed, it has to be. The cell is always hyper-paced for slow running and the sodium ion pump builds up a surplus of sodium ions outside of the cell membrane during extended periods of slow firing. After a period of slow running, the membrane becomes hyper-potentiated. Hyper-potentiated, it is hyper sensitive and it begins to oscillate. The cortical cell, with its thicker membrane, does not squegg. Instead, it fires a series of "one shot" self-excited oscillations to "burn off" the excessive accumulation of sodium ions. The "one shot" firing is repeated 10 to 20 times per second and the bursts of equalizing pulses will appear intermittently, and as often as necessary, until the cortex shifts back to high speed running. It shifts to high speed as minute to minute experience requires. The slow running brain is in reverie.

The cortex executes these extra firings; it is "exercised", and only after a period of slow running, for the specific purpose of equalizing the buildup of surplus ions across the membrane. The equalizing firings can be detected with scalp electrodes and their rhythmic patterns are useful in diagnosing brain dysfunction. Five groups of firings are recognized and each group is designated with a letter of the Greek alphabet. Frequencies vary from less than three cycles to about 24 cycles. (Slow waves, three cycles or less, indicate the lobe is dead under the scalp electrode. This is about the limit as an aid to diagnosis of brain dysfunction.) Eight to twelve cycle waves are common and called Alpha waves; the "alpha exercise" of the cortex.

The reason the firings take place at one frequency on one occasion and a different frequency some time later has been something of a mystery. I will pass along my opinion.

The sketch (Fig. 83) has a hemisphere of the cortex adjusted to a watermelon shape. The large hatched area in the area of the lobe being monitored by the scalp electrode. Hyper-potentiation has been going on for some time and the most hyper-potentiated, that is, the least recently fired, cells begin to execute their one-shot firings (in groups of 8 to 10 firings).

A first cell, or a few cells, will initiate the cycle of extra firings. These are the _least_ recently fired cells and they "nucleate" a wave front of firings which begins to propagate through the hemisphere. The drawing shows the surface component of the wave on its way from the site of nucleation to the monitored area.

The concentric lines represent the crests of a couple of waves to be followed with the next six or eight waves of the

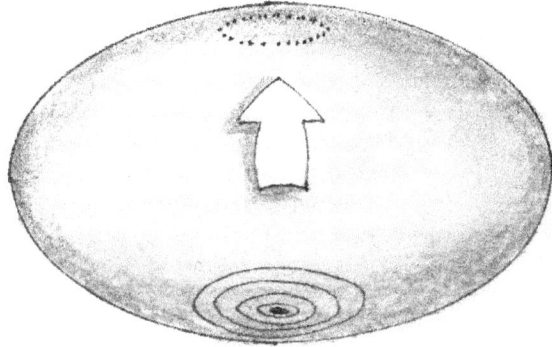

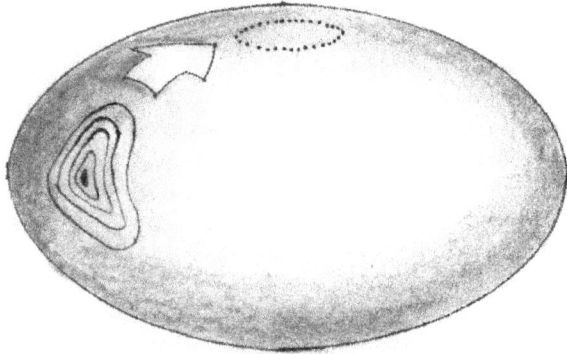

Figure 83

alpha burst. Pacing does not vary within the series of waves.

These are over-voltage firings because the cell membrane is

hyper-potentiated. The over-voltage pulse is communicated to an immediate neighbor cell by the "cross talk" process. (Cross talk coupling between cells can result from A.C. capacity effects; any D.C. conduction path will carry the pulse, or coupling can be made with the sudden removal of ions from a common pool of ions outside of the cells. Cross talk immunity is predicated for pulses of normal amplitude and the normal on axis movement of the signal. Even the electrotonic junction, in its normal service as part of the crosstalk immunity system, may, in a wrongly executed usage, contribute to coupling these pulses between cells.)

The least recently fired cells, those that initiated the first wave, will again be the first to build up hyper-potentiation and the first to begin a new round of firings. The wave front dissipates at one extreme of its travel only to be re-nucleated at the original starting site. Starting at the same site and traveling a uniform distance accounts for the rhythmic nature of the "alpha exercise".

The site of nucleation will move from one area to another because the site of the least recently fired cells will vary with the task the cortex has been working at. This presents a variation in the cortical volume the wave front must traverse and is responsible for "exercising" at one frequency part of the time and another frequency at another time.

(The cells in the lobe are connected with a "sync" bus and are committed to fire synchronously. The wave front probably nucleates and begins moving as we have it thus far, but, when the wave front reaches the nearest exalted data stage, the firing mode translates and all of the remaining cells in the lobe fire synchronously.)

The memory mechanism cannot be turned off during the equalizing exercise of the lobe because there is no way to distinguish between the "exercise" pulse and the control pulse. It would be ill advised to turn the memory off because the memory units are synchronized and they would all have to start operating at the same instant, following a shutdown, to prevent de-synchronization of the individual memory units. (The reasons are a little clearer after a look at the cortex in the sleep mode.)

Since the memory unit cannot be shut off, it must make an entry when the cell is fired and this includes alpha firings. When the exalter fires during the alpha exercise, the memory units make an extra copy (an anomalous copy) of the preceding data plane. Since the cortex is in reverie, contrasted with running in "real-time" with a "real" assignment, the extra and anomalous data plane will not adduce an operational problem.

The extra data plane places a fiduciary mark on the memory molecule. (Fiduciary refers to trust. The marks on a yard stick are fiduciary marks.) The extra data plane functions as a fiduciary mark because all of the individual memory units, collectively participating in a memory scan, will either stop on, or pass, the extra data plane synchronously. Here, we have marked a data position of the memory tape which will always receive uniform treatment by all memory units at the same instant. It will either be a uniform "pass" or a uniform "stop". "Passing" is the more likely case. The operational uniformity at this mark will tend to "pull" the memory units into synchronization. The mark draws an operational relationship between the information on the tape and the scanning process.

3. The chemical neurotransmitter cannot be permitted to move around, as it will, in the axoplasm of the nerve cell. In the upper left of Fig. 84, the chemical neurotransmitter was released by the synapse of the upstream cell, a routine process at the synapse. In this fictitious drawing, it penetrated the axoplasm of the downstream cell and is free to roam around at random and, in this case, it is adding chemical noise to the output of the downstream cell.

In the second drawing, the chemical neurotransmitter is manufactured by a hypothetical organelle within the cell plasma. This is also prohibited.

In the bottom drawing, the neurotransmitter is leaking, out of one electrophoretic apparatus and drifting in the cell plasma where it is a potential source of chemical "noise" if it found its way into another synapse in the same cell. The chemical current flowing in the electrophoretic mechanism is

306

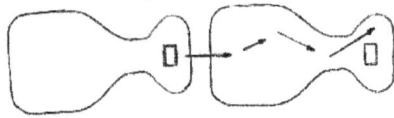

FORBIDDEN TERRITORY
FOR THE CHEMICAL
NEUROTRANSMITTER

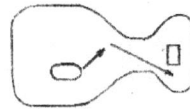

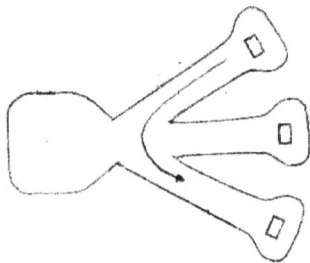

Fig 81

Figure 84

precisely controlled. The release of neurotransmitter is measured

in molecular quantities within the apparatus and stray

neurotransmitter, in the smallest amounts, would destroy the calibration of the synaptic mechanism.

Profound measures are needed to remove this problem. The enzyme known to dissolve the neurotransmitter is also known to reside in the cell axoplasm. This gets rid of the stray neurotransmitter but, in so doing, it prevents the manufacture of neurotransmitter within the nerve cell. The remarkable mechanism in Fig. 85 may keep free neurotransmitter out of the cell and at the same time supply the vesicular apparatus by a routine that is topologically outside of the cell. The neurotransmitter is manufactured by supporting cells and processes external to the nerve cell. The neurotransmitter chemical perfuses the interstitial serums and is "harvested" from the fluid surround by a process called "Pinocytosis". "Pinocytosis" is a combination of "drink" and "cell").

The short lines in the upper drawing are to suggest the membrane near the synaptic cleft is "normal" cell membrane, rather than the excitable kind. The cell membrane folds in and forms a pouch, and I do not think this can be done with excitable membrane without disturbing its calibration. The pouch closes at its neck forming a vesicle which is free to move in the cell plasma. Restrained in this manner, the neurotransmitter is insulated from both the cell enzymes and the electrophoretic gradient. The "come along" mechanism that loads the vesicle (or its charge) into the vesicular apparatus is unknown.

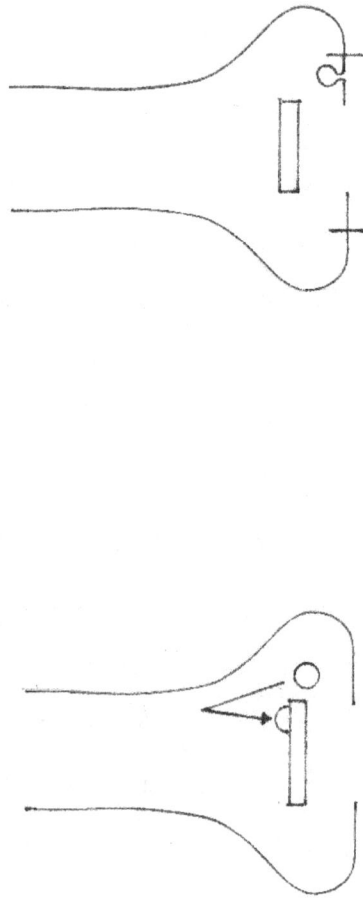

Figure 85

I am not qualified to manage the chemistry of neurotransmitter. I can pass along a few points that impress me. As many as 20 chemicals have been reported to be neurotransmitter. For signal

processing, we only need two, one with a positive or "excitory"
sense and one that is negative or "inhibitory". It is thought
sleep is induced by a chemical inhibitor that might inhibit at the
cortical synapse. One would think a special neurotransmitter would
be needed in this service which would account for a couple of
neurotransmitters on the list. I have a hunch about 15 of the 20
chemical are a part of a chemical noise immunity program and
perhaps alternately activate or neutralize the proprietary
neurotransmitter. They may function on a cyclic basis and, say,
protect the active neurotransmitter while it is in the synaptic
gradient and then immediately quench it after it has completed its
cycle as a neurotransmitter. (It cannot linger in the cleft. If
it did, one signal excursion would be inseparable from the next.)
A better understanding of the neurotransmitter is not a key issue
as far as moving the analogue signal down the data bus is
concerned. It is only significant to the extent the analogue is
given an additional translation, we hope a final translation, as it
moves from the output of the upstream cell to the cell next in
line.

If we can forebear more of my speculation than we already have,
an interesting conjecture comes up in connection with the special
routing or the neurotransmitter chemicals. Many recreational
drugs, "dope", the so-called psycho-active drugs, are chemical
relatives of neurotransmitters. Dope and neurotransmitter tend to
be built around a molecule (indole) with a common back bone and are
classified as chemicals of the indole group. The appalling truth
is they so closely resemble each other they cannot be separated in

the "harvesting" process. Dope enters the cell via the special routing reserved for the neurotransmitter and conveniently bypasses all of the several "blood/brain barriers". More alarming, the dope has direct access to the precise and delicate electrophoretic apparatus.

All it has to do is to damage one strand of memory molecule and the precision system is so far out of calibration it is useless as a memory site. (If the dope anomalized the memory molecule, ionic erosion would probably finish it off. I doubt if it could be repaired.)

The incompetent memory site is accompanied by both short and long term cortical disturbance. Cortical dominance authority, ranging from a small area within the lobe and expandable to the entire lobe, is frequently and rapidly re-assigned. Periodically each memory site is both permitted and expected to take an initiative and participate in writing a cortical instruction. A finesse of the exalter process tests all participating memory sites for competence at the instant before authority is delegated and authority is assigned, or canceled, on the basis of site competence. If a memory site is incompetent, the control system tries to restore competence by re-allocating authority, by trial running rates, or by trying either a new instruction or response. With so many sites incompetent, the cortex goes into a fruitless sequence of search, test, pass and search again. This uncontrolled, and uncontrollable, free scanning is drug adduced hallucination.

THE NERVE CELL AS THE ACTIVE ELEMENT

There are long term effects of drug insult to the brain destruction of the memory unit and an accompanying aggression against the memory throughput ledger. Here, the data that was stored in the damaged memory units is lost. Even if the damaged mechanism could be repaired, the old data it once carried cannot be replaced. If the memory unit could be repaired, it would be limited to making entries of information presented to the system on a contemporary basis. (This is about like a bingo player who dumps most of his markers and tries to get restarted in the middle of the game with a nearly blank card.) The older information, either missing or suffering technical damage, is unable to assume an initiative or to assert dominance on occasions when it would normally write the cortical statement and this is a condition necessary for the assured "exercise" of the data. Without "exercise" it is eventually deleted from the memory ledger altogether.

Aggression against the memory throughput ledger also damages intelligence. So much of intelligence depends not only on specific throughput information but also on a host of augmenter, associative and referencing habits, all of which contribute to, if not lionize, cortical intelligence. These habits are irreplaceable. They were built up in a continuum that started in infancy and progressed, without discontinuity, over the years of life. The ordered, step by step acquisition of the memory throughput ledger and its associations, the accumulation of the specific intelligence augmenter habits and their interdependencies will never be repeated within the context of contemporary experience.

The destruction of intelligence does not take place at, or even near, the hour of drug ingestion. Remembered throughputs and intelligence are inseparable and it may take a year or so for the assured movement of a damaged data plane to the distal end of the vault. It will be dropped from the ledger eventually; it is only a question of the length of time it will take.

During the interval when damaged data planes are being weeded out and ways are being found to compute around the missing site, memory will "rescue" fragments of missing and damaged data planes if they are recalled in the context of contemporary experience. I think of this process as the cortex "economizing" its inventory; it salvages the usable and jettisons the rest. The "economizing" cortex brings forward and re-enters early build-ups that are relatable to present experience during the economizing interval. This would have to be done before the memory molecule recycles or a very large part of the data must assuredly be lost. (Scanning normally passes damaged data planes. Even if computer time could be taken away from its daily assignments to the special purpose of reworking a damaged inventory, there is no technical way, other than random recall, to do this.)

Examples of drug damaged ex-dopers are not hard to find. They suffer from a special sort of impaired intelligence where the on-set of impairment came late in life. It should be recognized as different than a childhood impairment where the memory inventory does not build up properly to begin with and the hallmark of deficient intelligence is easily recognized.

THE NERVE CELL AS THE ACTIVE ELEMENT

Dope strikes the intelligent processes directly. It is not as easily recognized due to the special nature of damaged intelligence when the damage has a late on-set and because the economizing process brings forward whatever intellectual and behavioral habits that are salvageable. The ex-doper gets by because his iterative capability is still essentially intact and, with uncommon reliance on the remnants of his earlier intelligence the contemporary impairment is not as crippling as it would otherwise be. He reverts to thinking strategies that fit in with parroting, including parroting his earlier self, and whatever tidbits he can pick up from time to time and make use of.

"Economizing" is accompanied by a serious contraction of memory inventory and an irreversible crippling of associative skills. Following the drug insult to memory, he "isn't all there". He is able to articulate with, and appreciate, incoming experience only if it does not require him to expand on it with original imaginings or synthesis beyond his, by now, spare vocabulary. The trappings, the appearances and typology of earlier intelligence are still there, the restlessness and roiling of an underlying intelligence are not.

Intelligence is never suspended: it is diminished. With ex-dopers, a lingering "signature" of earlier intelligence and intelligent habits penetrates the murk, a feeble reminiscence of earlier capacities and ambitions. His persisting typology, kept more or less intact by egotism, makes it more difficult to evaluate whatever remains of his former intelligence. (I have no special view about making these evaluations. I do know one thing that may be interesting. I try to trace the source of his information and disregard the part he is obviously spieling from a "packaged" source. I look for his passed opportunities to advance an original idea and the operative value of the ideas he does attempt.)

Fig. 86 is the memory ledger again. It would be impossible to plot the millions of vertical lines in the ledger if one line is needed to indicate the relative reinforcement of each build-up. Fig. 87 is the same as Fig. 86 with a solid line suggesting the profile of build-ups in memory and showing token cognizance of the hills and valleys the ledger must surely have. The exact profile of the ledger is left to imaginings. The ledger builds up over the years accompanied by a continuous small drift in all of its proportions. The aspect ratio, the height to width ratio, is important to preserving intelligence. There should not be radical or abrupt discontinuities in the pattern of build-up. We will call Fig. 87 the normal ledger. As usual, the dashed line is the retention fade threshold.

Making entries is ceaseless. Asleep or awake, second by second, for the whole of life, the throughput ledger is expanded, first vertically by the iterative process, then horizontally by the associative process, in a sort of "log rolling" scheme, accomplishing switching modes in a pattern that preserves the aspect ratio of the ledger.

The iterative process does not transpire in isolation, a few trial associations accompany each entry. A few reinforcements are always made with each association.

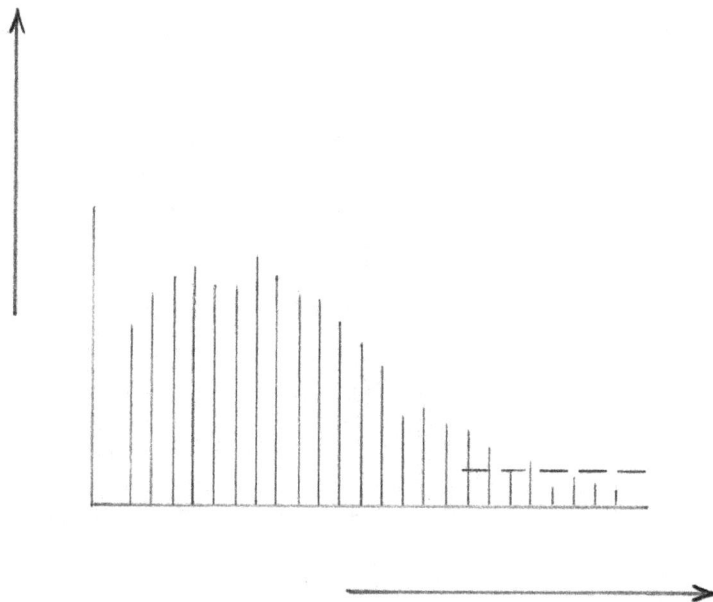

Figure 86

Proportioning of build-ups (vertical growth) relative to build-outs (horizontal expansion of the ledger) is a function of apportioning computer time between the associative and the iterative process.

Time apportionment sets the aspect ratio

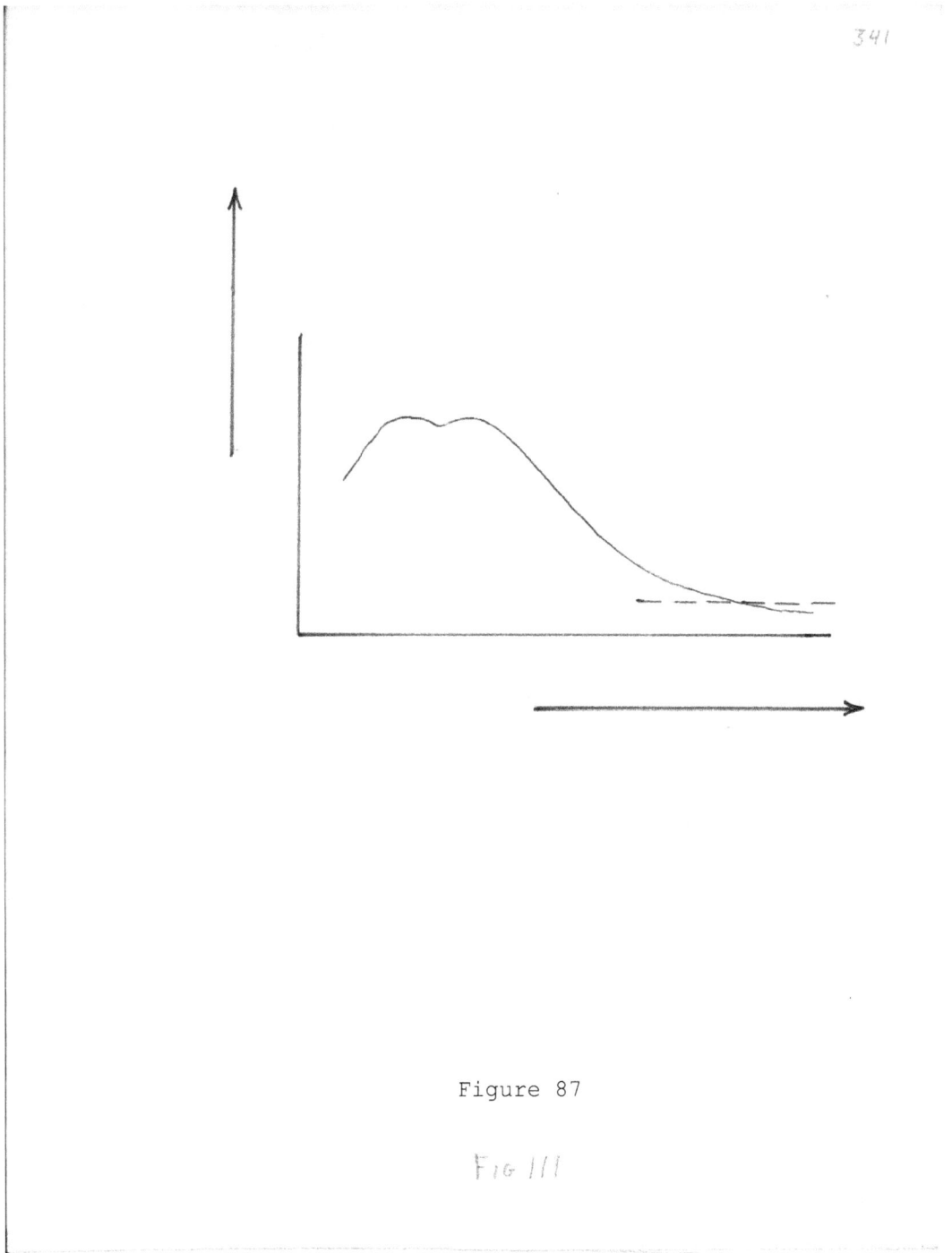

Figure 87

of the throughput ledger. The mode shift is made by speeding up or slowing down the firing rate (Fig. 88).

Trial throughputs generated by the cortex must be tested against

the requirements of environmental realities to

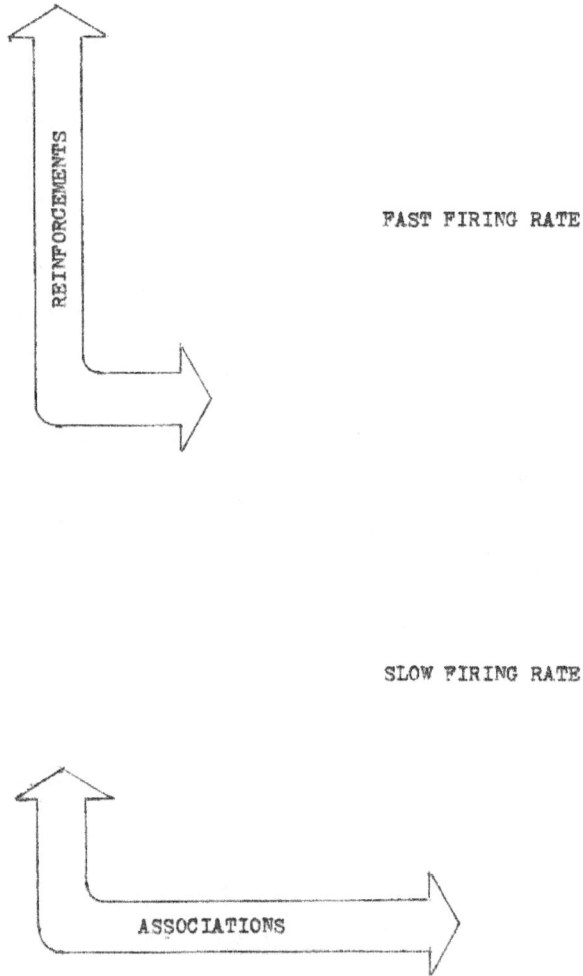

342

FAST FIRING RATE

SLOW FIRING RATE

ASSOCIATIONS

Figure 88

Fig 112

confirm the trial association will meet some sort of test for its validity. Acquiring (an input) or testing (an output) throughputs, taken together, are real-time operations of the cortex, and during this time the cortex is running in the iterative, high speed, mode. When it generates trial throughputs, it is in the slower, associative mode. This is essentially correct, though the two modes overlap each other.

The two modes share computer time and we have a question about the proper amount of time allocated to each mode. It turns out; a 50-50 division of time available is the most efficient operating point for the system. There is a difference between computer time and time measured by the clock. When the cortex is running in real time and in the iterative mode, it cannot run faster than the behaving events in its environment, so it has to wait for the passage of real-time before it can complete an input statement or test an output. Since it has to wait for its environment to make its contribution, it gets less real work done, in spite of its faster firing rate. Forming associations, even with its slower running rate, is faster than the iterative process because no waiting is involved.

If the cortex can form associations (say) ten times as fast as it can form reinforcements, then equal time apportionment would have the cortex run ten units of clock time in the iterative mode for each unit of time assigned to forming associations. A 50-50 division of computer time would agree with a ten to one proportioning of dwell times in each mode as measured by a stop watch.

Suppose we prevail upon an imaginary secretary to work at two tasks that must be performed serially. He (or she) must copy incoming information from a telephone that delivers information continuously. This is a real-time input. There would also be a real-time outputs, perhaps the secretary dictates outputs to another telephone. Attending to inputs and outputs, taken together, constitutes one of the two tasks. The other task requires internal works say, filing incoming information in as many places as possible or compiling information in preparation for dictating an output. It is not possible to attend the input/output traffic and do the internal work at the same time.

If we take the extreme case, if we allocate 100% of the time to internal work, then, oddly enough, internal work will be paralyzed because we are not accepting inputs and we need inputs to provide us with the internal information, the internal "currency" we need to carry on with internal work.

If our secretary should dwell a bit too long on the telephone, internal work is being neglected because input/output work is done at the expense of internal work.

While internal work is being neglected, the extra time devoted to inputs and outputs will enable the system to better process inputs and outputs. Here, more acquisitions are made, more outputs delivered and tested and input/output process is upgraded as a result of the longer dwell time.

On the other hand dwelling on internal work beyond the 50% time division will upgrade internal "noodle" work, albeit at the expense of slighting input/output traffic. The two processes are self-compensating. A small departure from the center operating point will upgrade one task at the expense of the other. Departures from the center operating point (the 50-50 point) are noncritical and self-compensating within limits.

The center point is set by the average firing rate and, <u>within limits</u>, small departures from the most efficient firing rate will not imbalance performance nor impair intelligence. There is a virtue built into a cortex with such forgiving parameters that the histogenic process is relieved of fabricating a cortex with a precision center rate. Without a tolerance for operating at rates slightly above or below optimal rate, the cortex would have been an evolutionary impossibility.

I should also note: "switching", as such, is forbidden in the nervous system. If there was a switch--it could involve millions of contacts-- and, if it disconnected one circuit and switched to another, the circuit just disconnected is left without the excitation it needs to keep it vital and calibrated. There is a point of finesse in making the mode shift from iterative to associative mode by speeding up or slowing down the firing rate because the process does not entail switching.

Our imaginary secretary is not doing things very efficiently if she is timing her activities with a stop watch. Her performance can be immeasurably upgraded if she will pay attention to the information appearing at the input. If it is redundant, if it is already in inventory, then ignore the input and use this time to get on with the internal work. There is no point in wasting time acquiring information already in inventory. This releases enormous amounts of time for internal work because copying the input is the slowest process and cannot be expedited because it is paced by the environment. If an incoming input is not in inventory, then take the time and make the acquisition while the input is still present, we can always do the "noodle" work at a later time.

A strategy such as ignoring redundant throughputs skews the efficiency picture to the extent the center point is no longer recognizable. While there is no maximizing strategy as far as the computer is concerned, we have a powerful augmenter strategy when we tailor the allocation of computer to conform to the specific information processing task at hand. Augmenter strategies such as this better improve the raw machine efficiency, surely well beyond a robot-like 50-50 allocation of computer time.

(A throughput statement is based on a guideline that either comes from the environment or is recalled from memory. Intelligent procedure fills in the missing or uncommitted parts of the statement not fixed by the guideline. Machine intelligence makes the fill-in on a trial and error basis. There is an important point at stake here. The cortical contribution to intelligence is not based on maximizable parameters, certainly not when chance is one of the parameters. Since the machine contribution to intelligence is not maximizable, it cannot be evaluated on a graduated scale of (say) zero to 100 units of intelligence. Intelligent procedure is the trial fill-in of the throughput statement and is itself, a strategy for managing problems that are otherwise unmanageable. It is merely a strategy that works, it gets a job done, beyond this, it is not a maximizable strategy.

I doubt if it can be said intelligence is an optimizable strategy unless we say it is the only strategy that fits the unique milieu of intelligent machination and therefore it is optimal. The computer is still most efficient at the 50-50 operating point. The acquired augmenter strategies make more discerning use of the efficiency available and, by reason of the very selective end use of the computer, do upgrade the overall end product of intelligent effort.)

Balancing the center point of computer operation between "real" and internal work is not critical within limits, small imbalances are self-compensating. If reasonable imbalances are chronically exceeded, then intelligence itself is at stake.

(Perhaps an exaggerated example with a couple of straw men will make it easier to see why this is the case.

There are men of "action" and men of "thought". To a man of action, knowledge is "working" knowledge. Knowledge comes from sources out there in the world somewhere and the only way to acquire it is through "mixing it up" with that world. Detached erudition may have its merit but he is a practical man and the only way to learn is to learn from experience.

The trouble with this guy: he is forever assailing the wrong rampart or tying one shoe twice and the other not at all. His is a life of adversity and it is adversity that quickens the eye and trains the hand.

He has never taken the time to cultivate a personal wisdom or to sharpen his critical faculties. When we listen to his thinking we find he is not thinking; he is either vacillating around the opinion of the last person he talked to, of fixed at the opinion of the first man that got to him. He reminds us of Eric Hoffer's <u>True Believer</u>: "a man who will lay down his life, and yours too, for the things he believes in, whatever they may be".

Rather than studying his last move, or his next--for that matter, he throws away whatever profit there may have been in all of this indiscriminate experiencing. Without this profit, he has to start from "square one" as he plunges into each of his mindless acts. If he wants to upgrade his performance, he has to upgrade his intelligence, something he will never be able to do unless he regularly takes time to think before and after he acts. His best strategy is to think half of the time and to act half of the time. If he is able to think ten times as fast as he can act, he should think one minute for every ten minutes of action.

The man of thought wants to avoid the heartbreak and bruises that must surely afflict the man of action. He doesn't make a move, even licking a postage stamp, before he has studied every possible ramification of the action he is about to take, assuming he will get around to action having used up so much of his time thinking about it.

He does the thinking all right, but is the thinking any good? He fashions ideas, one after another, and they have all been carefully thought out, at least in a technical sense. He still needs to articulate his ideas to confirm the soundness of his thinking amongst practical transactions with his environment.

With his attempts to maximize thought at the expense of action, his thinking becomes internalized. Genius that he is, he orders

his iced tea without ice because he gets more tea that way. He
wants to invent the locomotive, so he starts by inventing the
wheel. Inventing the wheel requires a pencil, so he invents it to,
along with the pencil sharpener, not having bothered to find out if
these things have already been invented.

His logic is atrocious. He moves on to his newest untested idea
without being aware of the failure of the last. He is reminiscent
of another of Hoffer's "True Believers": "a man guided through life
by an inner light and only an inner light."

He can improve his intelligence if he will get some rational
information flowing through his life, to do this, he needs to deal
with his real world, half in thought and half in action.)

On a smaller scale, and with much more frequent switching between
action and thought, the cortex has its own version of the action
versus thought problem. One cortical process iterates entries to
and from memory and the other process forms associations. If the
iterative process carried on without interruption, it would
eventually enter an unlimited number of reinforcements in memory.
(The brain would have to live forever and never forget anything in
order to do this.) In theory, the extreme limit of the iterative
parameter would approach unlimited reinforcement.

If the associative process ran without restraint, it would
associate everything in memory with everything else in memory
whether it was necessary to form these associations or not. The
associative parameter would become "infinitely discursive".

Both parameters are unlimited and open ended at one extreme of
the parameter. The other end of the parameter is found at the

point where the two parameters intersect. The point of intersection is the center operating point and is set be the average firing rate. Reinforcements are made more frequently when it is running fast, associations when it is running slow. (The item on the finesse of the exalted data stage explains how the character of the system is made to shift with changes in the firing rate.)

The iterative process is self-reinforcing and there must be forceful provisions to "close out" the possibility of unlimited, or "run-away", self-reinforcement. Operationally, the iterative and the associative processes are mutually perturbing. The associative process "closes out" the iterative processes by usurping half of the computer time during which it re-randomizes inventory, the normal outcome of running in the associative mode. There is a complementary aspect to this. The iterative process, with its high speed firings, closes out scanning (necessary for forming associations), so switching to the iterative mode "closes out" the tendency to unlimited discursiveness of the associative process.

All cortical processes must overlay and collaborate in a manner that does not contribute to either hyper-reinforcement or runaway discursiveness. The memory ledger profile in Fig. 89 has been skewed by the cortical vulnerability to hyper-reinforcement. The cortical environment is not responsible for this.

(It is very improbable the environment would ever make too many repetitious entries that a skewing of the memory ledger is a serious possibility, then too, the cortex ignores repetitive inputs. I think skewing the memory ledger through hyper-reinforcement does happen, and I think it is a protracted process attributable to chronically running the cortex at rates beyond the "forgiveness" built into the center operating rate. Here, the cortex is chronically dwelling in high speed running and this may be a factor in a type of schizophrenia called chronic schizophrenia.)

Hyper-reinforcement, an internal cortical dysfunction, expands the ledger vertically at the expense of forming associations and forming associations is the intelligent process of the cortex. The throughput ledger contracts, relatively, on its associative, or intelligent, axis (horizontally). Hyper-reinforcement damages cortical intelligence. Any aggression against the throughput ledger is at the expense of intelligence.

In Fig. 90 we have damage to intelligence and a skewing of the memory ledger when the cortex chronically runs slower than the lower limit of the center firing rate.

The throughput ledger (solid line) in Fig. 90 has been insufficiently reinforced (another potential malfunction of the cortex) and only the small part above the survival threshold will remain in memory. Here the cortex is running slow and, running slow; it dwells excessively in the associative mode and becomes wastefully discursive. It does the technical operations required for associations all right, but it forms too many of them. It forms associations that need not have been formed, associations that are meaningless and irrational and cannot be validated by the environment, associations so numerous there is not enough time to "exercise" them against the indicators of the environment or

319

associations so rarely useable there is little prospect for them to build up in the memory ledger. (They might receive one reinforcement at the time the association was formed and never used again.) The superfluous and discursive associations will never be given enough iterative reinforcement to raise them above the survival threshold (dashed line in the sketch). The computer has been wasting

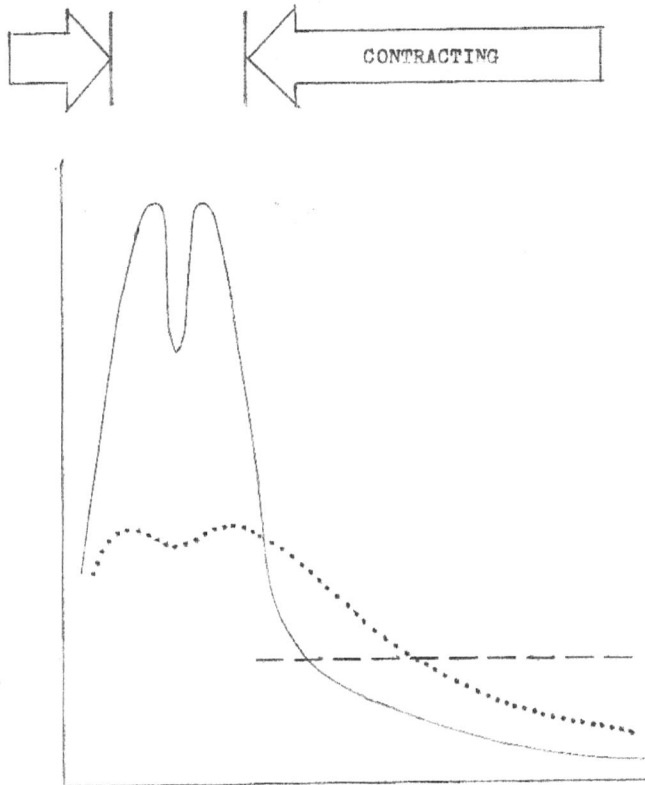

Figure 89

its time; it has been forming associations it will never use when

it could have been reinforcing necessary and useful throughputs.

The part of the profile above the retention fade threshold is the

part retained so there is a contraction

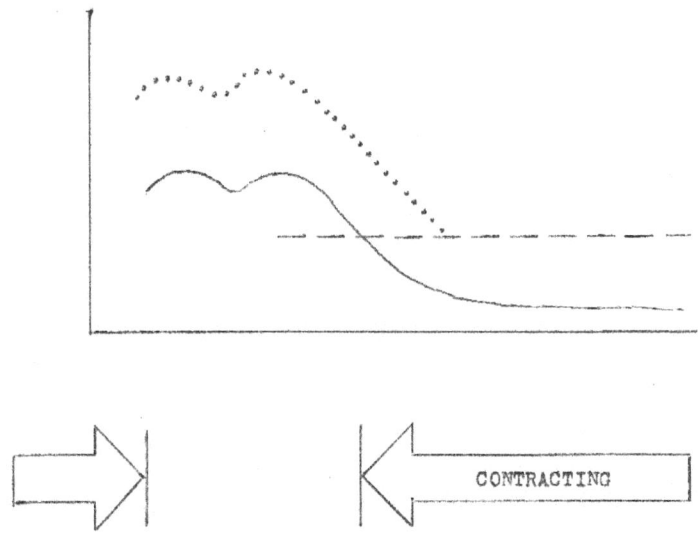

Figure 90

to the usable ledger both vertically and horizontally. The

horizontal contraction reduces the diversification of inventory and

constitutes impaired intelligence.

Fig. 91 is another cortical mishap where a small number of throughputs, all related to a very narrow range of subject matter, has been selected (fortuitously) and are building up a monolith in the throughput ledger. The drawing shows the monolith built up at, or clustered around, a single throughput. We would expect a selected throughput to have corollaries (paralleling and supporting throughputs) scattered throughout the ledger. If we show the selected throughput and its corollaries all at one place on the ledger, the drawing will suggest the anomalous build-up with better polarity.

Normally, a dominant lobe dictates instructions to a slaved lobe at a rate the slaved lobe is willing to accept. It the slaved lobe is running abnormally slow, the dominant lobe will chronically repeat the instruction. The cortical control system tries to maintain competence in both the dominate and slaved lobe and it "figures out" running the dominant lobe at twice the firing rate of the slaved lobe will do this. In effect, the retrieval instruction "sticks" and the throughput is given extra and unwanted reinforcement which can only aggravate the tendency to hyper-reinforce. Small monoliths may build up in memory from time to time, all selected fortuitously because the cortex does not have access to the subject matter of the throughput. Small monoliths in memory are nullified when the inventory is re-randomized in

363A

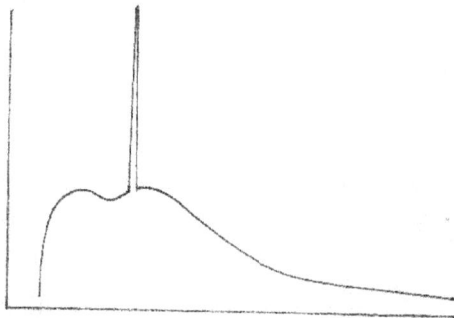

Figure 91

sleep.   If re-randomizations fails, the monoliths become permanent

and intelligence suffers.

I think it is correct to say: there are three basic cortical dysfunctions, each something of a collection of dysfunctions in itself. They are: epilepsy-several variations, amentia ("mental retardation", the primary form from birth, the secondary form from disease or injury), and two forms of schizophrenia.

("Schizophrenia" means "split-headed". "Schizophrenia" is an awkward and somewhat misleading label for this illness. The label would more factually apply to that facet of the illness wherein the patient seems to possess a "head" that never seems to lose its capacity to button buttons and mail letters and still another "head" that makes the patient say and do strange things. Novelists do not help matters when they present their schizophrenic having two "personalities", somewhat along the lines of Robert Louis Stevenson's Dr. Jekyll and Mr. Hyde)

There are two forms of schizophrenia; forms so different from each other, it is surprising they are both called "schizophrenia".

The "acute" form comes and goes in episodes. The episode usually lasts about a month and there is no predictable time interval between episodes. With bad luck there may be one or more episodes in a year with better luck, there may be remissions of several years between episodes. Most home medical dictionaries describe the symptoms of the episode. During the episode the patient may be agitated, at times unmanageable, irrational, occasionally destructive. There is depressed version of the symptoms where the patient is "withdrawn", "down", reports pain and fears not founded and, in extreme cases, catatonic.

I have several acquaintances who suffer from the acute form of this very distressing illness. Those I know show no symptoms whatever of the illness between episodes. They are sharp, forward looking, and cheerful as can be expected and there is no sign of cortical dysfunction or embarrassed intelligence between episodes. Between episodes, knowing they are not free of the illness is unnerving, sometimes alarming. Their specific recollection of the episode is quite weak.

The chronic version of the illness seems to be present continuously and its effects spread out over many years. The "signature" of the illness is impaired intelligence and bad judgment. While "impaired intelligence" and "bad judgment" are such broad and indefinite observations that they could include practically anything, the clinicians point out: broad and inclusive as they may be, they are nevertheless symptomatic of chronic schizophrenia.

Habituation over the years gives the memory ledger its profile. Over these same years, chronic cortical dysfunction has plenty of time to skew the memory ledger. Skewing changes the aspect ratio of the ledger and the preceding drawings of the throughput ledger explain how a change in the aspect ratio of the ledger is damaging to intelligence. "Sticking" ideas—monoliths--may be, probably are, a factor in chronic schizophrenia.

A specific etiology for schizophrenia is still in the future. If a list of possible causes is being kept somewhere, I would like to add either a cortical running rate dysfunction or a sleep dysfunction to the list for the chronic form.

(Contrary to the beloved and belabored formula of the fiction writer, schizophrenia is an organic problem and not induced by experience. There is no therapy for the illness. Lithium carbonate, a pseudo-metabolite, seems helpful with the acute form. Psychotherapy, on the wane in the clinic, lingers on as a fiction writers invention.)

Restraint must not only be applied to idiopathic hyper-reinforcement, a cortical dysfunction, but also to the normal iterative process to prevent nullifying intelligence. Iteration de-randomizes inventory at the expense of intelligence. The counterforce preserving intelligence is re-randomizing inventory when and where possible. Awake and alert, taking time out for a little random thought is one strategy. Ignoring redundant inputs and substituting reverie when they are present is another.

A discussion of what the cortex might be doing while it is asleep would not be hard to get started and it would probably be sprinkled with positive thoughts and affirmation toward the idea the cortex may do some useful work while it is asleep. For myself. I am more concerned with the things the cortex cannot, must not, do while it is in the sleep mode. It cannot, must not, hyper-reinforce the memory throughput ledger.

Factory made computers are turned off when they are not in use or otherwise enjoined so they will not play games with a memory inventory loaded with expensive, perhaps irreplaceable, data during an unsupervised opportunity.

The cortical smart engine cannot be turned off for at least two reasons.

1. The memory molecule does not have a physical "handle" that can be grasped by the control system enabling it to shut down the action of the memory unit. In the item on the nerve cell, the memory molecule is found in one of three states. It is either "following", "entering" or "delivering". The memory unit is supervised electronically and there are only three possible control signals and they are assigned to the three states of the memory unit. Furthermore, the cortical cell must be fired throughout the night to pace the cell's metabolic processes and preserve the vitality of the cell. A memory entry must be made with each firing; it cannot be prevented.

2. If the memory units could be shut off, a very precise provision would have to be made to assure they will all start making entries at the exact instant of awakening because the memory units must function synchronously or not all. Firing the cell throughout the night preserves synchronization of the memory units.

A data plane is recalled and, upon recall, a new copy of an old data plane is newly entered in memory: this is self-reinforcement. With the self-reinforcement capability, there is a nightmare possibility the cortex could run off thousands of unwanted copies of the same data plane, uncontrolled, for the eight or so hours of sleep.

The cortex free-scans in sleep and the throughputs most likely to be hyper-reinforced when the cortex free-scans in sleep are those that were entered from the experience of the preceding day. As the psychologists say: the experience of the preceding day has "recency". Being recent, it is already slightly hyper-reinforced by experience as it naturally occurred during the day. Recent and enriched with extra reinforcement, there is a favoring probability the preceding day will monopolize the free-scanning recall of the cortex when it is in its sleep mode.

There is no operating format whereby the system could specifically boycott these monopolies once they started to build up because doing so would require access to the subject matter of the throughput and this is ruled out for reasons explained elsewhere. (Hyper-reinforcement is a self-regenerating process. Once the monolith has started its disproportionate build up, the emphasized throughput turns up disproportionately on free-scan which builds it up even further.)

There is no way to deliberately "erase" anything in memory, (Deliberately or otherwise, it cannot be erased.) The preceding day may have made entries in the ledger that are to be retained well into the future, so for this and other reasons, erasure is barred.

Now then, the "recency" of these recently built up throughputs can be relatively "built down", so to speak, by building up something else in the ledger to equalize the favored throughputs before the system is allowed to free-scan. This way, recent entries lose their monopoly and become competitive with lesser reinforced throughputs in the ledger.

Sleep experts recognize five states of sleep, I think these are variations of basic modes of sleep. We will call one of these modes "noisy" sleep. (Here again, the noise is electrical noise and not an irritating sound. This electronic noise can be seen as black and white splotches or snow at the periphery of the recalled visual image with the eyes closed. In noisy sleep, the entire visual image is given over to noise. This image is all black splotches with no coherent information in it. Perhaps "black noise" would describe it.)

In the first stage of sleep, at the onset of sleep, the cortex is electronically configured so the exalted data stage is denied coherent data. (Suppressing the white arcuate fibers between the lobes would render the lobe incoherent.) In this configuration the exalter still fires synchronously because the sync system enforces synchronized firings. However, the entries it is making in this mode are black noise and not coherent throughputs. I believe the first stage of sleep is about a half hour of "black noisy" sleep. At the end of the half hour, noise has "recency" and the half hour of noise entries becomes competitive with the monopoly of the recent day's experience.

After a half hour of black noise entries, the cortex is reconfigured for "coherent" sleep. (Perhaps the arcuate fibers are allowed to function and the radial fibers to the body may be "inhibited". The cortex functions in isolation while asleep, yet there seems to be a provision to activate it by outside stimulus during sleep. It is not a simple scheme.) With the cortex operationally isolated, the exalted data stage is allowed to start making coherent entries. In this configuration, there is no real retrieval instruction in the network(s) and the cortex free-scans at random. The noise entries in the preceding half hour compel some randomization of the scan. True, we do recall a few scattered events from the preceding day, but this is entirely different than recalling, all, or even a large part of, the daily influx of redundant information. Forced randomization by noise build-ups prevents this.

After somewhat less than an hour of coherent sleep, the cortex reverts to black noisy sleep which re-randomizes the recent memory inventory again to the extent another half hour of noise will randomize it. Sleep is cyclic. The first part of the cycle is black noise, followed by coherent sleep, followed by black noise, and so on. I am not sure of the dwell times. There may be, say, a dozen of these sleep cycles throughout the night.

The cortex must be in a "safe" configuration in sleep. If the choice is between the cortex running off iterations or associations during sleep, it should run off as few iterations as possible. Sleep expands the ledger by the associative process, and there will be less aggression against the sense and proprieties of the throughput ledger because the low level of reinforcement for the associations formed in sleep will permit then to be forgotten and dropped from the ledger. Due allowance should be made for a few associations formed in sleep that are permanently retained. If sleep is going to make entries that are "mistakes", then it should make its mistakes in a format where the mistakes are more likely to be forgotten than retained. If, during sleep, the choice is between expanding the ledger vertically on the iterative axis or horizontally on the associative axis, expanding associations will preserve intelligence while iterative expansion is done at the expense of intelligence.

Hyper-reinforcement is a monopoly for a limited number of throughputs. Randomization "democratizes" the scanning process and obsolete and seldom used throughputs, throughputs that would not ordinarily be "exercised" by day to day experience, are now (in sleep) competitive with recently entered and more favored throughputs. Randomization makes it possible for them to be "exercised" and re-entered in sleep when there is little hope they would otherwise be retained in the context of immediate need. The sleep mode "rescues" older and seldom used throughputs where they would probably be removed from the ledger by the fade process.

Whatever functions sleep serves , it has to be a "safe" configuration for the computer so it will not skew the memory ledger of diminish intelligence. Whether sleep makes positive contributions to the ledger can be left an open question.

For a given throughput, there is a spectrum of corollaries ranging from "near" corollaries at one end of the spectrum to "remote" corollaries at the other.

The "remote" corollaries are irrational, bizarre, and will never be used in the context of rational experience, so they eventually fade from the ledger without being "exercised". "Near" corollaries are another matter. They are "near" enough to real experience so there is a possibility a retrieval instruction written by real experience could select a trial throughput, formed, "packaged" ready for use, but nevertheless generated while the cortex was asleep. There is no subjective way to decide if it was generated awake or asleep. This sort of thing may happen regularly and we are just not aware of it. There is no way to be sure. We do surprise ourselves, from time to time when we suddenly and unexpectedly dig into some small and unfamiliar task we have never tried before and without the thought and planning the task would seem to need, we manage rather well at that. Perhaps some of these small skills and perceptions are generated, if not generated, say, "polished", during sleep.

I have often wondered if there are, or if there have ever been, animals having no cortex or its equivalent. I think insects are that way and get by with neither conditionability of intelligence, notwithstanding an occasional report by an experimenter claiming conditionablitly in this or that bug. I am less interested in the specific animal, whether it was an ancient precursor of the earliest fossilized shell fish or if it is, say, a living segmented pond worm, and more interested in its brain as a theoretical archetype.

Even if a brain without a smart module is altogether a matter of imaginings, I see it as a classic brain functioning exclusively as a "fixed" or an "arithmetical" brain.

While we may never find our archetypal insect, one with a nervous system based exclusively on summator arithmetic, we can look into some of its limitations. For one thing, it has a critical dependency on a histogenic process capable of assembling a nervous system with a quantity and quality of "wired in" behavior that has to suffice for the lifetime of the animal and for generations of its species. Since the throughput has to be correct without variance, and built into the physical "wiring" of the nervous system, the repertory of throughputs cannot be very extensive or diversified.

There are other problems using fixed arithmetical instructions to control the muscles of the animal's body. Both the fixed instruction and the structure of the body must be precisely replicated generation after generation and the fixed motor instruction would have to match the kinematics of the body perpetually. If the physics of the body or the motor instruction are so inflexible they limit the animal, there has to be a provision to adapt the fixed instruction to fit the variables in the conformation of the body. I think the rules for forming synapses are sufficiently open ended and uncommitted to make small adjustments in the fixed arithmetical instructions to compensate for the small variables in the formation and growth of the body. (This should be understood as neural "accommodation" and not "conditionability" in the fixed system. It does not add new freedom or intention to the movements of the body; it merely compensates for misfit between the fixed instructions and the muscles of the body.) I think, initially, the cortex filtered out very early in animal evolution in the form of "cortical brain service". While the emergence of the cortex and its "smart" module was an important waypoint in a course of evolution that can only be guessed at, the cerebral cortex began as, and continues to be (in animals), an accessory, an augmenter computing service that overlays and augments the extant primordial thalamic (fixed) brain system. (The thalamic system integrates reflexes, attends to inner

334

body housekeeping, and dictates the animal's instinctive behavior. Physically, the thalamus is an enlargement and an elaboration of the upper end of the spinal nerve. It is divided into separate halves and is situated in the middle and floor of the skull. It is a brain system in itself: composed of white fibers, it is neither conditionable nor intelligent.)

There will be a lot less critical apparatus and fewer critical histogenic codes if the cortical "augmenter service" will "figure out" an inventory of motor instructions for a particular body after the critter has been born and contemporaneous with its growth and specific character. "Figuring out" is easily an improvement of a hereditary "programming" of thousands of routine motor instructions in the fixed wiring of the system.

In addition to histogenic economies, the emergence of the cortical module allows for a "plasticity" in the shape and form of the animal and a lot more flexibility and diversity in the way the body is articulated and moved.

Only the free, the uncommitted, component of the machine's output is intelligent. As the degree of freedom approaches unrestrained freedom, the output approaches infinite discursiveness and both the efficiency and the efficacy of intelligence approach nullification. At the other extreme, running in the iterative mode This relieves the hereditary code of an enormous encumbrance and vulnerability, for all that is needed with this system is a "core" repertory of wired-in instructions and "cortical brain service" will fill in the remaining details.

Instinctive behavior amounts to serialized reflexes. Generating as many reflex and instinctive routines as possible at points distal to the brain is an efficient way to organize the system. Not all subroutines can be computed distally nor as isolated routines. Higher thalamic centers either compute or integrate those instinctive throughputs that require a change in systemic hormone balance, or where the cue is picked off from an extant perceptual system (such as the retina where the cue has to be sorted out of a mix of cues), or where several systems are involved with related timing and sequencing factors, or where the enabling authority is more than a simple, "go/no-go", proposition.

(The more sophisticated instinctive throughputs, say those requiring sight or sound to be integrated with whole body behavior may be computed in a cushion shaped ramification of the posterior thalamus called the "pulvinar". This is the first place I would look for wired-in whole body routines, in any case. The nursing reflex, on the other hand, may be computed distally. The lower face is innervated by the trigeminal nerve and it seems to be collecting all of the perceptual information and the motor channels it would need to compute the nursing reflex as an independent and self-sufficient routine.)

These two systems, cortex and thalamus, with their abysmally disparate circuit philosophies, must be fully prepared to collaborate, and to do so without conflict, as the occasion requires. The procedures and mechanisms that inveigle the collaboration without the conflict are touched on in this item and: "The Finesse of the Exalted Data Stage".

Surely the corticated animal incorporates periods of free behavior in its life. During these periods, the cortex is "boss" and its behavior is behavior acquired by learning from its environment. Not guided by fixed instruction, the range of its interests and activities extends well beyond any possible repertory off fixed instructions. In these free periods, with the system in the cortical mode, the animal's behavior is conditionable and supported with intelligent contribution.

The amount of intelligence the creatures of the wild manage to incorporate in the behavior is certainly a topical subject. For the acquired, or for the "figured out" component of behavior it would be safe today there is an inescapable dependency on the way the environment indicates what that behavior ought to be.

If we stop and think about it, the problem here is the non-indicativeness of the animal's environment. The critter only has a perceptual grasp on the behavior of its surroundings. Its understanding of that behavior can only be "as perceived". Doubtlessly there are many occasions where there is a clear one-to-one correspondence between the perceptual image presented to the animal and the environment. The animal is out of luck when the perceived image is at odds with the sense of the underlying transaction.

The animal inherits a core repertory of instinctive throughputs. These are the "must do" skills essential to feeding, reproduction and care of the young. We can only guess at the way the raw instinctive reflexes would work in the absence of cortical augmentation. We can only guess at the number and kind of instincts that the animal has.

When the two systems, thalamus and cortex, are electronically configured for behavior in the instinctive mode, the thalamus acquires the cue and delivers the output or tells an appropriate subsystem to deliver its wired-in output. In this configuration, the animal is behaving essentially as an automated mechanism. The nearly automated throughput is a bare, inflexible and a "one use" stereotype. Supplemental computation from the cortical brain service will abolish the rigidity of the fixed throughput and adapt it to the situation at hand. Here, the thalamic systems are still the "boss" and the cortex is still in augmenter service. The foregoing is probably the common behavioral plan for life in the wild.

If we look at the animal's behavior the other way around, if it should try to make gainful use of its intelligence in the uncommitted periods of its life, it is confronted with an environment that is ambivalent, non-indicative or contra-indicative, or so inconsistent, the animal could, sparely and only with great difficulty, incorporate, intelligence in its volitional life over and above augmentation of its fixed repertory. If the animal had to depend on its intelligence to negotiate this milieu, the best outcome would be not much more than a half education in the school of hard knocks. Furthermore, it is wasting its time on trial and error negotiations and it can afford very few errors. It probably applies a small amount of intelligence to getting on with its life. Intelligent contribution probably enables the animal to better fit the small variables in its habitat, diet and life style and trims and tailors its net behavior to fit the times and circumstances. Overall, the animal's behavior is, and had better remain, an instinctive matter.

The human uses his conditionability and his intelligence in a manner so different from its wild usage, there are not enough points of comparability to make valid comparisons. Setting aside a few well known reflexes, including the nursing reflex and those related to sex (cued only after the sexual coupling has been established), it is essentially accurate to say the human is devoid of an instinctive repertory. The human repertory is entirely acquired from the human environment. The human is also vulnerable to the non-indicativeness of his environment, and if his sole understanding of his environment was "as perceived", the human would have been out business long ago.

The cortex is physically organized so the lobes that must continuously compute body posture and movement are arranged in one physical grouping. They are the frontal, motor, parietal and visual lobes. The functions not needed for maintaining the posture and movement of the body are grouped in on "off-set" lobe:the temporal lobe. I call it an "off-set" lobe because it is set off from the mainstream of data flow assigned to body tasks. The off-set lobe is free to think, to plan, within its own informational and timing regimen. The temporal lobe can accept or ignore, dictate or reverie, without concern for keeping up with the movements of the body. Both the auditory and speech motor cortex are parts of the temporal lobe.

The anatomy of the larynx and vocal cords is a mechanical marvel of muscle strands and pivots. Apparently there are separate muscle systems at work. One system, when tensed, will bring the vocal cords into opposition across the airway when the system is commanded to produce audible sound. I will call this system the "drone" system because it seems to do little more than position the cords so they intercept the airway, probably setting the net frequency of the sound emitted by the vocal cords.

There is another system of independently controlled tiny muscles which produce finely detailed variations in the character of the sound. I will call this system the "modulator". When the sound is audibly expressed, both modulator and drone contribute to generating the sound. If the drone system relaxes the cords, a motor instruction from the modulator can still be impressed on the vocal cords but there is no sound because, with relaxed cords, the sound is not respired. This is silent vocalization. (The two systems may be independently projected to separate areas in the cortex, the most likely case is not, the cortex "figures-out" how to make them function independently. The cords have been observed trembling and moving slightly in the silent vocalization configuration. The movement is volitional and theorists have regarded this silent vocalization a consequence of silent verbalization and a part of, probably most of, the verbal thinking process.)

We verbalize as we experience and as we perceive, a silent running annotation of the workings of the world around us. (We also contrive a verbal "subjective", a personal "spook" as a part of this silent commentary.)

This silent commentary is processed by the vocal cortex as a vocal motor instruction. The motor statement is an aid to memory, a mnemonic "flag", packaged and entered in memory at the same time the experience is entered. (Both the mnemonic and psychological value of motor activity in association with experience are recognized by the psychology people.) I imagine the enjoyment and anticipation of motor action, even if it is no more than vocal, makes up a lot of what we have in mind when we refer to, or try to define "subjective".

This silent vocal throughput, an add-on to the cortical statement as it enters memory, will better assure the retention of the entire cortical statement in the memory ledger. In addition to psychological factors, verbalization augments retention because the cortical statement is technically more competent: there is more to it and it has better referencing. The experience may be recalled by more than one "handle" so it has better prospects for building up in memory by both iteration and association.

To oversimplify a fairly complex scheme, an experience is assigned a verbal symbol (or symbols) and, from then on, it is manipulated, on a surrogate basis, by manipulating symbols. I doubt if anyone knows just how this is done. Maybe there is a sequence where the symbol is associated with an experience which is, in turn, associated with another symbol and so on. Here symbols are used as a sort of internal "currency" where a complete experience is implied with each symbol.

Having translated real experience to verbal experience, the human, using symbols, is able to artificially plan and test his own thinking (symbolically) without wasting time and energy in a blow-for-blow exchange with his environment solely to test his own thinking. Qualitative and quantitatively, new and broader dimensions for augmenting intelligence now become commonplace.

If we drew up a list of strategies that augment intelligence, silent vocalization would be near the top of the list. (Audible vocalization provides the same augmentation but it is a much slower process.)

Somewhere along the way, in an uncalculated history that may never be fully understood, the human vocal system, more sophisticated and freer of instinctive assignment than the sounds of our furred and feathered brethren, was diverted to the deliberate and patterned sounds of speech. With speech comes language and, with language ideational systems. Now the human is able to generate, to grasp and to traffic artificial information about himself and his surrounding world. Now he is able to expand the range of his interests and his transactions with his world, and to expand well beyond the spare capabilities of the cortex in its primordial usage. Now perception, per se, predicates only a small part of human behavior.

In this extra-ordinary milieu, the symbol is substituted for the event, perceptual identifications are categorical identifications, the outcome of a transaction either agrees with, or disagrees with, a prior classification of expected outcomes. The human acquires the habit of construing the behavior of his milieu with a greater

HABITS AND STRATEGIES FOR AUGMENTING THE RAW MACHINE INTELLIGENCE
dependency on concepts over percepts, classification over
observation, remembrances over empiricisms.

Experience from distant times and places is now a consideration
in his immediate thinking. With civilized living, ideas and plans,
institutions and philosophies, and arts and technologies are
indispensable to day to day living. The ideational system evolves,
even modernizes itself from time to time; and while it evolves,
ideas accumulate and an extant generation is able to make use of
the accumulated wisdom of the past, good bad or indifferent. It
isn't necessary for each generation, each individual, to start from
"square one", a tedium that would dissipate intelligence in a
treadmill of trial and error just to get the mechanics of living
started.

The human now lives in an ambience manufactured by himself and
unignorably cluttered with his own arts and artifacts. These
physical arts and artifacts amount to a virtual language and
mnemonic system. These physical reminders and a pattern of daily
rituals set out the guidelines for his day to day business on the
whole; intelligence, relieved of this tedium, is free to look after
other, presumably better, things.

Next on a long list of strategies that augment intelligence, we
must surely include environmentally induced intelligence: the
formal and informal training of the human, the environmental
encouragement toward cultivation of a personal intelligence, the
incorporation of intelligence in the work and play of life, and so
on. One psychologist sees 20 different areas of activity that tend
to expand intelligence. Intelligence begets intelligence, the more

343

it expands; the more it tends to expand. Everything we do, stipulating it is not a repetition of something we have done before, will expand intelligence. It is a provocative subject and best be exposited by experts who make a career of it.

Our list of augmenter strategies should also include thousands of small and less topical strategies which, being less conspicuous could be overlooked. I can stare fixedly at something I am watching or I can order my eyes to roam around and explore the image, gathering far more information with the roving eye than ever possible with passively looking straight ahead.

I can look down a rain barrel to see if there is water in it, and then I can feel the water to see if it is wetter, or warmer or colder, than some other kind of water. Here we have a behavior, habitual behavior, for the express purpose of seeking, detailing, verifying experience for both its informational value and the pleasure of experiencing its acquisition. With trivial strategies just such as this, and there must surely be thousands of them, we are expanding a personal repertory at a rate far greater than we could realistically hope for with an inactive body that carried us nowhere and a brain that merely "took pictures" of whatever happened to be in front of the eyes.

If there is a confusion of activity in my surroundings and the events I am looking at are all about equally interesting, or disinteresting, as the case may be, I can, ad hoc, chose one of these events as a "feature", arbitrarily posing it as more interesting than the rest. By creating this synthetic "feature", I am adducing a "behavior" within the events in my surroundings that did not exist as a naturally occurring event in the freely occurring stream of experience. Artificially exacting a "feature", or artificially suppressing a "surround", allows the cortex to step beyond the blindness of its passivity. The cortex now has an extra "handle" with which it can sort out an undifferentiated mass of experience giving chosen parts of it a behavior, a saliency and meaning, that would otherwise not exist without this strategy. Whatever may be said of emotionality, and a lot is said of emotionality, it is also a strategy that augments the raw machine intelligence. As an augmenter, it is an operational variation of the "feature" and "surround" strategy. The cortex can attach an internal "reward" to a throughput, doing this on an arbitrary or trial basis to begin with. When scanning, the "reward" (a "flag" of sorts) will relieve the cortex of sorting through an overwhelming mass of otherwise undifferentiated information in memory because it can now scan for, and give priority to, "rewarded" throughputs on memory delivery.

The number and kinds of internal "reward" schemes are not known and the problem is further complicated by both the cortex and thalamus issuing "rewards". Very little is known about these systems and they are not accessible to experiment. They make fascinating speculation, so I will pass along a couple of ideas solely for their suggestive value.

The limbic system has been suggested--and I think erroneously suggested--as the seat of emotionality. "Limbus" means "margin" and the limbic system is in the space, the "margin" between the cortex and the thalamus.

(The cingulate lobe, a part of the limbic system, is the control
system for the cortex. The sweeping fiber tracts of the caudate
formation, the fornix and the hippocampus compute the mode shift
from cortical mode to instinctive mode. There are enough fiber
bundles and traces of gray tissue as yet unaccounted for in the
limbic system, so, if there is still a need for "reward" tracts,
there will be enough apparatus to go around. The suggestion the
limbic system is itself a "source" of emotionality is based on
wrongly interpreted experiments. This is explained later. The
item, "Finesse of the Exalted Data Stage" accounts for many of the
functions of the limbic system.)

Internal reward systems are thought to exist in the middle
(thalamic) brain somewhere, nothing is known about them and their
loci is beyond guessing. It would help to know how many there are
and how they work. Even without knowing precisely how the reward
systems work, the operational value of a cortical reward system is
clear and unmistakable. The cortex does not have access to the
subject matter of the throughput. Allowing it does not have access
to the subject matter, the cortex can still attach a reward to the
throughput, and this will, nevertheless, provide the cortex with
another "handle" for manipulating the throughput.

(The cortex recognizes redundant (cortex tends to speed up)
versus irredundant (cortex slows down) experience. One
manipulation that immediately comes to mind occurs when the cortex
uses the emotional "handle" to reward either redundant or
irredundant experience. Here the cortex has made a "separation"--
that is, either an extrication or a classification of a parcel of

experience on some recognizable basis--in this case, on the basis of its redundancy. I take it, we are pleased at recognizing both old and familiar or new and interesting experience.)

Earlier we noted all cortical processes must overlay the iterative process in a way that does not contribute to hyper-reinforcement. The reward must also be issued to ir-repetitive throughputs to counter-balance the tendency to hyper-reinforce the repetitive kind.

The reward resolves and enforces the already extant machine operations, now an entry is <u>either</u> an iterative build-up <u>or</u> an associative build-up, rather than a featureless outpouring of data on memory delivery. The reward scheme augments intelligence because it enforces the machine parameters, giving artificial emphasis to the associative parameter and expediting habituation on the iterative parameter.

While it is true we can only speculate about reward systems, it is interesting speculation and well worth looking into. The chances are, there are reward systems that apply to the cortex only (conditionable) and some that are thalamic only (fixed) and there may be schemes where the cortex shares thalamic rewards. The reward system with the greatest potential for augmenting intelligence would be a free and uncommitted cortical reward which could be attached to a parcel of experience on a trial and error basis. Without access to the throughput subject matter, it can only be done on a trial basis. "Reward" emphasis of throughputs generated by cortical intelligence itself is a straightforward and profitable augmentation of intelligence. In all cases, the reward is a trial matter and experience alone eventually decides if the rewarded throughput is to stay in the ledger or not. Whatever reward schemes there may be, I am almost compelled to believe there is a cortical scheme of this general character.

Very little is known about the thalamic brain. It evidently registers its own efferents for pain, thirst, hunger, satiety and the like, and registers them in its own way. It also delivers efferents for say, momentary control of hormonal levels or whole body instinctive instructions such as the "fight or flight" reaction in animals. The animal repertory of instinctive and reflex needs further study. The summary of this item makes the point that instinctive behavior in humans, if it ever existed, has faded away some time in the very distant past. The repertory of reflexes managing the internal affairs of the body is much more intact in humans. Some of these reflexes are quite interesting and I wish more was known about them. For example, the thalamus is thought to originate an internal reflex that will compel a sick child to lie down and remain relatively quiet until the illness passes. Surviving the disappearance of instincts in humans, there is still something of a collection of these internal reflexes amounting to a sort of primordial internal wisdom so necessary to the survival of both man and beast.

The cortex, open to learning, will learn both the reflex and the instinctive routines of the thalamus and learn them by a "parasitic" procedure. The cortex, intimately captive in the same body with the thalamus and its fixed routines, learns and

HABITS AND STRATEGIES FOR AUGMENTING THE RAW MACHINE INTELLIGENCE duplicates the repertory of thalamic routines. More of this in the summary of this item.

(The crying of a very young infant and its mysterious cueing is evidently a hereditary routine in the first weeks of life. Time goes on, the infant grows and the cortex learns the crying reflex. A few months later we find it increasingly difficult to be sure of the crying behavior is still a reflex or now learned behavior. More time goes by, and soon there is no question a change has taken place and crying in now clearly no longer a fixed response to a set of "wired-in" cues. The cortex has usurped the "wired-in" routine and is now freely associating it with, learned cues.)

There are probably a number of emotions originating in the thalamus. Perhaps they are not so much emotions as they are "reports" with regard to this or that status of the internal body. I get the impression there is a "pleasurable" report, reporting a state of primal well-being and probably an opposing report: say, "distress" or "aversion".

If the cortex is able to usurp no more than these two thalamic reports and freely associate them, the possibilities for "emotionalizing" cortical throughputs is practically unlimited.

The sequence probably starts when the cortex selects one of its own throughputs (always on a trial basis) and trial associates it with a cortical variation of one of the thalamic reports. After the trial association has been made, environmental reinforcement will make permanent the relationship between the trial emotion and a particular twist of experience.

(Perusal of this line of reasoning ends with an opinion to the effect the subject matter of an emotion is a cultural matter for the most part. I suppose we could say the emotions of the thalami are "true" emotions. With thalamic emotions, we do note a very real physical cue must be present within, or in contact with, the body, in order to activate the emotion. The cortical version of the usurped thalamic emotion is "synthetic" and a "real" cue is not necessary to exercise the emotion. The thalamic emotion is transferred to cortical inventory and is open for free association from then on. Here and there, there may be credible traces of the original "wired-in" function of the emotion, but, after it has been worked over by the boundless association and mighty habituation of the cortex, the tracery of its original purpose is but a faint, a very faint, remembrance. Internally, a lot of specialized emotions are not needed, and I have a hunch pre-empted "pleasurable" and "distress" routines are probably at the core of most emotions, The pre-empted emotion takes on its new and topical "sense" because it is "signed" by the experience with which it is chronically associated. Cultural suggestion and cortical play with a couple of internal emotions--though, working at a distance and through many distortions--may well be responsible for the elaborate lexicon of fashionable emotion.)

Here, selected cortical throughputs are commemorated with a "signed" or "dedicated" emotion. They will take of a character and a saliency, a mnemonic and behavioral uniqueness, they would not otherwise have if they were just another entry in the memory ledger. The emotionalized throughputs will influence intelligence because they influence behavior. Whether all of this augments intelligence or not can be debated another time.

Drawing up a list of habits and strategies that augment intelligence would be quite an under taking, especially where trivial augmentation is about as important as the more deliberate and conspicuous kind. Augmenter strategies augment the raw machine performance. There are so many of them and they color the externally observed performance to an extent it becomes impossible to say with confidence we are able to recognize and isolate the machine contribution to intelligence separated from the acquired contribution. We begin to wonder which is augmenting what.

There is little dependable criteria for evaluating intelligence and even less for separately recognizing and evaluating the machine versus the environmental contribution. The raw machine strategy is not a maximizable strategy in the first place. Its output can not be evaluated: "good", "better", "best", or on a scale of that general nature. (Cortical intelligence is either "normal" or "impaired" and impairment is a cortical dysfunction.)

Intelligence is not easy to evaluate because two determinants have to be considered in four possible combinations;

1. There is the case where both the environmental encouragement and machine contribution to intelligence are OK. Here we have the best to both worlds. The happy possessor of all of this is getting on in life with an environmentally augmented intelligence which, if it is not noticed as a problem solving capability, will manifest itself as a personal knowledgeability and an effective and reasonable life style. He has not been alone. It is easy to see

the effects of the deliberate cultivation and exploitation of his innate intelligence. He is not only intelligent, he is intelligent about something useful, he is knowledgeable. He does not have to "figure out" each and every step to be taken, a process fraught with vulnerability to error and one that will ultimately undermine confidence in his intelligence. It is also a waste of time because his intelligence is tied up figuring out things he should have been taught by his environment. There is nothing quite like an encouraging and informative environment, and, whatever may be said of it, it does release intelligence from a treadmill of day to day mistakes and intelligence is free to go on to think; to plan; to explore and expand the repertory. The self-regenerating nature of intelligence in unleashed and each expansion of intelligence begets further expansion.

2. Here we have a case where the cortical computer is impaired but the environment is doing its part as well as can be expected. This situation needs discussion by people who are more knowledgeable about brain impairment than myself. There is one extraordinary aspect of this problem that cannot be overlooked. There are two cortical processes: one is intelligent and one is repetitive. Intelligent capability is weakened by organic dysfunction. It is never weakened to utter ineffectiveness, but weakened nevertheless. The iterative (repetitive) mechanism, on the other hand, is almost indestructible. Parts of the cortex must be missing or destroyed to suspend the iterative process and when this happens a gross function of one kind or another is clearly not there.

The human, with compromised intelligence, carries on with life, often doing quite well, with his cortex functioning mostly in its iterative mode. (The iterative mode is the parrot like, rote learning process only. In the summary of this item, I have a remarkable example of a retarded person who tries to get as much mileage out of his iterative capability as he possibly can.)

With diminished associative capability, it is a compromised performance to be sure, but the day to day pattern of life is pretty much a settled routine and its challenges to thinking are seldom so exacting they cannot be managed by someone with embarrassed intelligence. Understandably, the degree of impairment is the key factor and it can range from barely noticeable to incapacitating.

The problem of evaluating intelligence is a little more complex than it might, at first, seem. It is not only necessary to sort out the environmental component from the machine component; we must also separately evaluate the iterative (rote) component from the associative (smart) component. A proper technique for evaluating the machine's associative capability in isolation, is yet to come about.

3. There is the all-to-common case where cortical intelligence is just fine, but the environment does not provide the information and guidelines, the opportunities and encouragement, or whatever is needed to cultivate a viable personal intelligence. The problem here is not a matter of cortical inadequacy. With all due kindness, the problem here is stupidity. (The word "stupidity" is so overused for its insult value that it draws attention away from

a single pervasive fact: stupidity is a day to day reality and the biggest waster of our capacities and energies we will ever encounter. I am not sure the insult value of "stupidity" is as great as it is advertised to be; after all, we come by our stupidity by honest means: we are taught how to be that way by our surroundings.)

The cortex does not pick information out of the air, it all derives from very real sources. Intelligence is not able to transcend the informational substrate--the informational "currency"-- it must inescapably do business with. We try to bring forward personal thinking skills and a habitual personal wisdom, and success or failure at this critically depends on the soundness and applicability of the information we have to work with,--an environmental matter.

In the long run, it makes little difference what is responsible for stupidity; we just want to correctly identify and repair the problem if possible. We can hardly fault the luckless human and his cortex if his environment is not telling him the things he needs to know.

4. In the worst case--more of a hypothetical situation--the cortex is inadequate and the environment is a basket case. Due to the cortical inadequacy, this is a clinical matter. Mental health care cannot cure the problem, though it can mitigate the difficulty of living with it to some extent.

HABITS AND STRATEGIES FOR AUGMENTING THE RAW MACHINE INTELLIGENCE

SUMMARY OF THE ITEM ON HABITS AND STRATEGIES FOR AUGMENTING THE
RAW MACHINE INTELLIGENCE

The geometry and dimensions of the microscopic synapse are
determined entirely by electronic requirements. The memory unit is
a part of the synaptic architecture. As I see it, there is, and
can only be, one synapse, hence, one "smart" engine and it is the
same smart engine in all corticated species. For there to be one
kind of intelligent mechanism for chipmunks and another for
giraffes is beyond imagining; especially, since I am not able to
imagine yet another smart engine of any kind.

A cortical module is a cortical module; it can only work one way.
The modules are all alike, so no one animal is fitted with
hereditary intelligence superior to another. Given intelligence is
not a maximizable strategy in the first place, and, given the
identical nature of the modules, we can say the cortical
contribution to intelligence is the same for all animals and
humans.

An animal with fingers that do not grasp, thumbs that do not
oppose, elbows that do not rotate and eyes and ears that are
selectively tuned to sights and sounds only meaningful to instinct
will have less use for intelligence that an animal with less
binding peripherals. Where there are differences in animal
intelligence, it is not the computer, it is the peripherals, the
inputs and outputs, that make the difference. The human with his
marvelous peripherals, his high resolution seeing and hearing
systems, the special bones to articulate his wrists and elbows, his

sophisticated and adaptable vocal system, his freedom from
instinctive command, are so different, so better able to make use
of the intelligence he does have, that comparisons between his and
animal intelligence are practically meaningless.

It is often said there is a relationship between brain volume and
intelligence. There is an assumption involved that may not be
entirely correct. The number of active elements in the cortex
would be the issue at stake and we would have to know if all
cortical cells, including supporting cells, are the same size
before we can say a larger brain will contain a larger number of
active cells. The number of white fibers in the cortical "fan-in"
will be set by the complexity of muscle in the body, the number of
receptors in the retina and so on. In turn, the number of modules
in the Cortex will be set by the number of fibers in the fan-in.
The number of lateral cells will be set by a formula requiring
another layer of lateral cells for each fixed increment in the
number of modules. Adding modules will increase the possible
combinations within the data plane, which, in principle, expands
the number of possible associations. Given that we are trying to
compare reasonably similar cortexes, we should expect to find a
relationship, a small and distant relationship, a technical matter
more than a key parameter between the number of modules and
intelligence. I include this in the interest of technical
completeness and I do not think brain mass is a first order
criterion for judging intelligence.

We cannot have two captains at the helm for a lot of reasons and
we cannot have two instructions in the same data system when one

would be noise for the other. When the brain systems are in the instinctive mode, the thalamic system is "boss" and the system authority is configured along these lines:

1. The cortex cannot interfere with the instinctive (thalamic) throughput.

2. During the time the instinctive activity is in progress. The cortex must be able simultaneously provide supplementary computing service for the instinctive throughput.

3. The cortex is allowed to remain in service, on a fractional basis if necessary, and, being in service, it learns (or is forced to learn) the instinctive routine "parasitically". The feeding instincts of the herring gull hatchling have been studied. Briefly, and out of context with the study, we will use this as an example of a parasitic transfer of an instinctive routine to the cortex.

The parent herring gull has a more or less elliptical red spot near the end of its bill and somewhat toward the underside. The hatchling instinctively pecks the red spot and the parent regurgitates food. We cannot be excessively confident about the exact visual image the hatchling is seeing. The bill and the red spot seem to constitute the image. It is a unique visual image and will only appear in the chick's visual field when the parent is present.

The cue for an instinctive throughput is processed through a different system (thalamic ganglion) than a cortical throughput, though the fiber tracts are jointly used. The optic tract presents the thalamic brain system with a low definition electrical replica of the image. A high resolution image has as many elements of detail as there are retina receptors and a low resolution image has as many elements of detail as there are optic nerve fibers. There are 100 times as many receptors as there are fibers. For the fixed instinctive cues, the low resolution image is not only acceptable but desirable because it is projected against, or through, a fixed interpretive grid and a generalized assessment of the image, rather than a lot of detail, and is all that is needed for the instinctive cue. If a high resolution image was needed for the instinctive cue, the visual cue would be required to precisely fill in millions of sites where the tolerances would be so exacting the system would be vulnerable to rejecting perfectly valid cues. On the other hand, if the tolerances are not sufficiently exacting, the system is vulnerable to accepting cues that only resemble the proper cue. (The cue is presented to a cue grid, or cue "matrix", where it is verified as the proper cue. Students of bird song refer to the cue matrix as a "template". They believe hereditary bird song is not "programmed" as a vocal skill, as such. According to their view, the bird starts with a trial song, listens to it, and, if it agrees with a fixed auditory "template" (an input grid), the song becomes part of its repertory.)

The cue matrix makes the survival critical trade-off between exactness in the way the cue is replicated in nature and forgiveness in the amount of cue distortion the system can afford to accept. The cue matrix requires the cue to "fill in the squares", so to speak, enough of the cue must be present and in the correct physical sites before it is accepted as a valid cue.

The next step in the instinctive sequence can only be a guess. Possibly a valid cue in the input captures an interface between the input grid and a similar grid in the output and a wired-in instruction is sent to the muscles of the body. An "enable" authority is implied in the process.

The cortex can be allowed to stay in service while the foregoing transpires if it will behave according to a few rules. (As far as the allocation of authority is concerned, cortical perceptual systems can stay in service at all times with no problem, only an output can interfere with an instinctive throughput.)

The perceptual cortex lives in the same body with the instinctive brain, it listens with the same ears, sees with the same eyes, and learns a particular cue will predictably adduce certain movements of the body. The perceptual (posterior) cortex is permitted, (Perhaps "forced") to learn, and to learn "parasitically", the perceptual aspects of the instinctive throughput.

Of the several hundred muscles in the critters' body, the thalamus only needs to assume authority over those muscles directly involved in executing the wired-in instinctive routine. Large areas of the motor cortex can be left in service simply because they do not interfere with the immediate instinctive mode requirements. Having set aside the innocent areas of the cortex, only in those areas of the frontal lobe where there is a conflict between controlling muscles by the cortex and control by the thalamus will there be a need for an "over-ride" authority.

Now we encounter a couple of interesting rules. One rule, discussed elsewhere, permits the disputed areas in the frontal cortex to stay in service as long as they are competent. Another rule says the disputed areas will be taken out of service if they conflict with the instinctive instruction. The cortex carries on with its trial and error procedure, but, if it conflicts with a thalamic instruction, the conflicting areas will be over-ridden and taken out of service. With the systems in the instinctive configuration, the cortex has all of the freedom it normally has, but it either ends up agreeing with the instinctive (motor) instruction or it is vetoed. (This is a thalamic "over-ride". Only the conflicting areas are vetoed.) The cortex is compelled to "figure out" the motor aspects of the instinctive instruction if it wants to stay in service, which it does. It learns the specifics of the motor instruction "parasitically". Under the circumstances, there is very little else it could do.

Up to now we have looked at thalamic versus cortical authority from the thalamic point of view. There is also a cortical point of view. The cortex is allowed to assume dominance if it can demonstrate its competence, and, in the context of an instinctive instruction, it will only be competent if it can duplicate the instruction. If the cortex is competent, that is, able to carry out the normally instinctive throughput when the cue is present, the thalamic "over-ride" is suspended. (The remarkable mechanism that enforces or suspends the over-ride is the hippocampal formation. This mechanism and another of its procedures which permits the cortex to relinquish authority on those occasions when it is incompetent are discussed in: "The Finesse of the Exalted Data Stage".)

The cortex of the herring gull cannot be much of a cortex, about the thickness of a couple of sheets of heavy paper. There is enough of it to learn the cues and the outputs for the pecking routine from the instinctive system. In the animal's growth, a subtle transition in behavior is made wherein the cortex eventually takes over the entire feeding process.

If the transition could be separated into phases, they would probably go like this:

At the start, the animal is directed by instinct and functioning as an automated mechanism. At this stage the cortex itself is in augmenter service. The pecking of the herring gull chick is a fine example of the usefulness of augmenter computation. The cue, the red spot on the parents bill, will vary in size and change its shape as the parent changes the position of the bill with respect to the chick's sight. As the chick's cortex learns the pecking reflex, the cortex will also learn the cue seen from an odd angle is still the same cue, so, as more of the routine is learned, there is less need for the cue to be in exact agreement with the much stricter cue "template".

At the completion of the transition, the cortex, having served an apprenticeship as a supplemental cortical service, is now fully versed in all of the instinctive routines and capable of doing the whole task without the participation of the thalamus. The thalamus overrides only when the cortex "goofs". After the cortex has added its own embellishments and variation to the instinctive routines, after successfully "figuring out" how to avoid thalamic veto, after a protracted and captive conditioning, the cortex becomes very nearly "goof" proof. (The technical aspects of the take over procedure are in the item on the exalted data stage.)

The search for an instinctive repertory in humans has been studied intensely and competently for at least the recent 100 years and by some of the most knowledgeable specialists in this field of study. Their cumulative opinion argues against instincts in humans. If we set aside human reflexes, most requiring the cue to be in contact with the body, there is no behavior in humans that can fairly be called "instinctive".

Notwithstanding the frank contra-indications, speculating on the possibility of there being instincts in humans is one of our traditional entertainments. Up to now, instincts in humans have eluded both observation and experiments confirmation. Confirming instinctive behavior should meet the following tests:

1. The instinctive system is triggered by the minutia of a very definite and unique cue. One accepted test for instinct requires the response to appear each time the cue is present--same cue, same output. (The pecking instinct of the hatchling gull will vanish by the time it becomes an adult. There is no way to know if the reflex is hereditarily programmed to fizzle out or if the cortex takes over or just how it is dispensed with.

2. The first presentation of the cue must adduce the response and at a time in the animal's life before learning has a chance to acquire the behavior. Furthermore, the routine must appear spontaneously in animals raised in isolation.

3. The instinctive routine must be uniformly present in all members of the species.

HABITS AND STRATEGIES FOR AUGMENTING THE RAW MACHINE INTELLIGENCE

(Human thalami have not survived the drift of evolution and remained intact. At one time in the very distant past, there was a commissural fiber bundle (massa intermedia) interconnecting the left and right halves of the thalamic brain. It is physically absent in about 20% of the human population and I doubt if it is functional in the remaining 80%. The purpose of the bridge between the left and right inner brain can only be a guess. It may be responsible for collaboration of the thalamic halves for those instinctive throughputs that require left/right reconciliation of whole body routines. Instincts in humans extinguished in some very distant human precursor and the extant human probably never possessed much of an instinctive repertory, or so I would believe. In the human transition from instinctive behavior to acquired behavior, acquired behavior became increasingly central to survival and instinctive behavior was no longer survival tested each generation. With disuse and without constant testing, it was only a question of time before it disappeared from the thalamic inventory. The human became entirely dependent on his cortex and folk behavior. The modified end use of the human cortex, that is, the change-over from augmenting instincts to acquiring behavior, did not require a biological revision of the cortical design.)

Ideas about the brain come and go in fashions and I think the same Murphy who wrote Murphy's law is responsible for the fashions. One of these fashionable ideas: the idea of a "conditioned reflex", became a catch word and caught practically everybody for a while. The neurologists and experimenters concluded, many years ago, there are no conditioned reflexes. If there is any doubt left at this late date, I will add one more reason to their list or reasons regarding the impossibility of conditioned reflexes. Conditioning requires a memory mechanism and reflex fibers are white fibers carrying the pulse rate code which the memory unit unable to accept. The memory unit is found only in the D.C. (gray) cells of the cortex and as a reserved but doubtful possibility, the gray cells of the cerebellum (little brain).

I haven't studied the cerebellum and very little is known about it. I will pass along my impression of the system because it may represent an archetype of a neural computing system halfway between a fixed D.C. arithmetical scheme and intelligence.

The spinal nerve penetrates the floor of the skull about dead center. The cerebellum lies in the space just posterior to the spinal nerve and just below the posterior cortex.

The motor cortex instructs the skeletal muscles to move the body to a new posture and to move it at a certain rate. There is a whole body reaction to the movement of anyone member of the body. There are also left/right reconciliations involved and there are energy-economical/stress-economical ways to produce the movement. The cerebellum probably works an arithmetic where the pulling effort of a muscle (always under cortical instruction) is sampled, and if the cerebellum can economize the effort by allocating to other muscles, it does so by computing, or re-computing a supplemental cerebellar instruction. The cortex dictates the volitional "sense" and rate of muscle effort and the cerebellum assists in carrying out the instruction in a fashion somewhat resembling the power steering in an automobile. The circuitry of the system is arranged so the cerebellum can provide the same service for instructions dictated by the thalamic system.

The cerebellum is a computing service, forbidden to originate instructions; it follows through on motor instructions originating in other systems. The service is available for both cortical and instinctive instructions.

The cerebellum is a special area of study, I touch on it here because the cerebellar computer may incorporate intelligence in a special usage. It may use both trial and error procedure and conditionability to "figure out" the arithmetic of an efficient motor instruction which it permanently enters into memory intact. Even though it uses the "smart" process in arriving at an answer to a muscle effort problem, it is still a "dumb" process overall because it is "figuring out" targeted answers which can be confirmed within this same system. Once the instruction has been entered in memory, the instruction is iterated (only) as one complete, whole body, instruction each time it is used.

There is a spectrum of cortex/reflex authority and a position within the spectrum vested with an appropriate degree of authority for every possible configuration of the systems. At one end of the spectrum there is an authority no more than a "virtual" authority and, at the other end of the spectrum, an absolute "override" authority. There is a position within the schedule of authority for any feasible task imaginable and, under the circumstances, there can never be a contention over which system is "boss" and which system is over-ridden. As we examine a particular task, we may not know whether the cortex or a fixed system is "boss", but we can bet there is a definite provision for making the decision that prevents both systems attempting an instruction simultaneously.

One of the eye-blink reflexes may be an example of a "virtual" cortical over-ride. This example may not be the essence of precise physiological accuracy, but it gets the idea across. There is evidently a sensing mechanism which detects dryness on the exposed surfaces of the eye. The dryness cue triggers a reflex and a wired-in motor instruction lowers the eyelid, spreading tears and wetting the eye. (The cornea is respired by the dissolved oxygen in the tears.) The cortex also has access to the cue, and it learns a drying eye will be followed by a predictable lowering of the eyelid.

The cortex also controls the eyelid and it learns it can postpone the reflex eye blink if it blinks the eye voluntarily and at a time convenient to the cortex. The cortex takes over the eye blink routine by moistening the eye and, in so doing, abolishing the dryness cue. When the cue is removed, the reflex is abolished: no cue, no reflex. Here authority is transferred from the reflex system to the cortex by a "virtual" over-ride. No special apparatus is needed to make the shift from reflex to cortical authority however, it is almost a cinch a cell or two will be allocated to the technical need of preventing two instructions in the same data system. As long as the cortex is willing to keep the eye moistened, the reflex is suspended. If the cortex gets lazy from time to time, the reflex will make sure the task is not neglected.

Reflex systems are automatic and essentially protective: they preserve the proprieties and feasibilities of the body's internal workings and attend to the "must do" chores of the inner body.

(Cortical access to the internal body is another overblown topic. It reminds me of a yoga I saw in a side show about 10 years ago. He was a skinny fellow and he had trained himself to either displace or flatten his intestines. This left a cavity where his belly was supposed to be. Seen from the front, there was a large depression bounded by the rib cage at the top, the back muscles at the sides and the pelvic iliac and ligament at the bottom. The skin of the belly pressed against the sacral vertebrae and the vertebral prominences could be seen from the front through the skin. He could also voluntarily relax the intercostal muscles and voluntarily spread the ribs on his left side. He then prolated the upper pole of the heart so it protruded through the ribs. The forward leaning heart appeared as a distinct protrusion between the ribs and pulsed with the contraction of the heart muscle. He did all of this on a raised platform, in broad daylight, and less than an arm's length from the unaided eye. Seeing this, I figured the cortex probably has access to any system in the body, providing the cortex is not allowed to violate the body's essential organic feasibilities.)

Skeletal muscle reflexes forbid cortical violation of the skeleton's key feasibilities and rectitude's. Authority is allocated so the cortex is free to do anything it takes a notion to do, with the stipulation a cortical threat to the body will be over-ridden by an absolute reflex over-ride.

The cortex is a free system and is not pre-loaded with motor instructions or "packaged" instructions of any kind. The "smart" modules have to "figure out" which motor instructions the body will accept. When the cortex attempts a non-feasible instruction the reflex veto "inhibits" the cortical motor site involved and, at the same time, renders the memory entry incoherent. The "wrong" instruction is not entered in memory so the cortex is only allowed to enter "correct" motor instructions. Only non-feasible instructions are vetoed, so, in effect, the reflex system teaches the cortex how the body is not to be moved.

Fig. 92 is an absolute reflex over-ride path for the skeletal muscles. This scheme is not confirmable but I believe it is a part of the nervous system. A summation is made of the tensing effort distributed between a flexor and extensor muscle pair, and the outcome of the arithmetic insists the opposing tensions must not exceed a limiting value. If the cortex instructs these muscles to operate in a way threatening injury to the muscle--and this could happen, an anomalous cortical instruction is capable damaging muscles, breaking bones for that matter--the reflex system over-rides the cortex. The sketch shows the reflex over-ride path to the motor cortex, the control cortex (the cingulum) and cerebellar computing service. None of these systems will be allowed to "learn" a non-feasible motor instruction.

I have never met an "idiot savant", as they are called. We hear about them from time to time. The "idiot Savant" is obviously retarded, yet he is able to discover a mental manipulation that enables him to, say, name the day falling on a selected calendar

date for years in the past or future. How he does this remains a
mystery.

I have an acquaintance who has been retarded since infancy, He
reads a lot and he comes across as an authority on just about any
subject one can think of. He likes to talk a lot, very loudly at
times, and he never listens. He holds forth. He declares. He
advises. He is didactic, pedagogic,

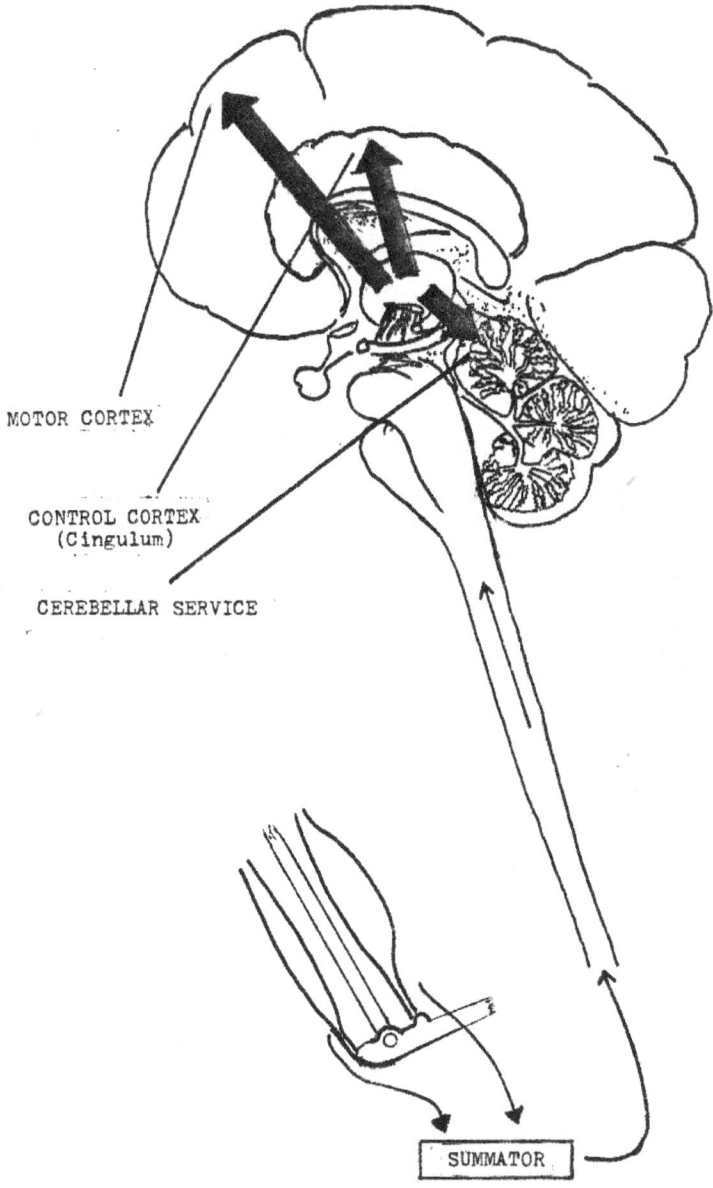

Figure 92

pedantic, demagogic and he is resounding, pompous, bombastic. He

is dead sure he is properly managing his thread of thought, a

370

thread of thought he is mechanically repeating from a book he read a short while ago. Alas, the refreshment of his own intelligent imaginings are not to be heard in this grave and ponderous monologue.

The unsuspecting listener gets the impression he is a seasoned intellectual, perhaps a lonely but talkative professor. He carries this off rather well, that is, up to a point where someone asks him a question. He doesn't like questions. If he cannot answer it, he appears pained, ignores the question and goes on talking as if nothing has happened.

The subject of his talk is an almost verbatim and parrot like repetition of the books he reads. If I ask him a question and the question was answered, as asked, in a book he recently read, he graciously, nay, gleefully, spiels off the lucky answer. If the listener gets the impression his answer was a result of his own thinking, it is an impression he does not discourage.

If he is reading a book about the North American wilderness, I will ask him a question such as: "Is it true both the North American brown bear and the wolverine are canines?" (I figure out fine questions to ask by listening to him.) If the question was not discussed quite this way in the book, he will attempt an answer by making a statement about bears, followed by a statement about wolverines. By a series of re-statements of the terms of the question, he will work his way back and forth from term to term and from question to answer. If his answer has to come from more than one source, he forms the necessary associations by a series of side steps and circumlocutions and sooner or later he will get there. A "yes" or "no" answer for a question would suffice if he knew what answer to give.

If he can't answer the question at all, strange and wondrous things happen. His performance breaks up. He becomes incoherent and he resorts to a kind of "word salad" or "idea salad". Sometimes he even grunts or snorts. He will use the word "incredible" every fourth or fifth word to smoke-screen his inability to get his answer together. Sometimes he loses his temper. It is a little breathtaking to watch all of this happen, especially right after he has provided erudite and polished answers to the two or three immediately preceding questions

THE DIFFICULTY OF SPECIFYING EXACT CIRCUITRY

If we had to depend on a study of the connections between cortical cells to guide us in order to diagram the cortical circuitry, we would be sparely advised indeed. Over the years, the histology people have invented all sorts of ingenious ways to visualize the microscopic nerve cell. The cells are stained for the light microscope and infused with electron opaque metals or plated with evaporated heavy metal cladding for the electron microscope. One ingenious experimenter uses metal cladding to fabricate a credible three dimensional model of a cluster of cortical cells.

Unfortunately cell studies do not bring forward the kind of information we need with regard to the cell's function in the circuit. Even if the histologist is successful isolating the nerve routing, we still do not know if the nerve is carrying specific data, ASC control information or supervisory signals. (Knowing the route of the nerve will not clear up as many disputes as we may think. I have an acquaintance who teaches anatomy and he tells me there is a nerve tract that will take me from anywhere in the brain I might be looking to anywhere I might want to go.)

In the item on the nerve cell as the active element, the somewhat labored discussion of the electrotonic synapse becomes an important factor in specifying nerve circuits. According to the way I have it, the electrotonic junction is not a signal processing junction. It is an accessory device. It is a component of an extensive stray-voltage/stray-current immunity program and is found everywhere in the nervous system.

373

Demoting the electrotonic terminal from a status of an active signal processing junction to an inactive (grounding) device is entirely my idea. The implications here are not to be scorned.

Up to now, the histologist has not made a distinction between active junctions and passive electronic junctions when he diagrams nerve circuits. He regards the electrotonic junction as a signal processing junction and includes it is his circuitry as such. There are billions of electrotonic junctions in the nervous system and they have to be systematically disregarded when laying out the active signal routing. (If I am right, and I am sure I am.)

Fig. 93 shows a fan-in fiber entering the underside of the cortical layers and penetrating the lateral re-organization in the outermost layer. (This is the ascending columnar cell. In earlier drawings it was shown as two cells for purposes of expository. The ascending columnar cell is the arborization of the fan-in fiber.)

The ascending signal is carried to the outer layer of the cortex where the lateral re-organization is carried out by the lateral fibers. In Fig. 93, there is a strange

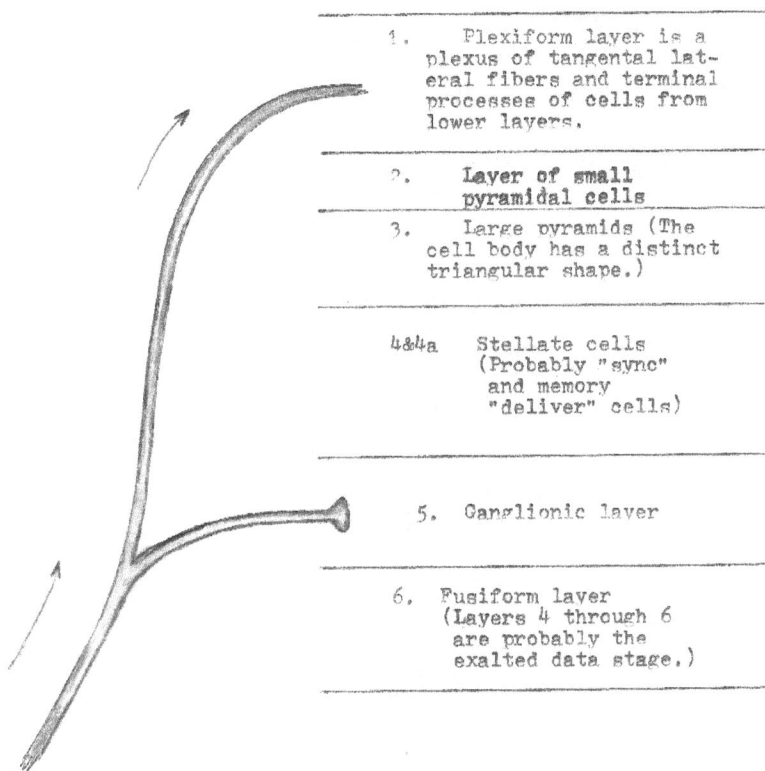

1. Plexiform layer is a plexus of tangental lateral fibers and terminal processes of cells from lower layers.

2. **Layer of small pyramidal cells**

3. Large pyramids (The cell body has a distinct triangular shape.)

4&4a Stellate cells (Probably "sync" and memory "deliver" cells)

5. Ganglionic layer

6. Fusiform layer (Layers 4 through 6 are probably the exalted data stage.)

Figure 93

collateral axon running directly to the exalted data stage (layer 5). I think of this as a "pushy" collateral because it seems to be in a hurry to by-pass the lateral re-organization of the data buses and rush directly to the exalted data stage.

The termination of the ascending cell in more than one layer is an odd way of doing things. I think I will be able to account for this later on. The histologist draws what he sees in his microscope and only a learned eye and steady hand stand between him and error. He is looking at a microscopic can of worms and it is not easy to disentangle each worm for a separate study of its routing.

The microscope, used alone, has probably told us as much about cortical electronics as can be expected, it is not an unlimited source of crystal clear information about circuitry. I think the next step for cortical studies is to figure out the electronics of the system and work backward to nerve circuits and the way they are laid out in the tissue.

Fig. 94, with its block diagrams and straight-line signal paths, will begin to devolve the layout of the computer. There is no problem fitting these, or any, block diagrams to the anatomy of the cortex. The appearance of cortical tissue is such that it would be hard to find a circuit so misfitted to cortical anatomy it clearly could not be used. The entrained computer is in the outer gray "bark" of the cortex and there are sweeping arcs of white fibers carrying instructions between lobes and radial fibers conducting

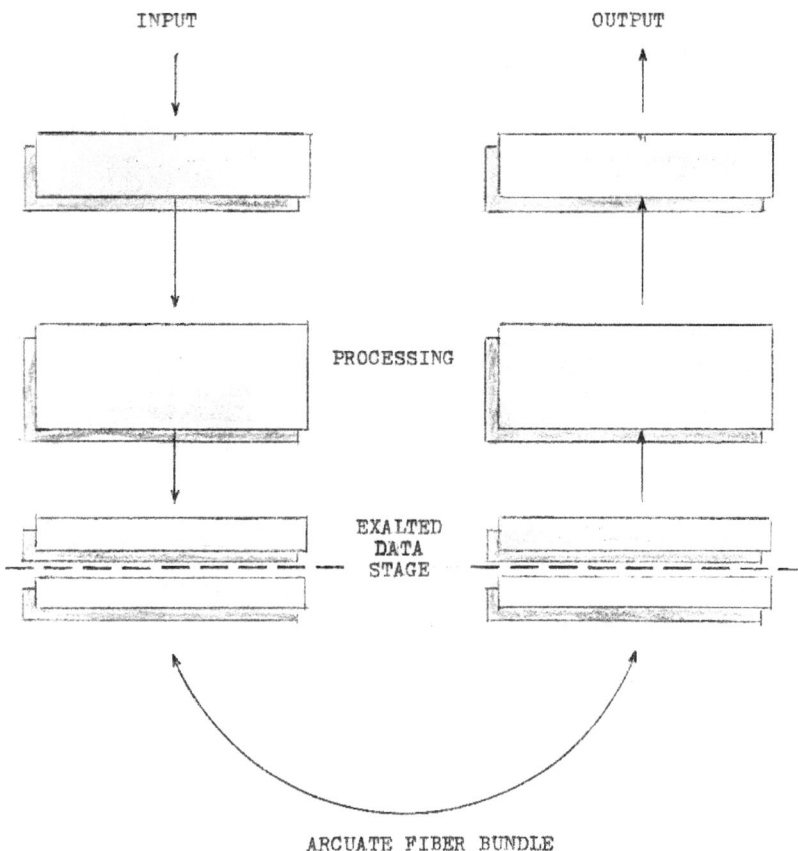

Figure 94

signal in and out. This arrangement is compatible, almost

compulsory, with almost any circuit that can be proposed.

Fig. 94 is a simplified and "straight-through" layout.

Perceptual systems are on the left, motor systems on the right.

In the cortex in situ, perceptual systems are toward the rear and motor systems immediately forward of the central sulcus, the central sulcus divides the brain into its frontal and posterior masses. White arcuate fibers carry retrieval instructions between the lobes. (Textbooks call the arcuate fibers "associative" tracts and the radial fibers are called "projection" fibers.) The arcuate fiber bundles carry instructions both ways.

The statement for the lobe is written in a language indigenous to the lobe and cannot be used to instruct another lobe because of language incompatibility. Comparator information is used instead. In the simple lash-up in Fig. 94, an instruction in comparator language would sound like this: The visual system is recalling its half of throughput no. 7328, the motor system must now recall its own half of this same throughput. The white arcuate fibers carry comparator information from dominant to slaved lobe and there is enough latitude in the way the retrieval instruction is written to permit the slaved lobe to respond with one of several "near" corollaries.

The block diagram in Fig. 94 is incomplete and probably non-feasible as shown. For one thing, it is only capable of functioning in real time. I do not believe there is a real-time (input) to real-time (output) coupling because, with the straight through arrangement, the motor system would be stranded without an instruction the instant the perceptual cue was removed. In a hand eye task, this would happen the instant the eyes were closed.

I am almost certain there cannot be straight-through real-time input to real-time output pathways. Ultimately, the retrieval instruction must originate in memory in order to avoid the pitfall of "instantaneous" experience. When memory participates in writing the statement it is "referenced" behavior: not only referenced to the continuum of events just preceding and just following but also referenced to an inventory of proven responses. In a larger referencing picture, there will be more freedom with respect to thinking and technical options.

Fig. 95 is a simplified schematic of the exalted data stage in Fig. 94. The comparator cells are accepting data events from six descending columnar cells in each lobe. A practical number ought to be about 100 in opposing pairs. 50 of the pairs in the dominant lobe and 50 at the other end of the white arcuate fiber. Half of the data plane is written in the dominant lobe and the other half in the responding lobe.

The arcuate white fiber can be looked at as a stretched out comparator cell. The arrows show information flowing both

320

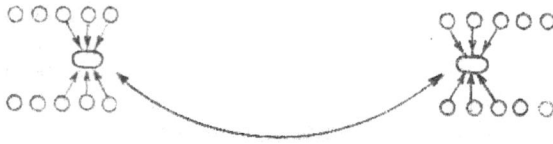

Figure 95

ways in the arcuate fiber bundle. Information can only flow one

way on a given nerve. The bundle is arranged so every other fiber

physically points in opposite directions.

The information carried by the arcuate white fibers is the
arithmetical outcome of comparing the inequalities, with some
averaging of the data events standing in opposing sites across the
comparator. The outcome of the comparating arithmetic will
uniquely fit a particular data plane. Each lobe writes its own
piece of the overall statement. Since each complementary piece is
unique, one of these pieces written in a dominant lobe will imply
its complementary fragment in the slaved lobe. The slaved lobe
will contain at least one response used sometime in the past.

The information carried by the arcuate fiber bundles is
supervisory information in supervisory language. The hypothetical
and straight-through example in Fig. 95 is capable of iteration
only, it does not free associate. With this limited apparatus, the
arcuate fiber instruction can only command the dominant and slaved
lobes to iterate their respective fragments of a common cortical
statement.

The retrieval instruction does not request specific data in
specific data language, it requests specific data planes and the
request is in supervisory language. This incredible finesse of the
exalted data stage obviates the need to translate, say, a visual
cue out of visual language and into motor language before the
cortex is able to instruct the body in, say, a hand/eye task.
Translations of this sort are a technical impossibility anyway;
making them simply cannot be done. (The arcuate fiber tract is
called a "fasciculus". they are conspicuous in cortical anatomy.)

The instruction from dominant to slaved lobe is written within
the "forgiveness" of the comparator tolerances. If there are

competing data planes (or fractions) in a given response, the first choice would probably be a nearly complete data plane that had been used with this retrieval instruction before, at least this much of a response is practically guaranteed. Second priority would be a competent data plane that can be delivered in the least time. With all other factors equal, the third choice would probably settle for corollaries, fractional data planes, and data planes minimally competent but can be located quickly. The ongoing test for memory response is the data plane having the most matched data events.

The circles in Fig. 95 are the descending cells and the lozenge shape is the comparator. All of the descending columnar cells in the lobe terminate at a comparator. The match of elements in the data plane is made by subdividing the decision into comparing the signal from small groups of descending cells with 100, perhaps several hundred, signals compared at each comparator. Here, the trade-off is made between the precision with which the signal amplitudes must be matched and the number of signals that must be matched.

There is "forgiveness" in both the number of sites (say, 50%) that must be matched and the degree to which the signal amplitudes must equate. The system will take on a variable, but controllable, forgiving regarding the precision with which the responding data must match the retrieval instruction. With tolerances set as tight as possible, the system runs in the iterative mode only. When forgiveness is set at its greatest, imperfect and incomplete data planes can be entertained as an adequate response and corollaries can range from "exact" to nearly "free" and still be within tolerance.

(The underlying finesse of the exalted data stage begins to emerge here, the exalter control system makes a trade-off between D.C. error and firing rate. When the system speeds up and switches to the iterative mode, error is a smaller concern. Switching to the associative mode, the error signal sets the firing rate slower and more time is allowed for forming associations.)

Both the iterative and a certain amount of the associative capability carry through the slaving path in Fig. 96, however, we will have to interdict in this straight-through and real-time circuit of Fig. 96 before it is "free" enough to freely associate. Before thoughtful contribution can be inserted in the otherwise robot-like, cue-then-output format of Fig. 96 the input and output lobes must be decoupled. The

324

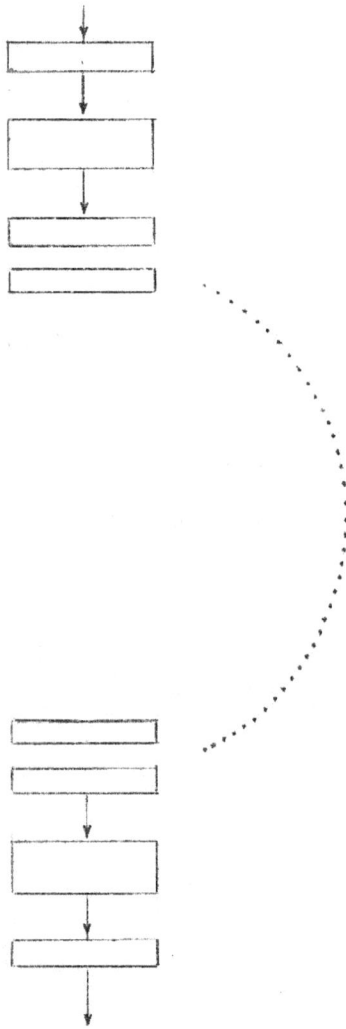

Figure 96

only scenario the circuit of Fig. 96 could manage would be "bursts"
or "instants" of experience, so in addition to de-coupling, a

384

memory for the lobe is needed to reference these "instants" of experience to a larger context of prior experience.

Beginning with Fig. 96, I have to devolve the circuit rationale a little. Fig. 96 differs from Fig. 94 or Fig. 95 only because it has an in-line data flow. The arcuate white fibers (dotted) between these two real-time systems must be interrupted and reconnected in a way that will let the lobes function independently and permit memory for the lobe to participate in the signal traffic between the lobes.

Fig. 97 is a block diagram of the lobe. While the data flow within the lobe is toward the interface between the memory and real-time division of the lobe (Fig. 97), the overall data flow is from an input lobe (perceptual) to an output lobe (frontal). I think Fig. 98 is the probable circuit. Pending an opinion from the anatomist, this is the typical arrangement and the perceptual lobe instructs the slaved lobe via the comparator and exalted data stage they have in common. (Anatomically the arcuate white fiber tract is a true fasciculus. The arcuate white fiber is either a comparator cell, as such, or one of the cells in the comparator circuit. I am not sure which.) The input and output lobes now "talk" to each other with referenced data by letting each resident memory for the lobe write its half of the common throughput statement.

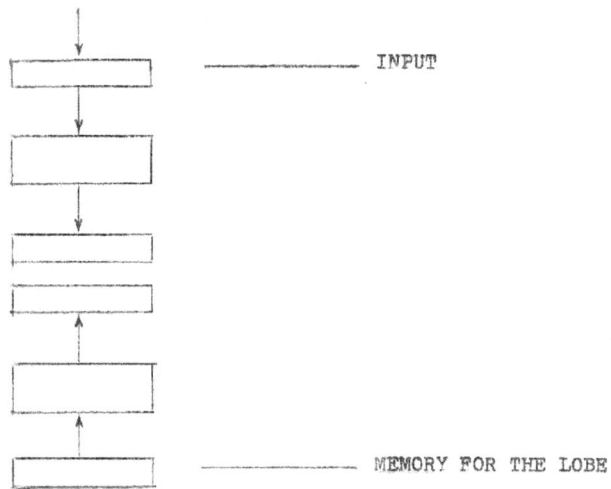

INPUT

MEMORY FOR THE LOBE

Figure 97

Fig. 99 further devolves the co₁_____ _____. The posterior lobes,

all perceptual lobes, are at the top of the drawing. There short

arcuate tracts between the separate posterior

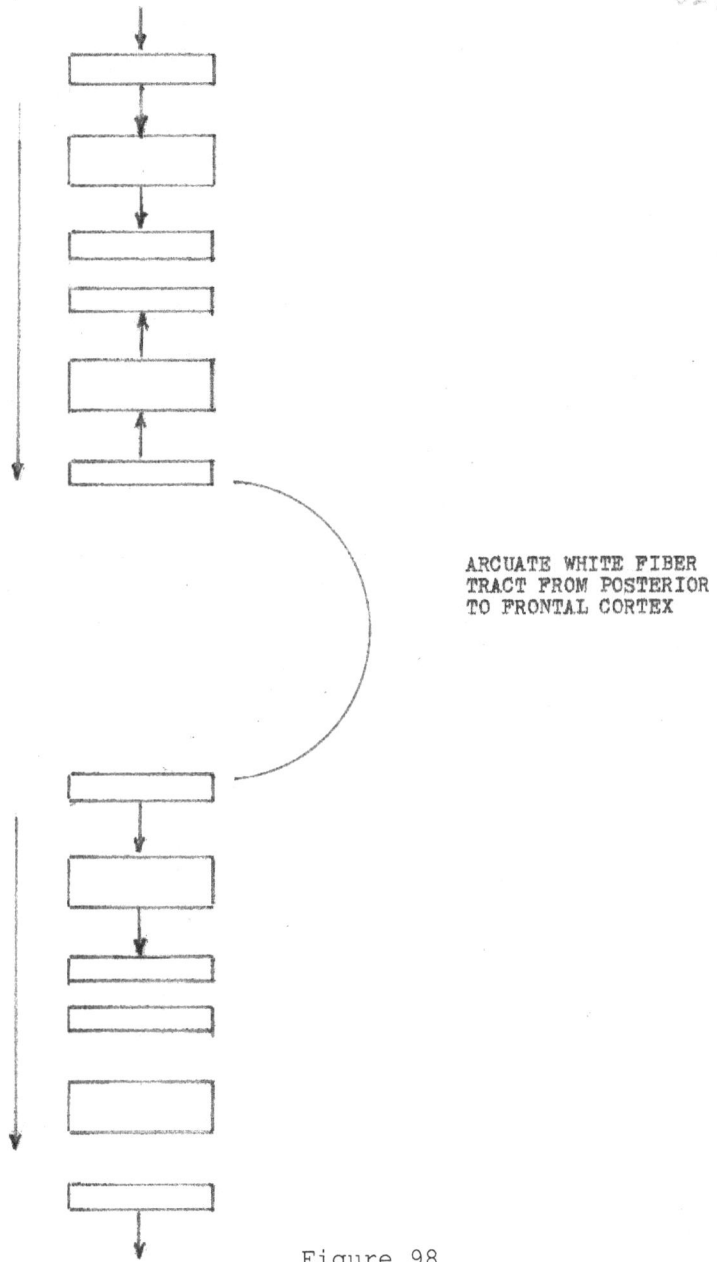

ARCUATE WHITE FIBER
TRACT FROM POSTERIOR
TO FRONTAL CORTEX

Figure 98

lobes enabling them to write a common analyzand or, if one is

dominant and another slaved, to write instructions for each other.

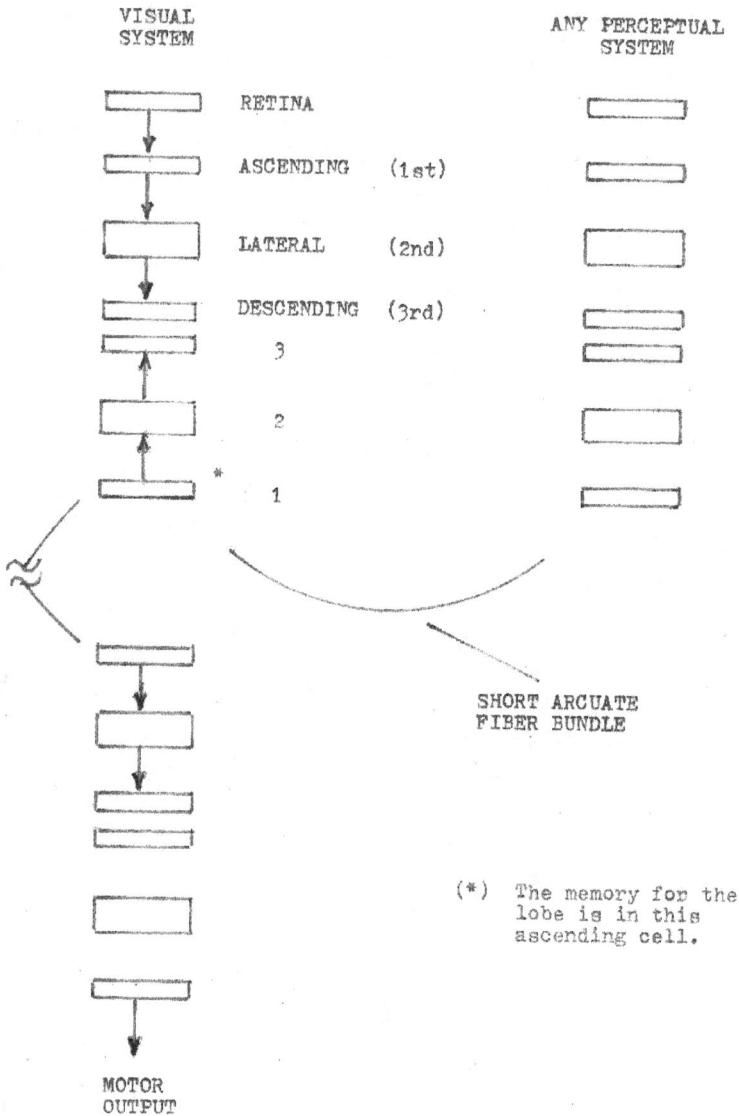

Figure 99

I have numbered the stages in ___ e module in the order of

data flow. Real-time stages are numbered, 1st, 2nd and 3rd.

Memory stages are numbered: 1, 2 and 3. (Fig. 100 is a semi-anatomical sketch and the dimensions of the flow path are impossibly exaggerated; the module could be seen only with a microscope. The real-time stages are not numbered.)

There is a short term technical, or buffer, memory in the real-time descending columnar cell (marked "3rd" in Fig. 99) This is a short term memory, measured in fractions of a second (possible a whole second at times), and I believe it is responsible for a fast moving form of the so-called hypnogogic hallucination, a sleep vagary discussed in the next item.

The real-time retrieval instruction, an electrical analogue of the visual image, appears at the interface between the two systems: the descending columnar cells in Fig. 99. The response for this instruction is "figured out" at a point slightly removed from the interface. It is figured out in the memory for the lobe: asterisk in Fig. 99. This odd flow of data is needed because it is impossible to make memory entries backward through the memory synapses. This is better explained in the next item.

The visual and motor lobes are capable of more sophisticated work than the simple hand/eye tasks which would be their limit if the arcuate fiber tract was the only link carrying instructions between the posterior and frontal systems. The performance of these systems will be expanded well beyond their "perceive-then-act" capability if the

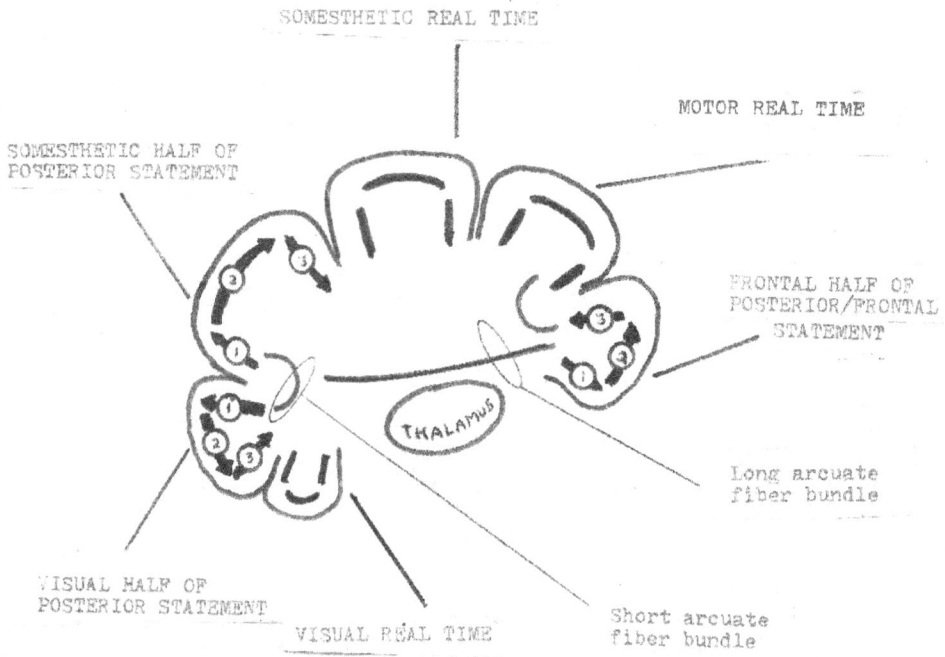

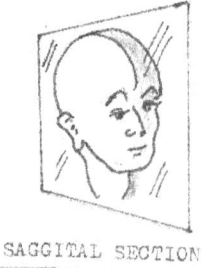

SOMESTHETIC REAL TIME

MOTOR REAL TIME

SOMESTHETIC HALF OF
POSTERIOR STATEMENT

FRONTAL HALF OF
POSTERIOR/FRONTAL
STATEMENT

THALAMUS

Long arcuate
fiber bundle

VISUAL HALF OF
POSTERIOR STATEMENT

VISUAL REAL TIME

Short arcuate
fiber bundle

SAGGITAL SECTION

Figure 100

posterior and frontal systems can be separated and let the off-set
system bring a little thinking into their unthinking ways.

THE DIFFICULTY OF SPECIFYING EXACT CIRCUITRY

The statement written in any specific lobe is derived from a real image of one kind or another. The language for this statement cannot be moved out of the lobe where it is written because the language is not compatible as an "addenda" when presented to the comparator, we can then say the outputs of the comparators constitute a "dedendal" statement. We now have a comparator language and it can be used as a sort of lingua franca to transmit instructions from one lobe to another. The instruction can be conveyed by either the dedicated fiber tracts or by the off-set routing. The long fiber bundles still carry instructions that will retrieve the addendal specific data for real-time operation and, for thoughtful work, the arcuate white fiber link is effectively replaced with a link that is both intelligent and conditionable. As a matter of fact, the link is operationally replaced with what amounts to a complete miniature cortex. The dedicated link is still functioning, it is supplemented to the extent it is effectively subordinate.

If the pole of the temporal lobe is pulled downward, a lobe called the "insular" lobe can be seen. Anatomy tells us nothing about the function of the "island" lobe so I will account for it as I am able. The island lobe is a "buffer" computer serving the dual function of permitting the temporal lobe to be off-set from the main axis of data flow and able to write instructions for the rest of the system, and de-coupling (operationally isolating) any of the lobes in the cortical system. Fig. 101 and Fig. 102 show the physical situation of the island lobe.

The island lobe, though histologically identical to the other lobes, accepts and delivers its inputs and outputs in supervisory (comparator) language. The island system accepts its version of the interlocutory statement in comparator language and delivers an instruction in comparator language as an output.

Operationally, the dedicated tract is subordinated and the island system introduced in the stream of data flow. The dedicated pathways are fixed and the island system is "plastic". The island lobe is, overall, a sort of controllable "ad hoc" substitute for any dedicated fiber tract (Fig. 103).

The work of the cortex can be fractionated into a number of relative independent, "straight through", systems as the task requires. The island system permits the independent and locally dedicated systems to function as a collaborating whole system. In addition to introducing plasticity in the physical routings, the island system, in its capacity as a buffer computer, permits, say, a perceptual system to function in real-time--its own real-time-- and, at the same

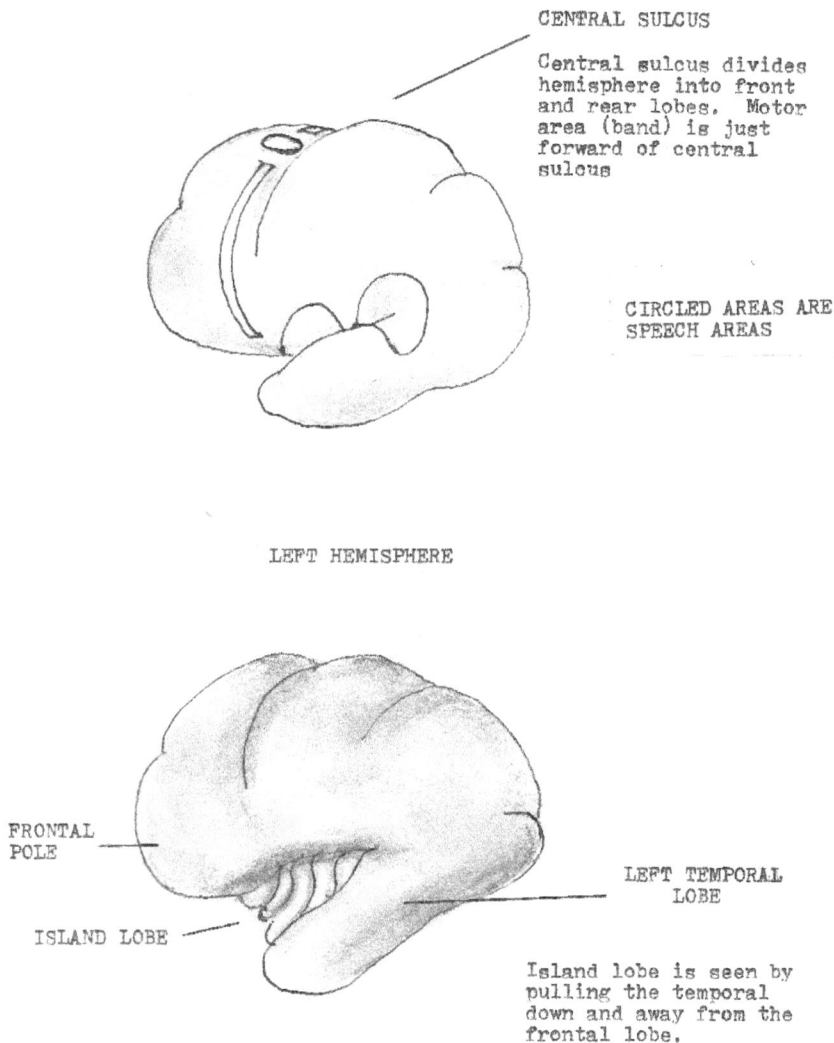

CENTRAL SULCUS

Central sulcus divides
hemisphere into front
and rear lobes. Motor
area (band) is just
forward of central
sulcus

CIRCLED AREAS ARE
SPEECH AREAS

LEFT HEMISPHERE

FRONTAL
POLE

LEFT TEMPORAL
LOBE

ISLAND LOBE

Island lobe is seen by
pulling the temporal
down and away from the
frontal lobe.

Figure 101

time, permits the slaved lobe to operate on a timing schedule

convenient to the output task.

Fig. 104 is an overall view where the island lobe makes it

technically possible for the temporal lobe to ingratiate

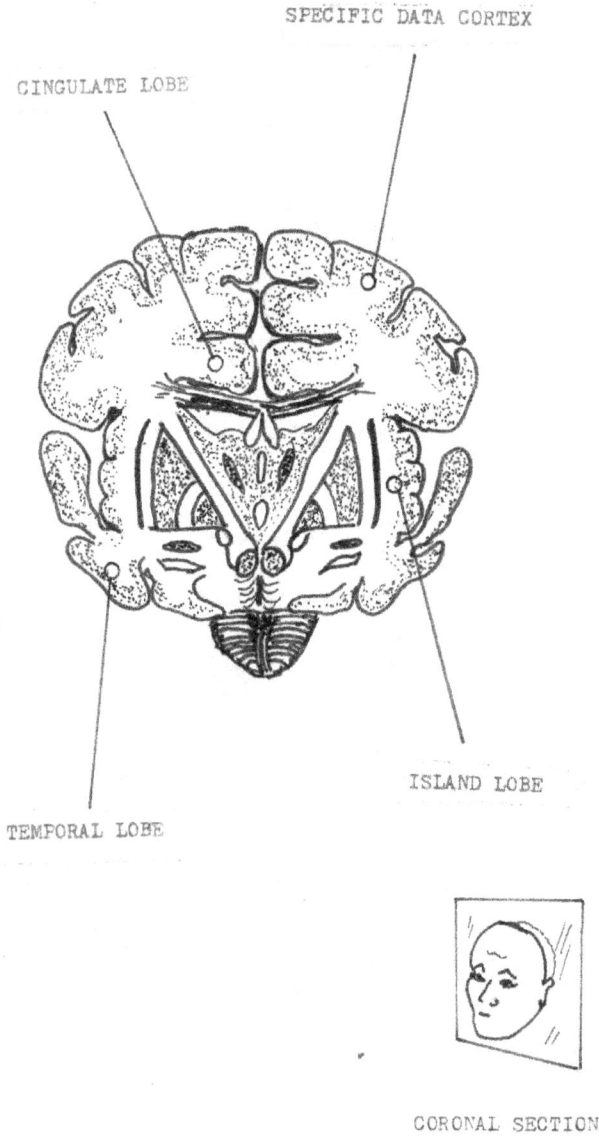

332

SPECIFIC DATA CORTEX

CINGULATE LOBE

ISLAND LOBE

TEMPORAL LOBE

CORONAL SECTION

Fig. 102

itself in any flow path in the cortex by volunteering to act as a

surrogate route for the dedicated path. The temporal lobe usurps

enough of the sense of the instruction in the

334

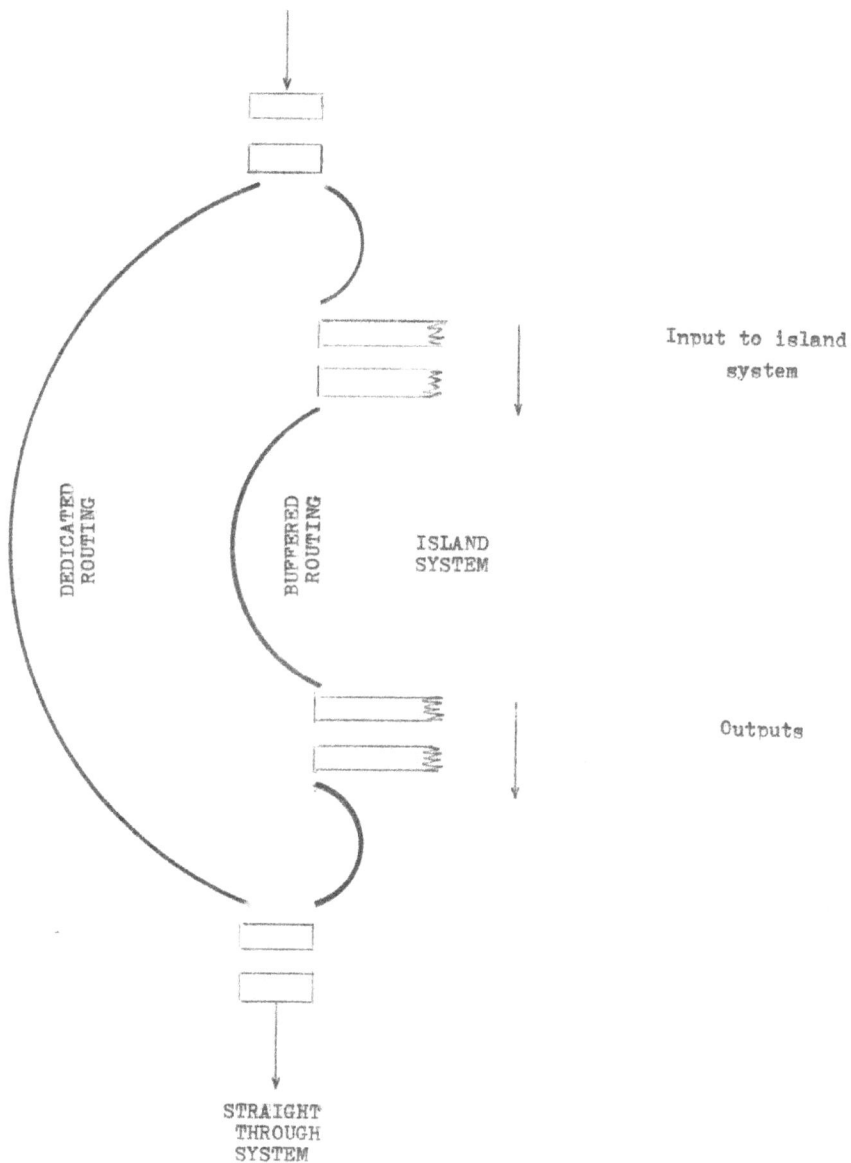

Input to island
system

DEDICATED ROUTING

BUFFERED ROUTING

ISLAND
SYSTEM

Outputs

STRAIGHT
THROUGH
SYSTEM

Figure 103

dedicated path so it is effectively re-routed via the temporal
lobe.

While the straight-through systems "act", the buffered temporal
lobe is free to stand off to the side and "think", adding temporal

395

thinking to any and whatever throughputs. It is free to both

verbally commemorate and to verbally

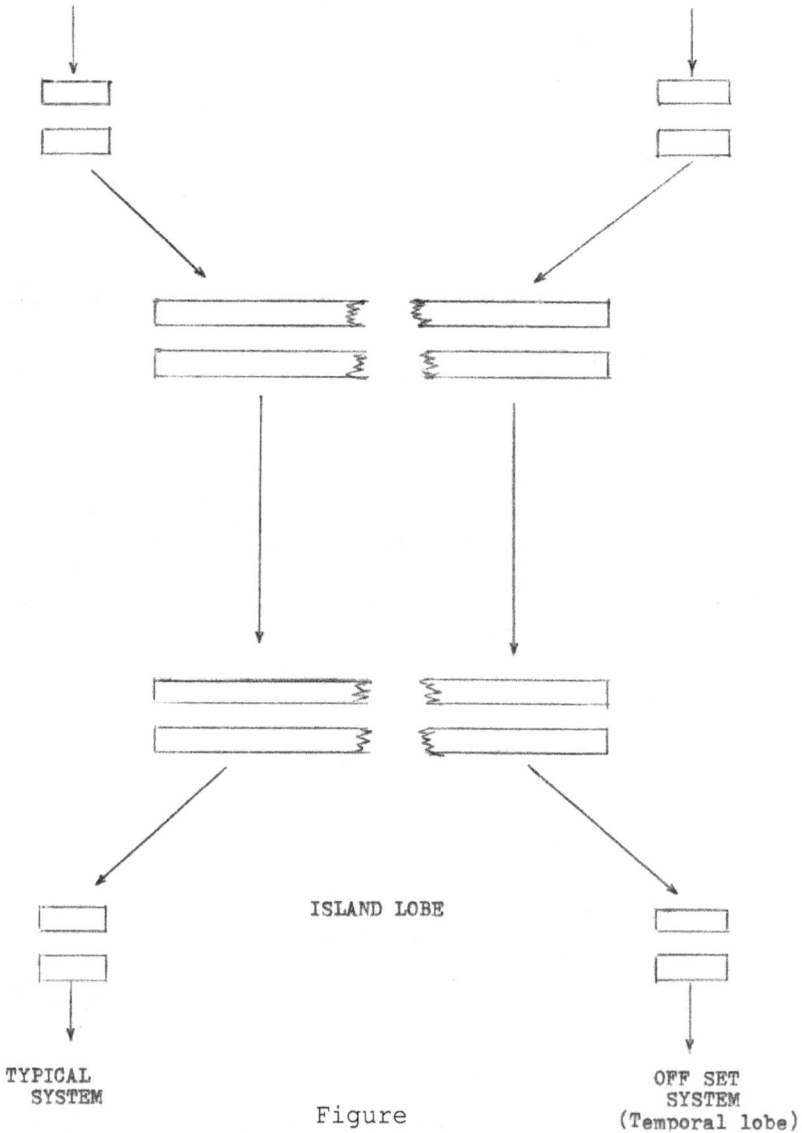

335

ISLAND LOBE

TYPICAL
SYSTEM

Figure
104

OFF SET
SYSTEM
(Temporal lobe)

surrogate experience, free to evaluate the last action and think about the next. The island lobe, the cingulum and the temporal lobe are all both intelligent and conditionable systems. They figure out a way for the temporal lobe to use a symbol to flag a particular experience so it is processable in the surrogate routing and the temporal lobe soon becomes able to insert its own instructions at will. Quickly it learns to dominate the flow of information through the cortex and habitual temporal dominance becomes one of the most deeply set habits in inventory.

Seen from the electronics point of view, the traffic between the lobes is one of the least accessible parts of the cortex to study. I think the coupling between the lobes can be worked out without protracted difficulty and the study will be set ahead with a better understanding of the way the arcuate fibers extricate the cortical statement from the lobe. As we saw earlier, there are no computing operations in the white fiber mass of the brain, so coupling between the lobes, as such is not a critical path issue.

The temporal cortex has been a study of long standing and will be for some time to come. The auditory cortex is in the temporal lobe and its circuit is probably about the same as the other perceptual systems. If the auditory cortex dictates an output at all, it would be efferent instruction to the organ of Corti to selectively nullify disinteresting parts of the sound image in order to better grasp the interesting parts, this was mentioned in the item on cochlear theory and, excepting this one efferent, the auditory cortex probably does not dictate outputs.

The output from the temporal lobe that we call "thinking" is a speech motor instruction, touched on in the item on augmenting intelligence. Contributions to speech motor instructions originate in three areas (sketch). The module, the throughput statement and technical procedures are the same in the temporal lobe as they are in any lobe. Studying vocalization, the process that underpins verbalization, will be less concerned with the technical manipulation of data within the temporal module and more so with the--I suppose; "parlays" --available to the temporal cortex. Freer and working in its own regimen, parlays for the temporal lobe would seem endless. For example, a short scenario of vocalization might have one length in one context and the scenario may be shortened or lengthened, ad hoc, in still another context. There may be strategies where one burst of speech is being expressed while the next parcel is being planned. With parlays, there could be further off-sets within the off-set system where one part will be dictating immediate speech while another section is rehearsing the next scenario.

I have a hunch some of these internal parlays will need a lot of thought to figure them out. The study of aphasia might be helpful here. Aphasia is a speech impairment, it comes in a number of forms. There is one version attributable to injury to a very long bundle of white fibers running from the temporal lobe to the motor cortex that is especially intriguing. After the injury, the neurologist holds up a spool of thread and asks his patient to tell him what it is, The patient replies, "That is the thing you wind thread on". He holds up a needle. "That is the thing you sew with". In every case, the noun that would name the subject matter is unexpressed and inexpressible. If we can forebear any more of my speculation, I think something like this may be happening, we are taught ways to think when we are taught language and we hold the "thing" (the subject) in the foreground of our thinking and we say something about it (the predicate). The cortex does not recognize the subject and predicate as such, due to the way the coded throughput statement is written, the cortex does not have access to the subject matter of the verbal throughput. There is another phenomenal "purchase" the cortex may be making use of. The cortex may recognize the emphatic-- and so often repeated--noun as a stable and invariant verbal operation, and it may recognize its variable "context", the things said about the noun that normally vary all over the place.

Is it possible the cortex learns a parlay where it artificially sets out the noun as a stable "feature" and the variable predicate as a changeable "surround"? The physiology of the cortex is compatible with working this way and the process may be enhanced with training and usage.

The cortex learns to store the "feature" (the noun) in the speech area of the motor lobe and the mobile predicate in temporal memory. Severing the fiber bundle interrupts this long standing habit and, when the temporal lobe tries to take over all speech computation after the injury, the noun is lost.

It is not so much a question of physiology or even the ability of the cortex to learn the parlay. The cortex normally uses "feature" and "surround" strategies with speed and elegance. The parlay must be suggested by the environment, the source of all learning, and the environment must suggest the parlay with sufficient force and clarity so the cortex will acquire the routine. This leads me to wonder if there was a convergence (or a fluke) in the way language evolved so its evolution takes advantage of an intrinsic tendency within the cortex to separate experience into "features" and "surrounds". (Do all languages place the same emphasis on the subject and predicate idea?)

The theorist in this area is less interested in the anatomy and function in the temporal cortex and more concerned with semantics, linguistics, computer equivalents of human performance and, most importantly, the end products of temporal computation rather than the computation itself.

The student of the speech cortex is confronted with the same scale of observation problems that apply to study of any throughput. The speech cortex processes the instantaneous minutia of a vocal motor instruction and the vocal behavior we hear is the end product of this burst of vocal instruction. From vocalization to sound, from sound to symbol, and from there on, it is a cultural matter: a pattern, an agreement with regard to which symbol will stand for which experience.

I enjoy reading the work of experts in this field and they report some progress from time to time. I do not think the verbal processes are so complex and esoteric they will elude exposure for any great length of time. It is a matter of plugging away.

From the information already available and from what I can reasonably infer, I am unable to think of a verbal procedure that would require a module more sophisticated than the one already outlined. The problem for the student of speech is the end use of

400

the module's computation and not the electronics of the module as such. The coder and finesse of the vocal lobe should be about the same as any other cortical procedure. The speech expert should begin with a rough idea of what the module is, and is not capable of doing and base his expectations of the speech process accordingly.

Before we can work out the language of the statement between the lobes, it would be helpful if the anatomist would give us a better picture of the roots and terminus of the arcuate fiber tracts. The slaving procedure itself is fairly simple and is one of the finesses of the exalted data stage.

There are a lot of arguments about the reasons so many people are right handed and the best thing to do with these arguments is to stay out of them. There are good psychological reasons for holding the work in one hand and manipulating the tool with the other, or on a finer scale, holding it with the small fingers and manipulating with the thumb and index finger. The fine work is set out as a "feature" and the drone tasks as a "surround". This artifice forces the feature to "behave" with respect to the surround. We have an extra psychological purchase we would not have had it not occurred to us to divide the task into feature and surround. "Handedness" is a variation of the "feature" and "surround" strategy and it is easy to see where it comes in handy and augments our performance.

A particular "handedness", say, right-handedness, is not suggested by the way tasks are presented to us by our environment. Students of this problem say the environment is neither right nor left handed. Right-handedness is of no advantage to the cortical computer; it can switch from either handedness without the slightest inconvenience.

The left temporal lobe is slightly larger than the right lobe in its inferior and medial aspects. The left lobe computes vocal instructions for the right half of the vocal system. While it only dictates vocal instructions, it is evidently an important factor responsible for right-handedness. Since the left temporal lobe is larger and there are a few more data elements in the left temporal statement, I can see where a larger left lobe might bias the dominance schedule toward chronic left lobe dominance. After a few fixed dominance requirements have been met, dominance authority then becomes democratic and dominance would probably be assigned to the lobe capable of writing a statement with the most data elements in it, all other factors being equal. Eventually the control system would habituate to chronic left dominance.

This line of reasoning may account for the anatomical tendency to right-handedness but does not explain the efficacy of right-handedness when the human brain could, in principle, just as easily alternate between right and left-handedness. Perhaps the larger left lobe and right-handedness are flukes of evolution.

One misunderstanding of the cortex comes from hanging the wrong inference on an observation of its left/right vagaries. The wrong inference is becoming entrenched, almost a legend. The temporal lobes write vocal motor instructions. Up to about age twelve, there is good reason to believe dominance between left and right lobes is about evenly divided as vocal skills develop. Before age twelve, the right lobe can take over if the left lobe is damaged. After age twelve. the right lobe cannot assume dominance and there is a speech impairment. Great empires of conceptualization have been floated on this spare knowledge, culminating in the claim the left lobe computes speech and the right lobe is preoccupied with more esoteric interests: abstract, complex and creative thought have been mentioned. While the physical evidence may beg inference, it does not beg the inference one lobe is processing one kind of subject matter and the other lobe something else. Calling them the way we see them, there is only one fact in evidence: the right lobe cannot assume dominance after the cut-off age has been reached, this and nothing more. No inference regarding the kind of information the lobes are processing can sensibly be attached to the physical observation, certainly not a finding as negative as this one.

The proposal the lobes are processing different subject matter is even less likely if we take a close look at the white fiber fan-in to the lobe. The fan-in (nerves to either sensors or muscles) carries information either to or from the lobe. The throughput statement is committed to the information carried by the fan-in. The nerve fan-in for the left temporal lobe carries exactly the same information presented to the right sides the only difference being: the input (or output) statements are mirror images of each other. If we toss in the coder technique, noting the lobe does not have access to the subject matter of the throughput, it is even more improbable the left temporal lobe is processing one kind of information and the right lobe another.

FINESSE OF THE EXALTED DATA STAGE

Two key factors dictate the circuit layout in the active stage in
the cortex. The fast rise rate of the signal excursion on memory
delivery may exceed the high frequency roll-off of the nerve cell.
The roll-off problem and the possibility of unacceptable phase
shift in the recalled signal prevent "piping" these precision
signals any greater distance than the synapse that contains the
memory unit. A second factor is the way memory must be
interrogated. The retrieval instruction is written in the form of
a data plane and can only be presented to memory. Memory delivery
must be made with (electronically) identical synapses facing each
other, vis a vis, with a comparator cell between.

Like any synapse, the memory synapse is unidirectional. The entry
path for a real-time entry in real-time memory is simple and
straight forward (left of center in Fig. 105). Now we have the
problem of making the initial entry in the memory for the lobe
(right synapse in Fig. 105) by a route that is against the normal
conducting direction of the synapse.

   (It may take a little noodle work to see this problem.
Regardless of the way the network might be wired, sooner or later
it will be necessary to confront a memory delivery with a retrieval
instruction, vis a vis. This dictates the way the systems face
each other physically. Data delivery is no

346

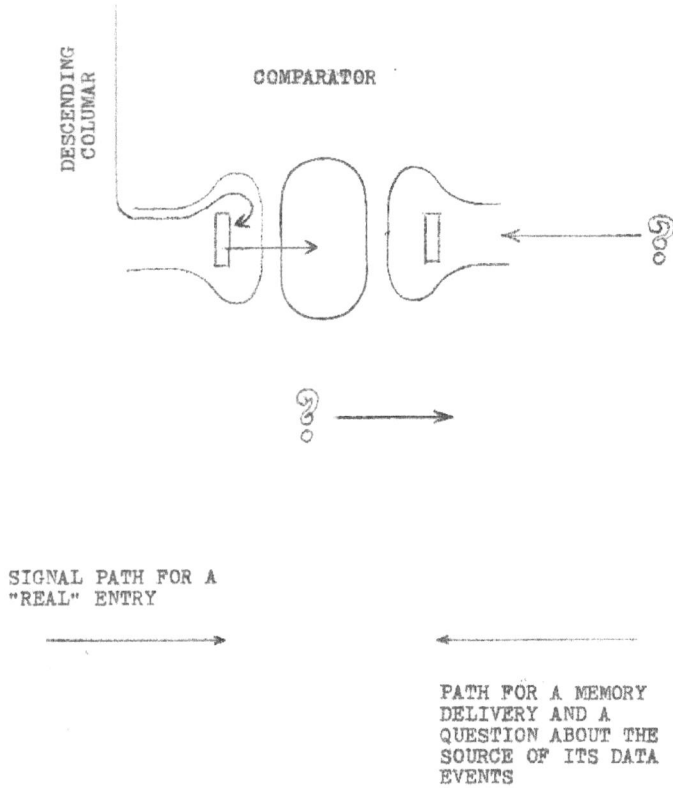

DESCENDING
COLUMAR

COMPARATOR

SIGNAL PATH FOR A
"REAL" ENTRY

PATH FOR A MEMORY
DELIVERY AND A
QUESTION ABOUT THE
SOURCE OF ITS DATA
EVENTS

Figure 105

problem. However, if the outflowing paths face each other, then

data from at least one of the faces, when it was initially entered,

would have to have been moved into the memory synapse, in effect, in a direction opposite the normal direction of conduction for the synapse.)

Fig. 106 is the module we first saw in the discussion of the smart engine and the comparator from Fig. 105 is in the center of this sketch. The trick here is to transfer the data event appearing at the real-time descending columnar (upper asterisk) to the memory for the lobe (lower asterisk). A trial data event is generated in the ascending columnar which contains the memory for the lobe (number 1). The smart engine in the ascending columnar repeatedly tries to produce a match at the descending columnar (number 2 in the sketch). Both the real-time comparator and the memory for the lobe are in exalted data stages and the exalted data stages are locked-in so a match at site 2 will fire both exalted data stages. (A successful match at site 2 will fire both exalted data stages.) The memory for the lobe is trying to "figure out" an amplitude for its data event that will produce a match for the "real" data event on the opposite side of the comparator (opposite site 2) and it is trying to do so notwithstanding the lateral re-organization of the network in the intervening lateral cells. Firing is delayed until the match is made. Under the circumstance, the trial in the "trial and error" procedure is largely eliminated. With a match, an indigenous data event is made at the respective memory sites.

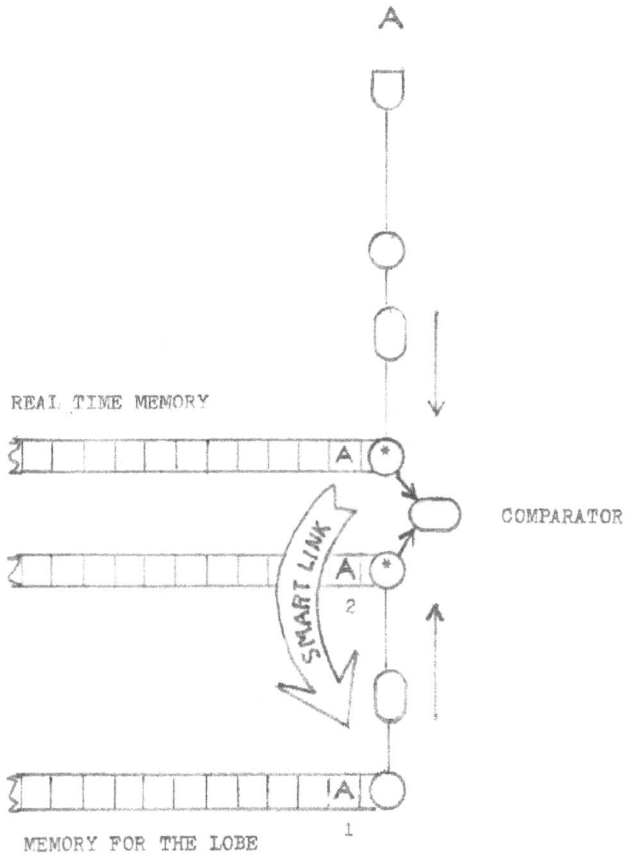

REAL TIME MEMORY

COMPARATOR

SMART LINK

MEMORY FOR THE LOBE

Figure 106

While this may look like a Figure 106 way of doing things, it is

not. The system is not doing anything it does not ordinarily do

anyway. The smart engine is extant and available and it is being

used in an internal service that exquisitely underlies its normal

usage with no extra burden. This plan is especially attractive
when the lateral reorganization of the network is taken into
account. This vis a vis presentation of the retrieval instruction
versus the response, with intelligent procedure "figuring out" the
response, rather than an impossible dual routing of signals, is
probably the only scheme that holds any prospect of working, given
the nerve cell as the active element.

The memory synapses are physically vis a vis with a comparator
between, and this standardizes the circuit layout for all exalted
data stages in the cortex. This basic layout makes the exalted
finesses possible, and the key problem of data flow into the memory
synapse has been satisfied. Many of the exalter finesse have
already been mentioned. Here are some additional finesses squeezed
into this simple apparatus:

1. The solution to the language translation problem between lobes
is now in sight and with no more apparatus than we already have.
The data plane in the dominant lobe stays in the language
indigenous to the lobe. It is compared to a memory response and
the outcome of the comparison is effectively used as a retrieval
instruction to request specific data planes in the slaved lobe
without attempting a language translation. Without this
simplification, the language translation problem would have been an
unbelievably complicated rigmarole in the cortex.

2. The specific data cortex is controlled by a control cortex
made up with the modules and same general plan as the specific data
cortex. The physical circuit of the exalted data stage makes the
control finesse possible. The marvelous finesse of the control

system comes to light shortly, and the control finesse, virtuosity
at its own assignment, also provides an interface and switching
authority between the cortex and the reflex and instinctive
systems.

3. The real-time system, using standard components, also serves a
second function as a "chopper"; the chopper is the rate-of-change
coder. The same basic exalter procedure is used in this special
"chopper" function as is used throughout the rest of the cortex.
These recursive and overlaying usages of the same standard
apparatus profoundly simplify the histogenic process.

4. The exalter finesse also takes care of a hodge-podge of
technical problems, none of which are trivial. For one thing, the
exalter "cleans up" the data plane by making sure all of the data
elements in the plane are in position before the plane is fired.
It also acts as an electronic "buffer" preventing noise and data
anomalies from blasting through the exalted data stage and on to
memory units elsewhere in the network.

Fig. 107 is the circuit which forces synchronized firing of the
cells in the exalted data stage. If the descending columnar cells
deliver signals with mismatched amplitudes, the comparator will
recognize the mismatch and generate an error signal which is sent
to the control system. The error signal is a D.C. signal with a
D.C. amplitude. The amplitude is a function of the degree of
mismatch.

The error signal is negative in sense (i.e. inhibitory) and
inhibits the firing of the sync cell. The error signal tries to
delay firing of the sync cell which will allow more time for

scanning and, in turn, improve the match. The control system tries to speed up firing in order to get on with necessary business. An agreement is reached by subtracting the "delay firing" signal from the "fire" signal and the firing rate the sync cell set accordingly.

I think of the sync cell as an octopus like cell with thousands of tentacles laid out in the physical plane of the exalted data stage. (The radiating branches of the cell have also given it the name "stellate" or "chandelier" cell.) The histogenic code for the sync cell can be simplified as the forming cell is programmed to form junctions with and fire any cell it can reach in its vicinity. Firing all of the cells in the lobe at the same time contributes to cortical noise immunity.

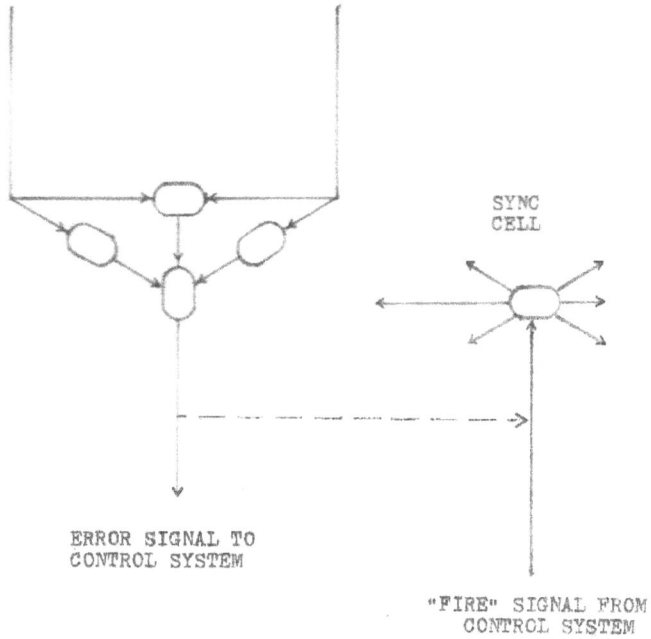

SYNC
CELL

ERROR SIGNAL TO
CONTROL SYSTEM

"FIRE" SIGNAL FROM
CONTROL SYSTEM

Figure 107

It would seem only cells conta   units should be, or need

be, fired when the memory entry is made. There are cortical cells

upstream of the exalted data stage and, though D.C. cells, they

must fire to preserve their cell vitality, ion balances and

411

metabolic power supply calibration. If these upstream cells are
fired at random, there is a possibility they might fire in the few
milliseconds preceding memory entry and their firing would be
superimposed on the D.C. analogue signals. This problem is
eliminated by forcing all of the cells in the lobe to fire
synchronously and only when the memory molecule is being advanced.

Physically the sync cells are in the physical plane of the
exalted data stage. The plane is distributed over the span of the
lobe and, allowing for a few convolutions, the plane should be
found at the junctions of the white fibers and the gray cells of
the cortex.

The output synapses of the sync cell are the "brute force" type
and, when the sync cell fires, all cells connected to its tentacles
are fired by brute force at the same instant. The sync cell also
synapses with other sync cells. When the agreement to fire has
been reached, the sync cells will forcibly fire each other, further
assuring all cells in the lobe fire at the same instant and further
assuring synchronization of all memory units in the data plane.
(There may be places in the exalter circuit where it seems positive
cells are driving positive cells in an manner that infringes the
"delta" circuit prohibition. The sync cell is a supervisory cell
controlled by an external source. Most of the time it is held in
cutoff where it could not transgress any rules whatever. During
the enforced firing interval, the sync cells all fire a "one-shot"
firing at the same instant, then back to cut-off. All of this is
under positive control rather than the uncontrolled self-excited
oscillation that disregard for delta circuit rules would hazard.)

The D.C. amplitude of the error signal is a direct function of the comparator mismatch; a greater mismatch will increase the D.C. error signal amplitude. The sense of the error signal is "inhibitory" and the sense of the sync signal is "excitory". It is interesting to note the circuit in Fig. 107 would self-sufficiently work as a exalter, after a fashion, if there was a direct connection between the error output and the sync cell (dashed line) and the control system eliminated altogether. The sync cell would have to agree to fire at a fast residual rate which the error signal would slow down. (I toy with the idea there may be brain systems that are conditionable (only). There is a small chance the cerebellar brain may be one of these. Here, the exalted data stage is not controlled but fires on a "plebiscite", that is, when errors are as small as they can be made, the stage fires automatically and no control system is needed. The "plebiscite" arrangement may have been an evolutionary precursor of the cerebral cortex.)

All we have to do with Fig. 107 is to conceptually remove the dashed line and insert a miniature cerebral cortex with its input terminals connected to the error buses and its outputs controlling the sync cells. According to me, the cingulate lobe of the cortex does this. It is illustrated later.

The format for the exalter control is simple. The control cortex accepts a D.C. error signal at its input. It delivers a D.C. error correcting signal at its output. The output from the control system is a D.C. excitory signal and its amplitude sets the firing rate of the sync cell. (The control system does not dictate the individual firings of the sync cell.) A slower firing rate corrects errors by allowing more time to scan for the most complete match of the retrieval instruction. Looked at another way, the control system accepts a firing rate as an input and delivers a firing rate as an output. This miniature control cortex figures out by trial and error, the D.C. value of the output signal that will correct the error, and the control system "learns" how to get rid of errors by adjusting firing rates. Both slowing down and speeding up firing rates to eliminate errors when dominant and slaved lobes are involved.

The rate at which the retrieval instruction is delivered can be adjusted by speeding up or slowing down the dominant lobe and a rate more favorable to the responding lobe can be found by working out a best compromise speed. If a lobe is forced to speed up, there must be a corresponding sacrifice of matched detail in the response because of the shortened scanning time. Running faster, "remote" corollaries are not considered so fewer responses of all kinds are entertained. This is a trade-off made to keep things moving when the system is keeping up with real-time. Fast running shortens the time available for the trials and errors of intelligent procedure, so fast running is at the expense of intelligent contribution to the throughput.

(It is easier to compute motor instructions for a body in fairly fast movement because it is not necessary to compute all of the detail of the small accelerations and rebalancing's of a slowly moving body. The acquaintance, I mentioned in the item on intelligence: the "all letter" savant, walks quite rapidly with an almost elephant like "planting" of one foot behind the other. If he is about to climb some stairs, he will position himself in the middle of the steps before he takes his first step. Strategies such as these reduce his vulnerability to cortical errors.)

Slowing the firing rate eliminates errors by allocating more time to scan for better matches at the comparators. Very slow running de-stabilizes the retrieval instruction which adds errors and, at the same time, entertains a much broader range of admissible corollaries. Slow running, the system free scans. Switching from task to reverie, the control system will "figure out" a running rate for the cortex that, will reduce errors given the assignment and time slot available.

Running rate is also a test for competence of the lobe. A lobe is competent if it tends to run fast. If it is running fast, or if it is willing to speed up on command, it is evidently having no trouble finding responses in memory to match the retrieval instruction, therefore it is competent.

The cingulate lobe, like all other lobes in the cortex, does not have access to the subject matter of its throughput. The finesse of the exalter procedure first interrogates a lobe to determine its competence with a trial speed up, this is not a separate operation and takes place as a part of assigning dominance. Having selected a competent lobe, it lets it write the retrieval instruction by making it dominant. (A slight speed-up of the lobe or area of the lobe makes it dominant.) It then selects another lobe, and this must be a feasible instruction routing, and lets it be the slaved lobe. The control system learns to speed-up or slow-down the dominant lobe, or speed-up or slow the slaved lobe, or to reassign dominance in order to maintain competence in as much of the cortex as is possible. It "figures out" ways to adjust firing rates in order to start, sustain and restore competence in the lobes involved and to expand this process to include all of the lobes in the cortex.

If there is a fixed hierarchy of dominance authority for the lobes of the cortex, it cannot be very complex. Probably all that is needed to satisfy the fixed authority is the observation of a few necessary and sensible feasibilities so instructions flow in the right direction and that sort of thing.

After the fixed restraints have been satisfied, the schedule of authority becomes democratic. An area that is competent and capable of writing an instruction will dominate. If two areas are qualified for dominance, the area that is capable of writing an instruction the quickest will dominate. If dominance is still not resolved, assuming all other factors to be equal, the lobe, or area, that is competent, fastest and able to write an instruction with the most elements in it will dominate. If the control system wants an area of the cortical data plane to assume dominance, it speeds up that area.

The control system "polices" the cortical data plane, speeding it up here, slowing it there, reassigning authority or shifting both timing and authority elsewhere, all of this, to establish or restore competence in all (or most) areas of the data plane. The area of the data plane can be subdivided into: the lobe, an area within the lobe and a subdivision as a small a few comparator cells. All divisions receive the same treatment from the control system.

The input signal to the control system can be looked at three ways, it is a D.C. signal, it is a firing rate and it is a statement of the competence of the area in question.

For a given task, the control system locates a competent lobe and a lobe able to "slave". It adjusts firing rates (by trial and error if this is the first attempt at this task) of both the dominant and slaved lobes to complete the task, If the control system does this correctly, the cortex will remain competent and the task is carried out. If the control system is wrong, the cortex will become increasingly incompetent, "balk", and the control system looks for another instruction or starts another effort to re-establish competence in all of the cortex if possible. This is done with a minimum of apparatus and without access to the subject matter of the throughput: one of the system's slicker finesses.

A wealth of implicit logic can be wrought from this simple control finesse:

1. If there is no error, the exalter is having no difficulty finding a match for an incoming instruction. If this condition persists, the system is obviously processing repeated information; since the control system is not being asked to slow down to extended scanning time, the exalter must be forming matches between present data planes and data planes that were recently entered. Rather than waste memory space making entries it already has, the control system relinquishes the real-time instruction, slows down,

and permits memory to free-scan. The system has now switched from building up the throughput ledger by the iterative process to building out the ledger by the associative process. The absence of an error signal cues the control system, telling it the input is redundant and the mode shift is due.

2. If the preceding gives the exalter control a "handle" for managing redundant throughputs, it also provides a handle for managing irredundant throughputs. If the D.C. error signal is near maximum amplitude, the data error is large and there is a good chance memory inventory does not contain matching data planes. Perhaps they were never entered in memory. Rather than risk assigning dominance to a doubtful lobe (or area), and, since the outcome of scanning cannot be predicted, protracted scanning will not make it less doubtful, this "handle" alerts the control system to an oncoming cortical "balk". With early warning, the control system is able to reassign dominance to less doubtful areas to head off the balk. The need to do something about "balk" before it gets out of hand is a little clearer in a later discussion of the mechanism that makes the shift from cortical to the instinctive mode.

4. The exalter finesse permits data errors to be corrected to the extent they can be corrected. If we say 50% of the sites must be matched as a test for a competent data plane, the exalter finesses can make a tradeoff between D.C. signal amplitude errors and site errors in order to obtain the match. Any area of the data plane can be expected to erect a technically competent contribution to the data plane and assume dominance from time to time. If it

contains noise or data anomalies, it will be subordinated and begin to lose ground staying above the memory survival threshold. The exalter finesse continuously improves the signal to noise ratio of the data in memory by permanently subordinating noise which is equivalent to dropping it from memory. (This was mentioned with reference to dope aggression against the memory ledger. The exalter finesse is one of the mechanisms that enforces the "economizing" procedure where defective data is thrown out and technically competent throughputs saved.)

The next three drawings show the effect movement in the visual image will have on signal amplitude. Fig. 108 is a practical drawing. A bright spot in the visual image is being swept past a photoreceptor and the outcome is the same if the spot stands still and the retina moves. The receptor output is plotted at the bottom of the drawing. The output is a positive signal amplitude excursion, rising as the light spot approaches and begins to illuminate the receptor. This is followed by a raised plateau as the spot makes its transit across the receptor, followed by a trailing off of signal amplitude as the stimulus passes. Output is then restored to the original static (background) illumination that prevailed before the disturbance.

Fig. 109 is a greatly simplified cortex with the receptor on one end of the data bus and the descending columnar on the other. A moving subject matter will superimpose a dynamic signal (AC) on the steady background signal (DC). If the optical image and the retina are stationary with respect to each other, there is no movement within the visual image and there is no dynamic component (AC) in the visual statement.

Fig. 110 is the same as the preceding sketch only the lateral re-organization of the network is included. The light excursion at a single receptor is reported at hundreds of descending columnar cells. (Regardless of it being a static or dynamic signal, the exact identity of the receptor has been "buried" in the lateral reorganization of the network. The "burial" began at the retinal coder, well upstream of the cortical reorganization. At the descending columnar, the spatial component of the image is not separately extricable. At the descending columnar, the A.C.

360

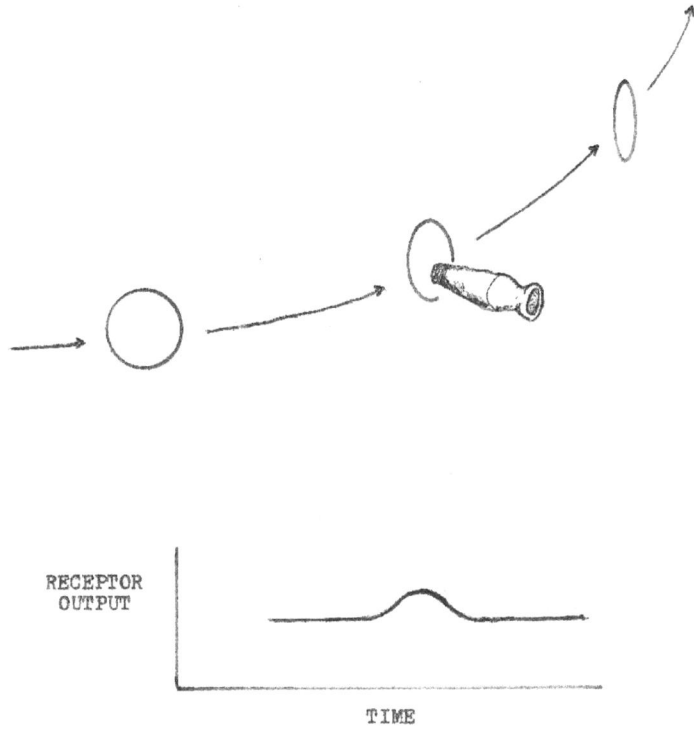

RECEPTOR
OUTPUT

TIME

Figure 108

and the D.C. components of the signal, as such, are the only events

in the visual image that can be used to make a record of movement

in the visual image,) The descending columnar carrying those areas

of the visual image where there is

421

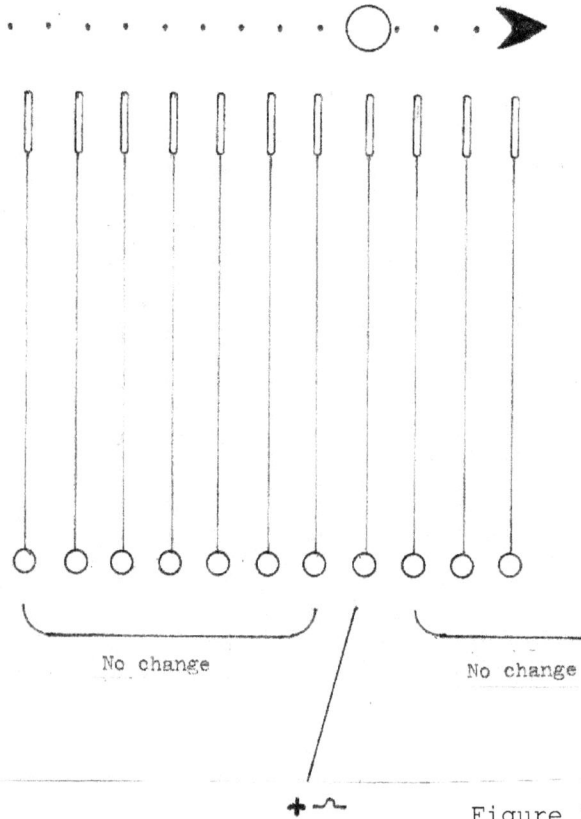

362

Figure 109

movement will be carrying a varying (AC) signal: the "mobile" in
Fig. 110. Descending columnar carrying signals from areas where
there is no movement will be carrying an unvarying (DC) signal: the
"stabile" in the same sketch.

If the visual image does not move across the retina, there will
be only one of these signals, the "stabile." The mechanism for
recording motion in the image works best with

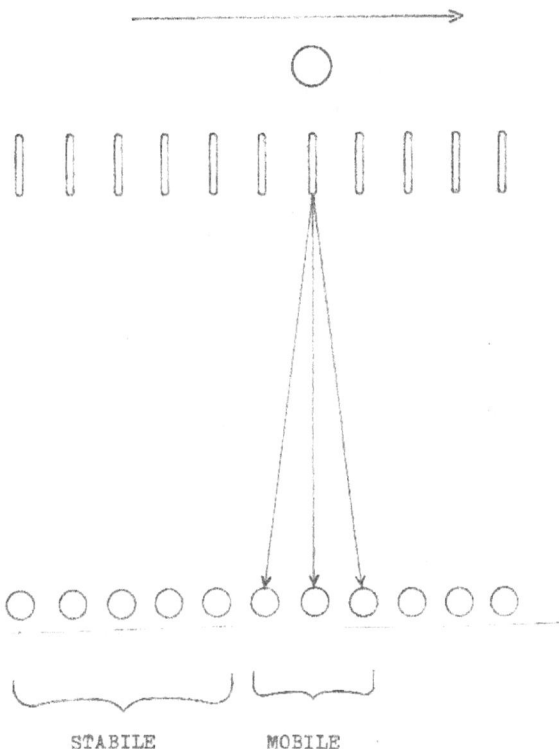

Figure 110

an image where something moves within the image, preferably a

moving "feature" which moves with respect to a stationary

"surround". Rather than passively waiting for movement in the

visual image to come along, the eye aiming mechanism can always take positive action by moving the eye to adduce movement in the image. On the other hand, if there is an interesting something moving across the visual field, eye aiming can "freeze" the movement by adjusting the motion of the retina so it matches the speed of the object, making it stand still on the retina, The moving object now becomes the fixed "stabile" and the heretofore stationary visual background becomes the "mobile" because it is now in retrograde motion with respect to the foveal retina. The cortex does not sort out the subject matter of the visual image; to do so would require a mechanism of staggering complexity and trillions of nerve cells the brain does not have.

The cortex does things in a much simpler fashion, it makes phenomenal "separations" by isolating and processing, in separation, the separable phenomena is the visual image. I think the visual system makes the following "separations:'

1. The specific data signal which is the black and white detail in the image.

2. Three color statements which are arithmetical "add-on" signals to the specific data signal.

3. A coded statement recording the rate of change of moving events in the visual image; let's call it the "speed coder". It will be easier to understand the speed coder if I explain it as it applies to the visual system. I imagine the motor lobes and all other perceptual systems have similar speed coders, each with its special adaptations and "feature" extrication schemes. (Without motion in the image, the rate of change coder is defeated and there is one less psychological "purchase" on the image. I doubt if this

happens naturally, at least not for any great length of time; even then, there is a tonic tremor in the rectus muscles of the eye which always leave some dynamic component in the image. Removing the speed coder cue has been simulated in the laboratory. A visual image is stabilized on the retina with an optical apparatus mounted on a contact lens in a way that prevents movement between the image and the lens. This defeats the speed coder and, after a short interval, visual performance becomes almost totally unraveled and the image breaks up, disappearing piece by piece.)

4. A control statement which, while it is processed in the control cortex, always accompanies its particular visual image. By recording the coded phenomenology of the visual image rather than its subject matter, these formats should be able to specify everything about the visual image that can be specified and should be capable of reconstructing the visual image on recall.

Fig. 111 is the real-time section of the module with the fan-in fiber and ascending columnar wrongly shown as two cells to make the two functions easier to see in the drawing.

367

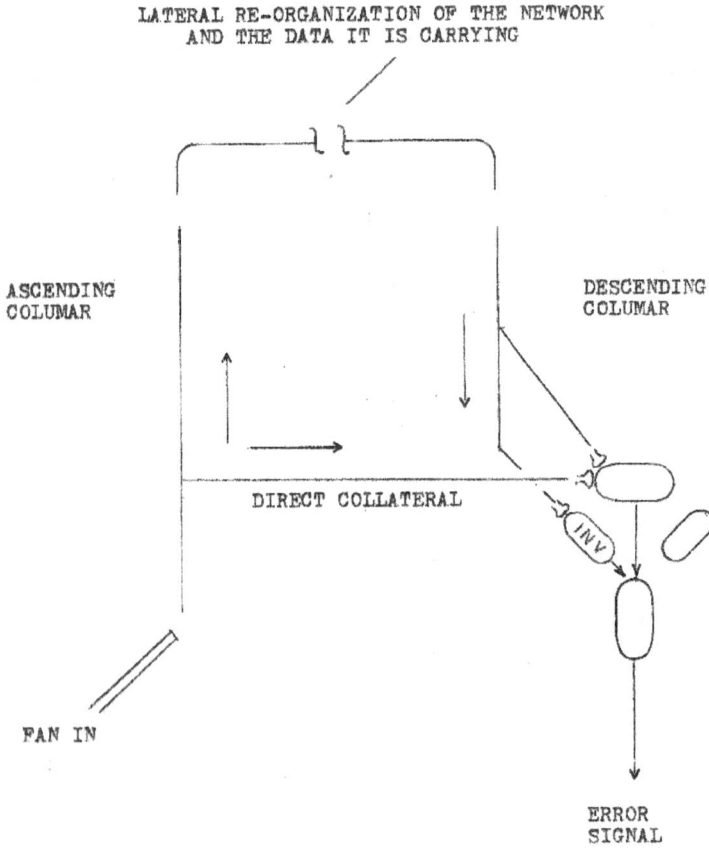

LATERAL RE-ORGANIZATION OF THE NETWORK
AND THE DATA IT IS CARRYING

ASCENDING
COLUMAR

DESCENDING
COLUMAR

DIRECT COLLATERAL

INV

FAN IN

ERROR
SIGNAL

Figure 111

The only thing new in this sketch is the direct collateral branch

of the ascending columnar which seems eager to go directly to the

exalted data stage and shunt the lateral re-organization that takes

place in the outer layers.

426

FINESSE OF THE EXALTED DATA STAGE

The rate of change coder uses standard circuits and the finesse of the existing exalted data stage adapted to the special service of recording movement in the image. The only apparatus needed is the extra direct branch of the ascending columnar branch in the real-time section of the module. This collateral is the raw "on-axis" data bus and it is carrying the information carried on one optic nerve fiber. This information is a low resolution signal, more a sampling than a signal, of the stimulus on 100 photo receptors in the vicinity of the retinal end of the optic nerve fiber. An instantaneous "picture" of visual experience will be "chopped" out of the uninterrupted flow of information coming down the optic tract, this is necessary to erect the visual statement in the form of a data plane. A decision has to be made about the frequency of these visual "pictures". If the control system will fire the real-time exalted data stage at a specially controlled rate, that is, if the real-time exalted data stage will act as a "chopper", the <u>control signal can be used as a means to code motion in the visual image</u>.

On those occasions when there is no movement between the image and the retina, the real-time system is processing the "stabile" in Fig. 110. Here, each "picture", each data plane, is identical to the one preceding. <u>Since there is no exchange of information between data planes, the network carrying a "stabile" can be fired at any convenient rate. This also applies to fractions of the area of the retina where there is no motion between the area and the image</u>.

Somewhere in this circuit there will be a strategically placed inverter, so connected that a sampling of the re-organized signal and the direct signal are added arithmetically. With a "stabile" (all DC) present in the circuit, the arithmetical proportioning is such that the two signals just cancel. When the signals cancel, there is no error output signal from the comparator.

If the D.C. signal on the raw bus and the unvarying (DC) signals on the descending columnar just cancel when the circuit is carrying a "stabile"--all D.C. on all buses-the signals will not cancel when the circuit is carrying A.C. signals.

With a "mobile" in the circuit, the amplitude of the D.C. signal on the raw bus will be arithmetically incorrect to balance the descending signals. The descending signals will not balance because they carry superimposed A.C. signal components derived from the nearby retina where there was movement in the image. (Here, the foveal retina was fixed on the image and the background was in motion.) With movement in the image, there will be an error output signal, it will be a D.C. analogue signal and its amplitude will be a function of the error. The error output signal is also an analogue of motion because the error in the arithmetic is caused by motion in the image.

The D.C. error signal is fed to the control system and the control system tries to get rid of the error by speeding up the "chopper" firing rate. The idea is something like speeding up a motion picture camera to "freeze" motion within the image (if not "freeze", then slow to a near stop).

Fig. 111 is the "chopper". Chopper firings are an adaptation of normal exalter firings, technically the same, save for the special firing rate applicable to chopper service. The chopper firing rate is controlled by a D.C. control signal from the control system, the speed up is a function of error and error, in turn, is a function of movement in the visual image. <u>Therefore the amplitude of the D.C. control signal that controls the firing of the real-time lobe—the "chopper" is an analogue of motion, per se</u>. This rate-of-movement is stored in memory like any other specific data signal, though, I think it is stored in the control cortex (the cingulum) rather than the specific data cortex.

There is a buffer memory in the descending columnar of the real-time lobe. As sleep approaches, this visual real-time memory will occasionally free-scan and it generates a fantastic display, a veritable river of fast moving/fast changing, brilliant and intensely colored images. The images are often geometric or floral patterns which repeat themselves, forming an overall pattern in rapid movement across the visual field. These images are the fast moving version of "hypnagogic hallucinations", as they are referred to.

There will be a short burst of one image and a rapid switch to another. I interpret the duration of the "burst" to be the time duration of the visual scenario. The eye chases the optical image in very rapid-measured in milliseconds-forays called "saccades". We are not aware of the saccade on recall because memory entries made during this short interval are technically incompetent. Rich with unique data vagaries. the three or four data planes of the saccade are the "scenario index" in the summary of the item on the "smart" engine.

Once the scenario index is specified, the rest of the scenario will follow. Both the specific data cortex and the control cortex have their own versions of the scenario index. There is a "virtual" coupling between the two systems. On recall, the control system dictates its own index and the recall cycle begins. The control index stipulates which sites in the specific data cortex were matched and mismatched and the time interval between data planes that prevailed when the entry was originally made. These are unique data anomalies common to both the specific data and the control index. There is almost a certainty only one, at most a few, data planes will have anomalies that correspond to the anomalies in the control index and, if it is more exactly specified, the anomalies must turn up at a particular instant in the scan, the probability of an exact response is almost exclusive. The virtual relationship between these anomalies will decide if the response is accepted or passed. Data plane by data plane, starting with the scenario index, the specific data cortex and the control cortex match data planes and firing rates until the last data plane in the scenario has been delivered. If it all comes out of memory the same way it went in, and there is no reason it will not, the lobes will remain competent. Incompetence cancels the attempt.

There are times when twilight sleep will also bring forward a slower moving version of "hypnagogic hallucinations". A "still", or slowly moving image is recalled with surprising clarity-the more surprising because we never realized we were observing it in such detail when the entry was originally made. I think careful interpretation of these images can give us some insight into the inner workings of the cortex. For example, the chromaticity of the recalled image exceeds the coloration of the natural image. When processing the "real" image, color is related, arithmetically, to the black and white reference signal. With the eyes closed or in sleep, there is no real reference signal and the chroma component is exaggerated.

I think real-time memory, working alone, recalls the fast hypnagogic hallucinations. The entire visual cortex probably generates the slow variety. They can be "still" or they can include the movement of the content of the image in about the same timing we would expect in the original entry. The slow image shows natural movements, rotations, and "trees-and-forest" effect. The image "pops" into the scene complete, centered, right side up, and with no antecedents. Here, both the visual "saccade" and the visual "scenario" are at work. The image is displayed only after its movement has been "stopped", fixed in both time and on the retina. The few data planes that immediately preceded the "stopping" of the image are so fast and anomalous they cannot be subjectively appreciated so the recalled scene seems to be suddenly "turned on" without continuity or prior history.

I also get the impression a moving subject matter in the image does not have a preference for entering the field of view from either "stage right" or "stage left", arguing for an environment innocent of "handedness". The image does not show (normal) shadows and this argues against habitual preference for light sources in certain positions with respect to the objects we are looking at. The image is seen at eye level, possibly looking slightly down at a target 15-20 feet ahead of the viewer. The center of the recalled image is properly lighted, technically rational, and always centered in the middle of the visual field. The periphery of the image is usually black, and, if a rare image suggests a direction for a light source, it is usually from above. The colorfulness of the image persuades us it is highly detailed: is less detailed on recall that it was when it was entered because there is no "real" instruction in the lobe. Even here, with these recalled images, it is clear the cortical computation is a small part of visual experience, most of the meaningfulness of the image is environmentally suggested.

I think a true cortical routine can be visualized while the cortex is awake. Suppose I close my eyes and attempt to recall the letter "A" in the foreground of the recalled visual field for an extended period of time, say a goal of 30 seconds. After several seconds the image will become unstable and fade away. It will be replaced by another image which, in turn, fades. In the early phases of this game, the images may be corollaries of the letter "A", but before long, the images are obviously selected from memory at random. Images follow images, and, after a short time, I find I am recalling anything but the letter "A" and it is becoming increasingly difficult to recall it at all. Evidently the cortex will dwell on a redundant throughput for a limited number of recalls then it is compelled to drift off and refuse the redundant throughput altogether, possibly a tactic to prevent hyper-reinforcement.

The memory "deliver" cell is added to the exalted data stage in Fig. 112 (shaded cell). This cell commands those cells containing memory units to initiate memory delivery. This is also an octopus like cell, physically resembling the sync cell, and it to, connects with as many cortical cells as it can reach in its nearby surroundings. Its output terminals are of the "avalanching" type and, unlike the sync cell, the sense of the output is "inhibit". This is a brute force "inhibit" that cuts off potassium ion conduction in the cells under its command. Ion current is cut off; membrane voltage goes to -70mv and the memory unit delivers while the -70mv is across the electrophoretic apparatus.

There has to be an exclusion scheme so the control system will not be commanding "scan" and "fire" at the same time. There are probably a half dozen arrangements of cells that would contain this exclusion in their truth tables. The exact circuit is a bit too speculative at the moment. For purposes of expository, I will show the circuit in the sketches; if the job can be done with fewer circuit elements, I would not be surprised.

Fig. 113 is the firing rate control circuit. The error "inhibit" signal is an analogue of comparator error and it could be sent directly to the sync cell to hold off firing

375

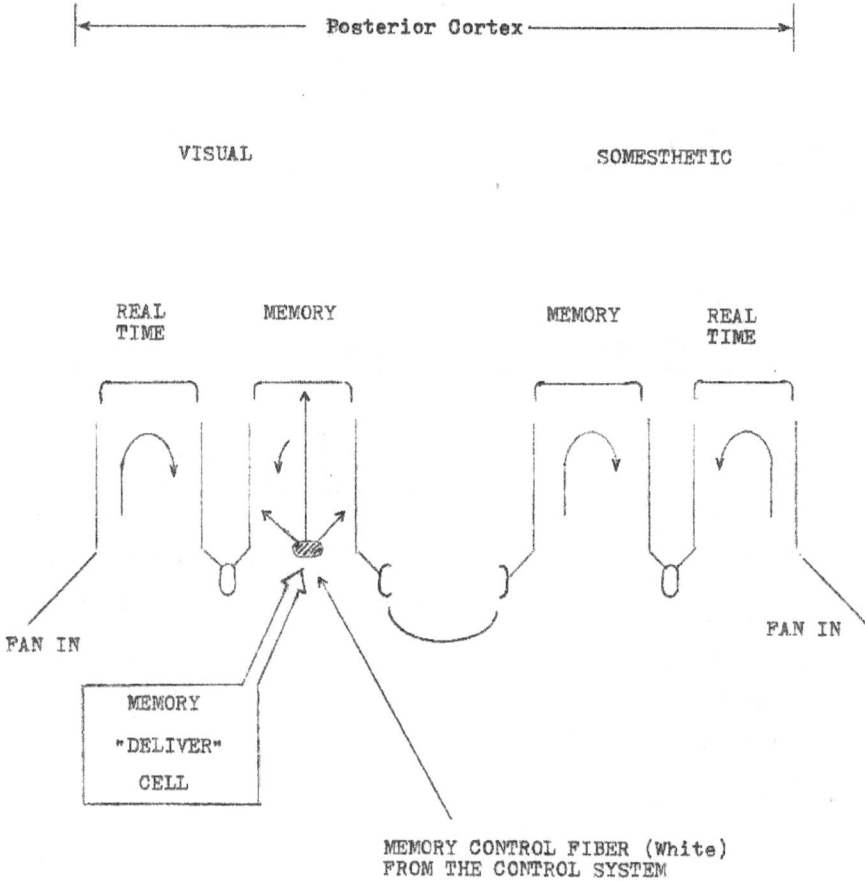

Figure 112

until the match is improved. The control system accepts the amount

of error as an input and "figures out" an amplitude for its output

signal that will keep error within limits and at the same time

434

speed up firings so throughputs can be

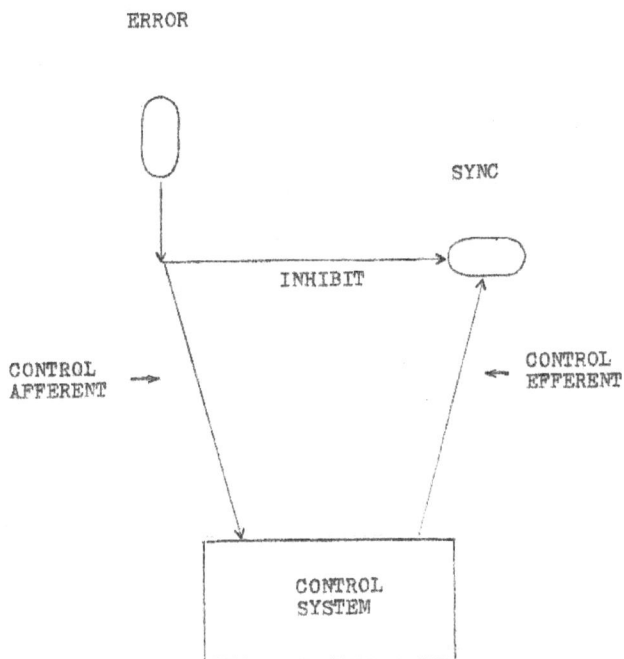

376

ERROR

SYNC

INHIBIT

CONTROL
AFFERENT

CONTROL
EFFERENT

CONTROL
SYSTEM

Figure 113

Fig 103

managed in the time slot available. Here, a tradeoff is made

between error and firing rates: the relative amplitudes of the

error signal (inhibits firing) and the control signal (advances
firing rates) make the tradeoff.

Fig. 114 is a circuit for memory control. The exact circuit
cannot be shown without more exact findings from the anatomist.
The dashed line speculates on a direct path from the error bus to
the memory delivery cell. I doubt there is such a path but the
drawing suggests an error system able to request more scanning time
with error present. The routing is through the control system.
Delta circuit rules are no problem here because these are all
"inhibit" (negative) circuits.

The control system learns how to maintain competence in the lobe
and will evidently do this even when there is a dysfunction in the
lobe. I think a visual dysfunction called eidetic imaging may be a
case in point. The memory lobe and the real-time lobe collaborate
when making an entry, there is probably a fixed authority that
requires either the real-time or the memory lobe to write the
visual statement but not both at the same time. When this
propriety is not preserved, I think eidetic imaging is the result.
With eidetic imaging, two visual images are seen superimposed. One
image is real and present in front of the eyes another image: one
from memory, is superimposed on the real image. If the eidetic is
watching a fire in a fireplace and then turns his head and looks
toward a blank wall, the fire and the fireplace will be recalled
and will seem to have moved to the wall he is looking at. If he is
looking at a sack of groceries and is

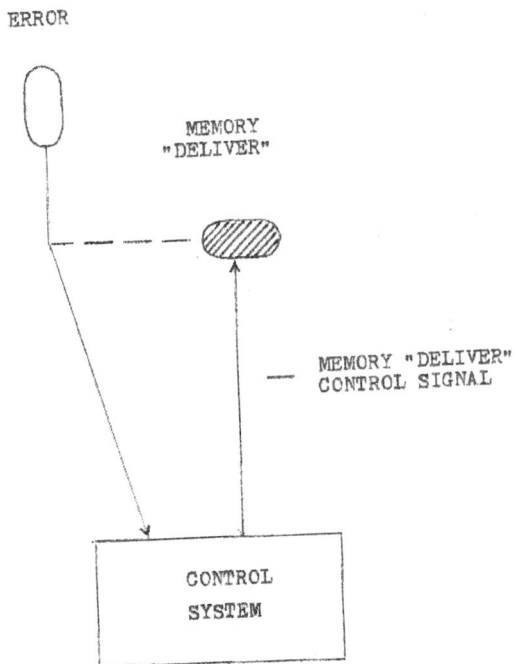

377

ERROR

MEMORY
"DELIVER"

MEMORY "DELIVER"
CONTROL SIGNAL

CONTROL
SYSTEM

Figure 114

recalling a chair, he will do some mental juggling and "park" the
sack in the chair so the interference between the two images is
brought into manageability. Eidetic imaging, more prevalent in
children, tends to clear up as the child grows older.

437

Like the specific data cortex; the control cortex has no wired-in programs and, in addition to being freely conditionable, it also incorporates intelligent capability. Predictability for control system management of a throughput is not much of an issue. The control task is relatively circumscribed. It maintains cortical competence by trial adjustment of firing rates. If, on occasion, it should fail to manage a particular throughput with perfection, it will try a different tactic the next time the same problem comes up. The control finesse trades off a little in the matter of predictability, which it doesn't need, and gains an enormous repertory of tactics, all acquired, all perfuse with intelligent contribution and all making the control finesse far more capable, more flexible than remotely possible with fixed procedures.

I will not try to guess at the potential control repertory. One strategy comes to mind. The control system may "figure out" it can maintain competence handily if it will speed up the dominant lobe so it is running at twice the rate of the slaved lobe, in effect repeating the instruction, so it can squeeze in a few trial corollaries while the task is in progress. Having learned a repeated cortical instruction is possible without loss of competence, the control system also learns it can repeat the instruction for the specific purpose of up-grading inventory.

The way this gambit works is sketched in Fig. 115. In the initial state, a fraction of an older data plane is at a distal position on the tape (small arrow). The tapes are synchronized so the system has no way to "slip" or to "slide" the distal fraction to a new position. After a number of deliberate repetitions of the retrieval instruction, intelligent procedure begins to "figure out", with trial values, the amplitudes of the data events it will need to duplicate the missing fraction of the data plane. If intelligent procedure is successful, a duplicate of the distal fraction will eventually be associated with a recent entry (end situation, Fig. 115). The distal fraction was synthesized, "manufactured from scratch", so to speak, rather than being "slipped" from one position on the tape to another.

The next sketches look at cortical anatomy. The views of anatomy are my idea so caution is advised. In Fig. 116, the control lobes (cingulate lobes) are arranged so its inputs and outputs will physically face the exalted data stages they are to control. The sketch is a coronal section and I have marked the "corpus callosum" (C.C.) because it is a very distinctive landmark. As I see it, the cingulate lobe computes control for the (outermost) specific data cortex.

380

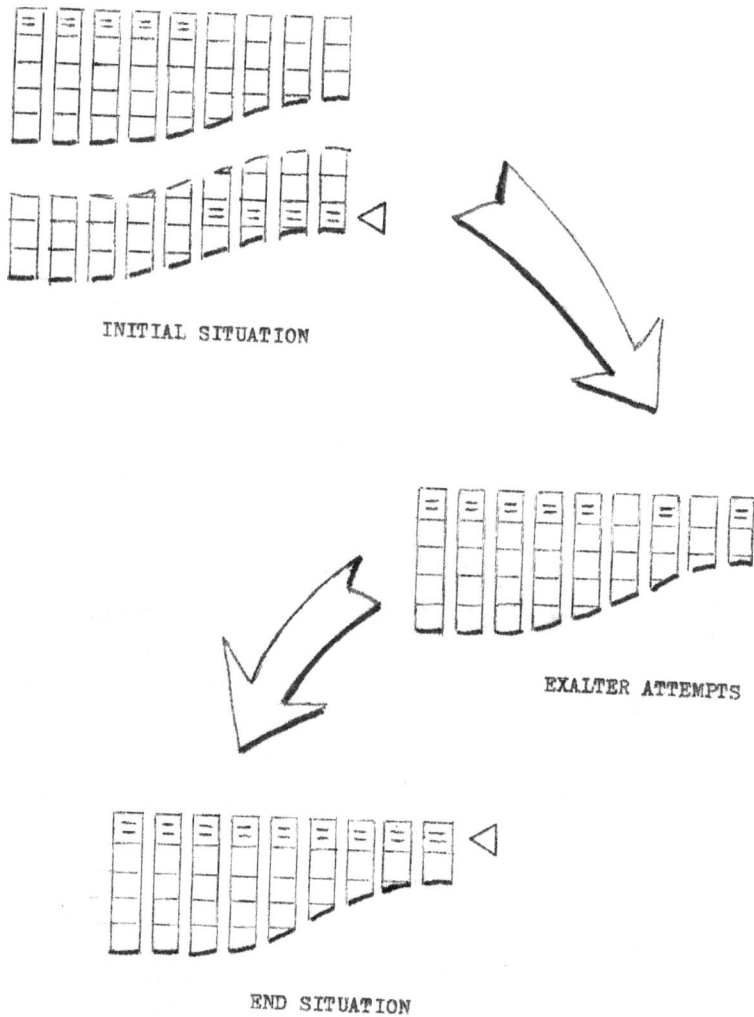

INITIAL SITUATION

EXALTER ATTEMPTS

END SITUATION

Figure 115

It is called the "cingulum" because it resembles a girdle. In Fig.
116, the cingulate lobe is "U" shaped it goes back (into the page),
down (in its rearmost curve) then forward again where it emerges in

the temporal lobe. I am not able

382

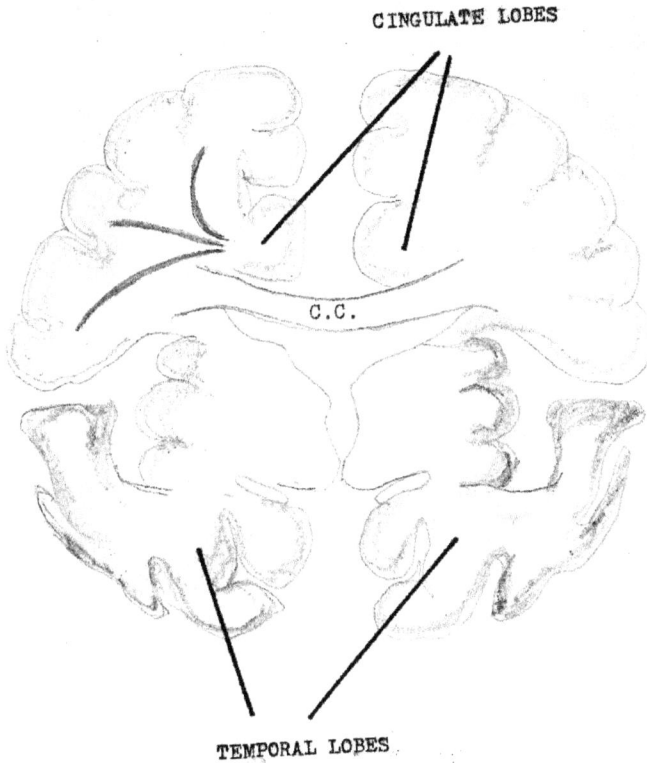

CINGULATE LOBES

C.C.

TEMPORAL LOBES

Figure 116

Fig 106

to say with confidence how the temporal and the island lobes are

controlled.

Fig. 117 is a semi-anatomical sketch of the upper left corner of
Fig. 116. The outer cortex is the specific data

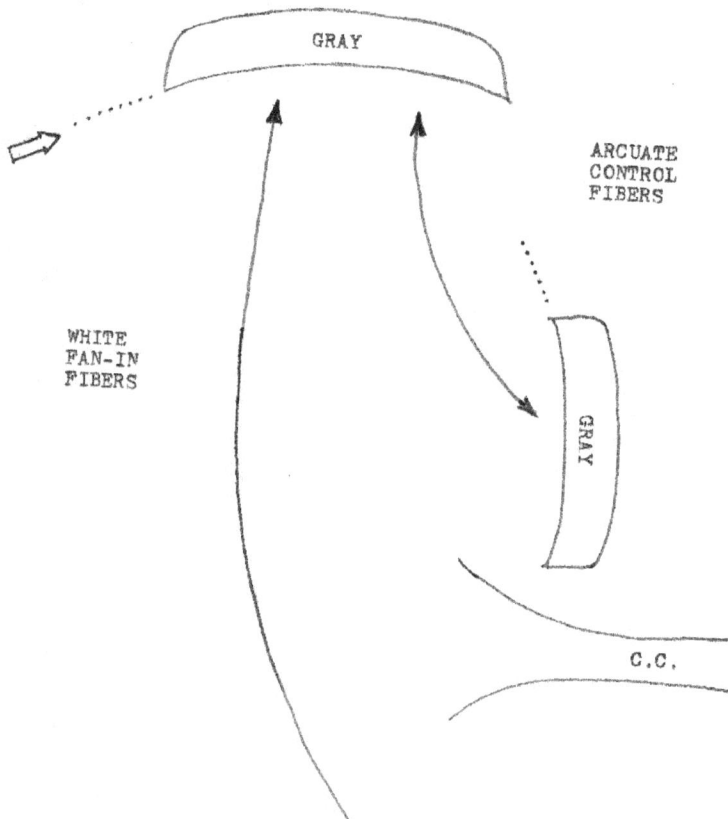

Figure 117

cortex and it is physically arranged so both specific data (fan-in) fibers and arcuate control fibers have access to its exalted data stage. The dotted line is the physical plane of the exalted data stage for the specific data cortex (top of Fig. 117). The control cortex also has its own exalted data stage. There may be some white fan-in fibers for the cortex originating on the underside of the thalamus possibly carrying reflexes "over-ride" signals.

(The arrow pointing along the plane of the exalted data stage brings up a factor that may help account for the peculiarities of the EEG trace just before and during the epileptic seizure. At the onset of the seizure, there is an organic dysfunction of the lobe attended by data anomalies and a pause in exalter firings. The control system cannot compensate for an organic dysfunction of the lobe, so it cannot resume the normal pattern of synchronized firings. At first there are intermittent pauses and the control system makes wrongly directed attempts to restore firings in a local area of the exalted data stage. At this phase, the EEG trace is registering the easily distinguished wave shape of the grass-like spikes of the "aura" that precedes the seizures.

The "spikes" are high speed attempts to restore coherence in the lobe and the sync cell suffers fatigue, intermittently refusing to fire at all. The sync-cell re-paces during these intervals of refusal. The now re-paced cell is hyper-sensitive and the situation deteriorates when the control system attempts to re-start normal firings with the hyper-sensitive cells in the circuit. Instead of restoring synchronized firings in keeping with data processing requirements, the hair-triggered cells fire precipitously and nucleate a wave front of uncontrolled firings which propagates _along_ the _plane_ of the exalted data stage. Neither the data anomaly nor the performance anomalies have cleared, and by now they are surely worse, so there is a pause and more attempted re-starts. I believe all of this generates the short spikes in the EEG trace during the aura.

The lobe remains incompetent and the sync cells are left even more out of calibration by the re-start attempts. The exalted data stage suspends firings, and, if it is a "grand mal" seizure, the victim may faint.

The control system itself probably gets involved in the incompetence; by now, it is improperly paced. Alternating between pauses and fast, senseless firings, with most of the sync cells in both the control and controlled lobes over-paced and hypersensitive, on the next attempted restart, the entire lobe fires the very large, over amplitude, "paroxysmal spindles" of the full blown epileptic seizure.

Fig. 118 is a sagittal section of the hemisphere with parts of the limbic system marked. The limbic system (limbus, margin) is both physically and operationally at the margin between the thalamic and cortical system. Operationally, it resolves the status of authority and prevents conflict between the cortical and limbic systems.

Sometimes the terminology used to describe the limbic system tends to suggest organs and organelles. Any of this terminology refers to either nerve tracts or ganglionic masses.

The limbic system is deep toward the midline of the brain. It is not amenable to experiment and the effects of lesions to the components of the limbic system tell us very little about the way they work. I will take it upon myself to set out the following account of the way I think the limbic system works.

It is something of a challenge to explain how the limbic system is laid out. I will do the best I can with the layout, but it may take some imagining to figure it out. These are intriguing systems and worth a little patience.

There are three fascinating "U" shaped fiber tracts in the limbic system. (The "U" is a "lazy U", it is lying down.) We can also say, with a certain amount of truth, the "U" shaped formations are (very loosely) "nesting", one within the other. Each half of the brain is a mirror image of the other half and the "U" shaped fiber tracts are represented in both hemispheres.

Fig. 118 is a sagittal section of the brain divided at the midline. This is a superficial view and the ribbon-like "tail" of the hippocampus ("sea horse", which it resembles) is in the cleft between the cingulum and the corpus callosum

387

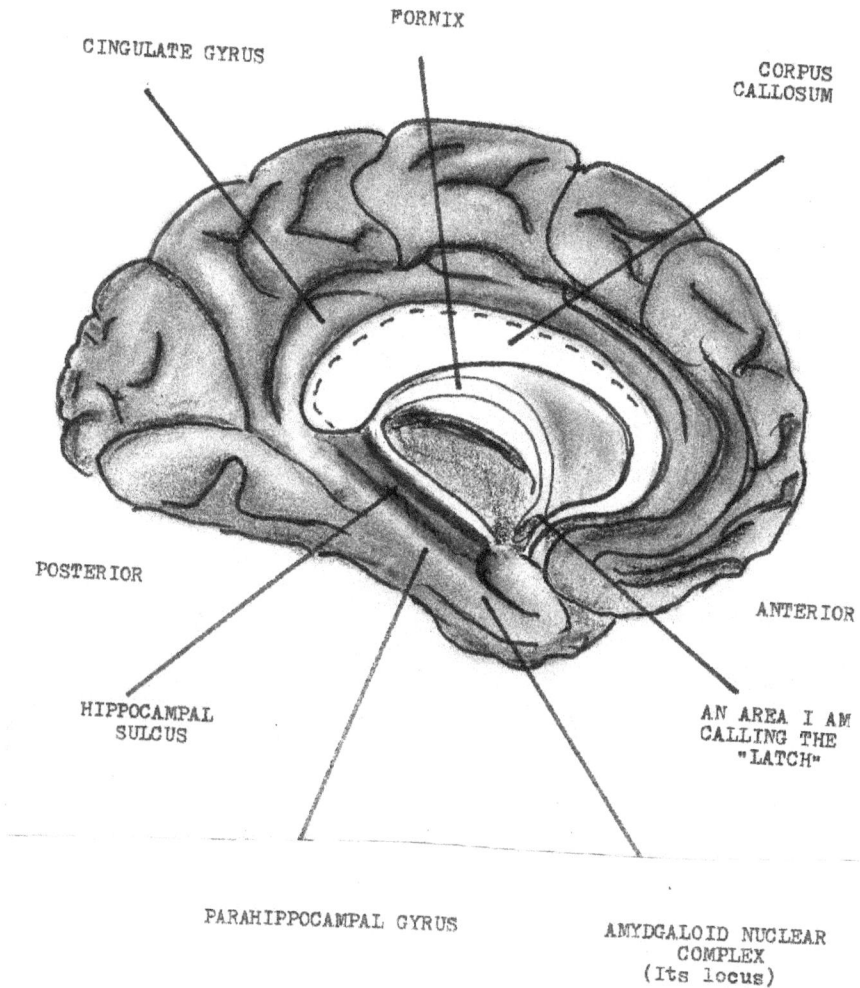

Figure 118

and would only be seen as a thin line in this view. The

hippocampal formation is the longest of the three "U" shaped tracts

and it follows the inner margin of the cingulate gyrus, courses its entire length and the length of the lower continuation of the cingulum: the parahippocampal gyrus. The dashed line is slightly to the center of its normal course.

Fig. 119 is the caudate formation ("caudate", resembles a "tail"). This is the left half. The head of the caudate tract is well toward the middle of the innermost brain. The caudate nucleus is slightly lateral with respect to the center line of the body and it carries information well lateral, out, almost to the poles of the temporal cortex.

The white cortical "fan-in" fibers running between the lower brain and the cortex pass through the caudate formation via a pathway called the "internal capsule"--the truncated and sculpted wedge in the center of the drawing. The internal capsule is "clasped" between the two large nuclei of the caudate formation, the other large nucleus is behind the internal capsule in the drawing. The "tail" of the caudate formation carries information gathered from the fibers of the internal capsule out to the amygdaloid complex. The "wire" model shows how the two assemblies are positioned with respect to each other.

Fibers running to the cortex will be taken out of service for any of the following reasons;

1. The cortex is dictating a non-feasible instruction and the reflex system is vetoing it.

2. There has been a reflex "over-ride". The reflex system has momentarily taken over to execute a reflex, say, an eye

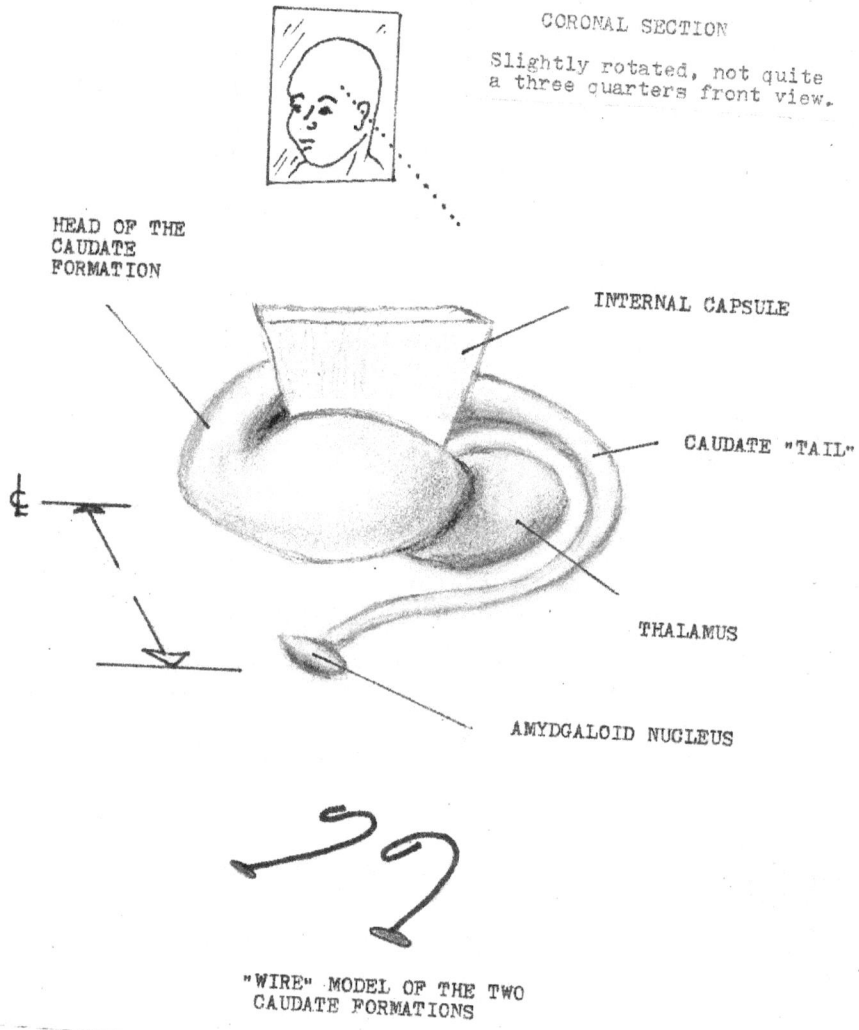

Figure 119

blink. The reflex system only "over-rides" those small areas of the cortex that are in conflict with the reflex; the remainder of the cortex can stay in service while this is going on.

3. A cue is present and authority is being transferred to the instinctive mode system.

The caudate formation reports to the amygdaloid system certain cortial fibers are temporarily under an authority other than the cortex. They are out of service, or under another authority, for known, good and sufficient reasons and are thus accounted for.

Judging from the mass of the caudate nuclei and the small cross section of the "tail", it is almost a cinch the caudate formation is a multiplexer and its report to the amygdala is a multiplexed statement. A multiplexer picks up information from a large number of sources and converges it so it can be carried on a smaller number of data buses. Without multiplexing, the caudate mass would be a large part of the brain mass. The caudate statement to the amygdala is a technical report regarding the status of the fibers in the internal capsule.

The innermost fibers of the "U" shaped tracts in the fornix (arch), in Fig. 119, loop up and over the thalamus. Almost all of the thalamus is left out of the sketch, it would be at the center of the sketch. The lower end of the fornix terminates in a couple of distinct protrusions on the underside of the thalamus called mammillary bodies. The columns rising from the mammillary bodies are the mamillothalamic tracts which are inside the mass of the thalamus.

This point of entrance is not far from the posterior pituitary gland. The signal from the fornix is probably capable of initiating both the excursion in systemic adrenalin concentration and triggering the specific "whole body" instructions associated with the so called "fight or flight" reaction, which probably includes the back arching, hair raising and snarling aspects of the reaction.

The fornix originates in the temporal cortex and it gets its signals from the hippocampal formation via the "fimbria" or "fringe" which connects to the hippocampus in the region where they run side by side.

If the specific data cortex is competent, it will not slow down or worse: "balk" the control cortex. The cingulum (control) is always competent as long as the specific data lobes are competent. In principle, the control cortex does not need supervision. It fires when it is competent and it is competent when a majority of the areas of the specific data cortex is competent. We will say it has a majority when 50% of the specific data cortex is competent. I have a feeling most of the 50% has to be in the frontal lobes.

The hippocampus collects a report of competence within the cingulum and this is, by implication, a status report of over all competence within the specific data cortex. I think the dentate gyrus, a part of the hippocampal formation, continuously assesses the cross section of the hippocampus, averages the statement of competence in the cingulum and forwards the statement to the amygdala.

The amygdala is the "switch" which makes the decision to switch the animals' behavior from cortical mode to instinctive mode. When the amygdala makes the mode shift a "flight or fight" subroutine is triggered and authority is abruptly transferred to thalamic system and instinctive behavior. The rather dramatic shift to "wired-in" behavior during mode shift gives the impression there is a lot of emotional activity under way. It is not cortical emotion, at any rate.

It is entirely compatible with all other reflex and instinctive procedures to permit the (frontal) cortex to disqualify itself, to take itself out of service and to transfer authority to the thalamic brain system. Why and when should the cortex do this? The cerebral cortex reports itself incompetent when the animal, and in certain cases, the human, is confronted with an experience that is so unfamiliar, one for which there is so little precedent in cortical inventory, that further efforts of the cortex would not be sufficiently reliable to make continued cortical attempts worthwhile. If the cortex, through confusion or lack of information, is no longer able to come forward with the second by second instructions the body needs or if it does not have a precedent to carry it through a heretofore unknown experience, authority had better be transferred to the tested and proven reflexes or antiquity.

(With no precedence in inventory and surrounded by unfamiliar experience, the animal ought to clear out. The TV conjury of a wild animal relying on intelligence to see it through the most harrowing and bizarre situations, of investing itself in one incredible threat to survival after another, and doing this for no reason more than surviving the episode, is asinine. If the animal has a problem and no solution in inventory, it should run first and figure things out later.)

The "balked" cortex mode shifts from cortical to instinctive mode. There are several ways to cue the mode shift. In a compulsory mode shift, a specific cue is recognized by the instinctive cue recognition system, and the thalamus overrides the cortex, forcing the switch from cortical to instinctive mode. A mode shift to instinctive mode in also made when the cortex disqualifies itself. The time to disqualify the cortex arrives when it cannot muster a 50% competence. The amygdala counts cortical competence and the count makes special allowances. If and when certain areas are taken out of service by the reflex system, the amygdala will be so advised by the caudate report which is fed to the amygdaloid complex. These votes will be excused.

The parahippocampal gyrus is a part of hippocampal formation, it is a small cortex and I think it, or the dentate gyrus, tries to figure out a way to transpose hippocampal procedure so it can re-establish a report of hippocampal competence after the disqualified areas and excused contributions have been accounted for. The dentate gyrus continuously monitors, and may correct, the hippocampal cross-section for the 50% competence requirement and this report is counted by the amygdala. The amygdala accepts both the hippocampal report and the caudate report and, allowing for the disqualified areas, makes the decision to "mode shift" accordingly.

The fornix is a fiber tract which monitors the hippocampus and accepts hippocampal signal as an input to the fornix. If the hippocampus is unable to muster a 50% competence after the amygdala has made its corrections, the fornix delivers the "mode shift"

signal to the underside of the thalamus and the thalamus takes
over.

I am not sure, but I think the fornix also delivers a signal to
the area I call the "latch" in the drawing. If the fornix sent a
signal to the frontal cortex (perhaps via the corpus callosum)
which rendered it _further_ incompetent, there would be an assurance
the "smart" control systems will not "figure out" a way to restore
cortical competence before the mode shift to instinctive mode has
been completed. The latch enforces the mode shift and assures at
least a brief instinctive take over before a shift back to cortical
authority can be permitted.

The sketch is very rudimentary and leaves out a lot of the
amygdaloid complex. The amygdala accepts a number of inputs; it
seems to be abundant with connections to the olfactory system. The
amygdala also has its own efferent; one of these: the stria
terminalis, is shown in the drawing (S.T.). (The amygdaloid
complex is in the tip of the temporal lobe. The temporal lobe has
been cut away in the drawing so it appears to be a sort of
protuberance here.)

It plainly stands to reason, if the cortex runs out of "smarts",
some provision must be made for the animals' next move. The
confusing cues, the unprecedented experience, balk the cortex and
it relinquishes command. The exalter control system will do what
it can to restore cortical competence. If the specific data cortex
is balked and stays balked, the control cortex will also be balked
and there is an immediate shift to instinctive mode. If there

cannot be two captains at the helm, there cannot be a confused and hesitant captain there either.

I think this "mode shift" business is commonly seen in the behavior of animals only we do not recognize it for what it is. A visitor to a park will be setting on a bench with a sack of peanuts. A squirrel will come down out of a nearby tree: this is an inexperienced squirrel, say a yearling. It approaches to within, say, 20 feet of the human figure. As it moves closer, a point is reached where its cortex does not have this experience: this business of being so close to a human, in inventory. Having overextended its cortical inventory and run out of "smarts", the animal's behavior mode shifts to instinct and the animal runs back up the tree. On its next approach, it now has, though just entered, a working knowledge of what it is like to be within 20 feet of a human, so it comes still closer, say, to 10 feet. It runs out of smarts again, "mode shifts", and scrambles back to safety. Adding to its cortical inventory a little bit at a time, it ends up eating out of human hands. On its retreats, we tend to say the squirrel is frightened. It is not; it's odd behavior is attributable to switching back and forth from cortical to instinctive authority.

While it is my own speculation, I get the impression humans also "mode shift" when flummoxed by a baffling experience, one which they are not informationally prepared to cope with. When this happens, the cortex disqualifies itself and the shift is attempted to instinctive mode. Since there is nothing in the human instinctive register, the shift is not captured by the thalamic system. The systems hold in the instinctive mode for a split second (the length of time the "latch" will hold the systems in the thalamic configuration), whereupon authority is returned to the cortical mode. The systems do not stay in the thalamic mode for long. They are, however, able to repeat the switching event a number of times on end.

Our lives are enriched with amusement, perhaps some comedy, when we insist on proceeding as though things are normal on those rare occasions when experience is so confusing, so bizarre, that our cortical performance is marginal or lapsed altogether. With an extra-ordinarily unfamiliar experience and a little bad luck, it may be responsible for digging an untimely grave here and there. I have often thought cortical balk may be involved in those stories we hear where a householder successfully escapes the flames of his burning house and, in the fright and excitement of the moment, runs back into the fire to rescue his Scrabble board or something of the sort.

The cortex becomes rough acting when it is balked, quickly switching from one mode to the other in a series of rapid but senseless mode shifts. I think this happens rather commonly but we fail to notice it or recognize it as such. If someone is trying to talk with a balked, or marginal, cortex, his speech may deteriorate into a sort of "word salad". He may have to start and stop repeatedly in order to say anything at all, even greater exertion to restore deliberate speech that agrees with what he is trying to say.

I believe a cortex with a slow running temporal lobe (say, one cortex in twenty) may add its own colorful embellishments to the balked cortex syndrome. I have often thought the "talking in tongues" rigmarole of some of the "holy roller" cults might be induced, in those individuals where it can be induced, by a combination of excitement, unfamiliar exertions and a cortex that is only marginally running in its proper timing regime.

I know nothing about hypnosis. I understand it is about 95% stagecraft and, unfortunately, the stagecraft obscures whatever validity there may be. In the interest of looking at hypnosis objectively, a balked cortex may produce some of the manifestations of hypnosis and, if it does, it is probably a slow running frontal cortex that does it. The subject has a slow running frontal cortex to begin with. He is persuaded to "slow down", more so than he already is and his frontal cortex is no longer dependable, intermittently dropping in and out of service. He is confused, diffusely motivated and exhibits enough of the advertised symptoms of hypnosis to say he has been hypnotized for some short period of time. I cannot see how it have a lasting effect or influence behavior any more than any other short transient experience.

www.ingramcontent.com/pod-product-compliance
Lightning Source LLC
Chambersburg PA
CBHW051114200326

41518CB00016B/2505